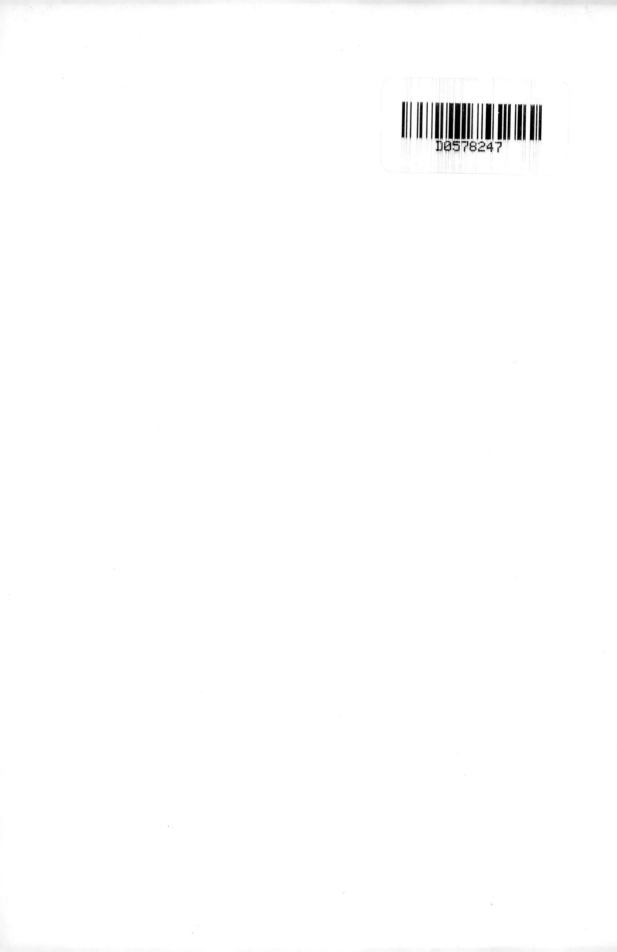

MINOR TOOTH MOVEMENT IN CHILDREN

Minor tooth movement in children

JOSEPH M. SIM

B.S., D.D.S., M.S.D.

Associate Professor of Clinical Dentistry and Chairman,
Department of Pedodontics, Southern Illinois University
School of Dental Medicine, Edwardsville, Illinois; formerly
Assistant Professor, Department of Pedodontics, University of
Alabama School of Dentistry, and Director, Dental Clinic,
The Children's Hospital, Birmingham, Alabama

WITH 528 ILLUSTRATIONS

THE C. V. MOSBY COMPANY

SAINT LOUIS   1972

Printed in the United States of America

International Standard Book Number 0-8016-4615-4

Library of Congress Catalog Card Number 72-81114

Distributed in Great Britain by Henry Kimpton, London

VH/VH/VH   9   8   7   6   5   4   3

With all my love
to my wife
Patricia
and
Murray, Shelley, and Joe

Preface

The ideas set forth in this book are presented in the hope that they will fill what has become a pressing need in the offices of most dentists who treat children—a deeper and more complete understanding of the techniques, procedures, and materials for accomplishing tooth guidance measures that can and should be handled by the interested general practitioner or pedodontist. One has only to look at the list of clinics presented at recent state, regional, and national meetings to gauge the heightened interest in this area. The emphasis in dentistry for children is clearly shifting toward an increased awareness of prevention. This prevention includes not only protection against caries and gingival problems but also the prevention, interception, or correction of many types of developing malocclusions.

These interceptive or minor corrective measures in the past have been referred to as *tooth guidance, preventive orthodontics, interceptive orthodontics,* or *pedodontic tooth movement.* As presented here, these clinical techniques collectively will be called *minor tooth movement in children.*

The need for such care is increasing in our society, a society that is gaining both in affluence and the recognition of the benefits of comprehensive dental care for younger children. At the same time, the general population curve is outstripping the number of dentists serving this population.

It has been estimated that one third to one half of all children treated in dental offices have some sort of malocclusion. More than 60% of all the children exhibiting discrepancies of occlusion could be classified as having Angle Class I malocclusions. The majority of the remainder would be classified as Angle Class II, and 3% to 5% would fall into Angle Class III.

Only Angle Class I malocclusions will be discussed here. Furthermore, only those cases will be described whose etiology is reasonably clear and explainable and for which the time and effort necessary to reduce the malocclusion satisfactorily is reasonably short term. These limitations appear to be severe, and very properly so. This is not a complete catalog of tooth movement techniques nor a book on "orthodontics." Rather, the text describes a limited number of successful techniques sifted from orthodontic, pedodontic, and general dental practitioner sources. Eight basic appliances are discussed, half of which are of the removable type and half are fixed.

Wherever possible, persons have been

given credit for their research ideas, appliance methods, and treatment procedures. However, much of our expertise in this area is the result of the contributions of so many dentists that in some instances credit for original ideas may have been inadvertently omitted.

The chapters are presented so that an organized flow of experience unfolds as one reads through the book. There are three sections. The first section is on theory and diagnosis. This is followed by the section on selection and treatment of minor malocclusions in the primary and mixed dentition age groups. The third section comprises chapters dealing with the detailed fabrication of the eight appliances. These last chapters may be used by the dentist to train his dental assistant or dental technician to fabricate these preventive orthodontic appliances. All chapters begin with the easier procedures, which may serve only as a review for many practitioners, and work forward to more advanced techniques, which in most cases are merely simple techniques added together to make a new whole.

Every effort has been made to present practical, clinically oriented techniques. When all of these are absorbed and practiced until facility comes in their use, the attentive dentist will find that he has added an interesting and necessary dimension to his office practice. And many of his young patients will have smiles that will reward him amply for the time taken to acquire these new skills.

As does each professional individual, I remain deeply in debt to many teachers who have shaped and guided me in my quest for knowledge and clinical skills. I also owe thanks to many persons for the ideas that appear in this book. Some of these people I know personally; others only through their books and articles.

Authors such as Moyers, Graber, Barber, Tweed, Salzmann, Adams, Moore, and Hitchcock have opened wide the gates of learning in this area of preventive orthodontics. I have felt free to borrow from them because they have been so generous in publishing their ideas and techniques.

Minor tooth movement techniques, however, become only a panoply of inactive ideas if they are not bolstered by specific suggestions concerning the instruments, attachments, and components used to fabricate the appliances described here. After a struggle with my conscience I resolved to present detailed lists of these necessary materials, primary and alternate sources, order numbers, and approximate costs, despite the fact that this might open opportunities for criticism. My sole defense is that I have tried to present as honestly as I can the sort of information that I found virtually unobtainable during my seven years of general practice.

Six men in particular have personally motivated me toward writing this book: Dr. John R. Rogers, an orthodontist who continues to explore new paths of early treatment; Dr. David B. Law, who opened many doors for me in expanding my graduate training in pedodontics; Dr. Sidney B. Finn, my teacher and colleague who urged me to reach for broader horizons in teaching pedodontics both at the undergraduate and the postgraduate levels; Dr. Harry C. Shirkey, whose skills as a pediatrician, author, speaker, and warm human being have helped me to believe I could in some small way follow his example; Dr. William A. Daniel, Jr., a pediatrician who taught me to see adolescents as very special people and whose knowledge of clinical photography was so wholeheartedly shared with me; and Dr. Thompson M. Lewis, who taught me by example that the child *and* the parent must be treated together if success is to follow pedodontic therapy.

Special thanks must also be extended to the pedodontic interns and residents at The Children's Hospital Dental Clinic, Birmingham, Alabama, who so patiently shared the burden of my experiments in teaching: Drs. E. L. Donaldson, C. Bernard Johnston, Allen D. McCaghren, Stanley A. Sheppard, Stanley C. Simons, William M. Bishop,

Karen Fox, W. Thomas James, Thomas K. Myers, Luis R. Regattieri, Paul Castellon, Jerry L. Parker, Jack S. Llewellyn, Alan Goldman, George E. Vezina, Stephanie K. Gonsoulin, Larry R. Roska, James F. White, Jr., and James F. Campbell.

These individuals endured a program that included studying dozens of varying clinical and laboratory methods of making and using minor tooth movement appliances for children. The stimulation provided by their comments after reading many of these chapters and their eagerness to forge new treatment goals in pedodontics was of inestimable value in giving a sense of worth to my ideas.

The artists, Mrs. Marlene Rikard and Mrs. Linda Donaldson, deserve the highest praise. Any inaccuracies contained in the illustrations are the result of my errors, since both artists were guided by my penciled sketches.

Most of the illustrations were made from colored slides either taken by me or photographed under my direction by one of our pedodontic interns or residents at the University of Alabama in Birmingham. Grateful acknowledgment is extended to Dr. Theodore R. Oldenburg for use of his excellent photographs demonstrating treatment of posterior cross-bites and the distalizing of 6-year molars.

When a clinician is the sole author of a book, he needs the balancing opinions of other practitioners who have a deep clinical interest in this area. I was fortunate to have excellent assistance from the following knowledgeable dentists, each of whom was at once both a friend and frank critic: Drs. C. Walter Andrews, Donald W. Englebert, Hollis N. Gieger, C. Cornell Hill, Jo Anne Jackson, Roy R. Kracke, William M. McDonald, Orland L. Rice, Bob L. Roebuck, and Larry R. Shannon, all members of the Birmingham Pedodontic Association.

My appreciation also goes to Drs. David L. Russell, Joe P. Thomas, Frederick B. Smith, John F. Simon, Jr., Theodore R. Oldenburg, and Col. Robert Gardner, who were among the many pedodontists who contributed valuable ideas, and to Dr. John R. Orr, Jr., who in his remarkable practice continually demonstrates the art of the possible.

To all my colleagues at our new School of Dental Medicine at Southern Illinois University–Edwardsville I wish to extend my appreciation for the warm welcome offered to my family and me. Special thanks go to our dean, Dr. Frank J. Sobkowski, and to Drs. Frederic Custer, Philip M. Hoag, and John Angelillo for helpful suggestions in the final manuscript.

For the seemingly endless typing of the manuscript, I am warmly indebted to Mrs. Barbara Smith, Mrs. Peggy McCaghren, Mrs. Karen Tombrello, Mrs. Darlene Clark, and my wife, Patricia.

Joseph M. Sim

Contents

Part I   THEORY AND DIAGNOSIS

1   What is minor tooth movement? 3
2   Normal and ectopic eruption of teeth, 16
3   Recognition of abnormal arch patterns, 28
4   Using the diagnostic quadrangle, 48
5   Selection of appliances, 69
6   The case presentation to parents, 86
7   Tissue response to natural and biomechanical forces, 96

Part II   SELECTION AND TREATMENT OF MINOR MALOCCLUSIONS

8   Preservation of arch form, 109
9   Treatment of lower anterior crowding, 126
10   Treatment of protruding upper incisors and anterior open-bite, 142
11   Treatment of anterior cross-bites, 162
12   Treatment of posterior cross-bites, 175
13   Treatment of mesially drifted 6-year molars, 195

Part III   FABRICATION OF APPLIANCES

14   Selection of instruments and appliance components, 213
15   Fabricating fixed and removable space maintainers, acrylic inclined planes, and oral screens, 238

16   Fabricating Hawley and palatal expansion appliances, 256

17   Fabricating lingual arches, 277

18   Fabricating heavy and light fixed labial arches, 290

19   Fabricating extraoral force appliances, 303

EPILOGUE

20   For the parents, 313

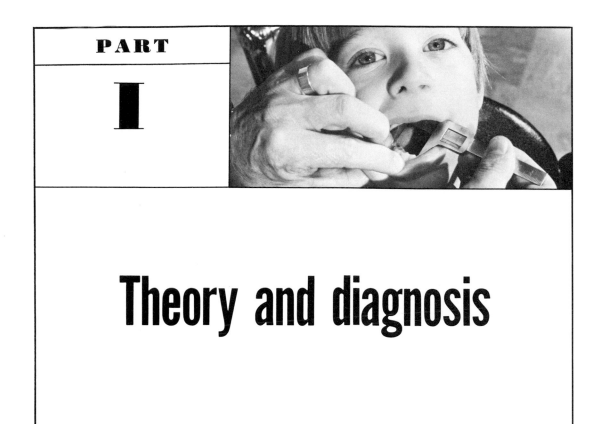

PART

I

Theory and diagnosis

1 | What is minor tooth movement?

In spite of the increasing numbers of specialists in the various disciplines within dentistry, the general practicing dentist rightfully continues to assume the largest and most meaningful responsibility for each family member's oral health care. And in the foreseeable future, as he assumes a greater role in preventive dentistry for his child patients, his responsibility will not be lessened. Indeed, the indications are clearly on the horizon that his expertise will be broadened to include more often the preventive treatment of minor malocclusions in children.

A fair amount has been written recently about how much we are *not* accomplishing in modern dentistry, as witness the galloping accusations of "Paul Revere, D.D.S."[4] It is deeply impressive, however, to review the giant strides dentistry has made during the past decade in positive directions toward better dental education, better techniques and instruments, a more highly developed group feeling among dentists, and an increasingly efficient delivery of dental care to each patient in a vastly more comfortable fashion. Dentists have rightly come to believe that they have a more and more important contribution to make toward the total mental and physical health of each member of the families who make up their dental practices.

This book concerns one important area of a general dental practice—how to knowledgeably guide the developing dentitions of children 4 to 10 years of age in ways that prevent them from straying too far from the path we have come to call "good occlusion." It is hoped each dentist who explores these chapters thoroughly will find that he has shared in a highly personal "teach-in" concerning the management of minor malocclusions in children. These experiences, complete with diagnostic puzzles to mull over, "practice pearls," and the laid-out elements of eight fixed and removable appliance techniques, should prove to be of immediate value in his daily practice.

CHANGING CONCEPTS AND PHILOSOPHY IN DENTISTRY

Certainly, as the years pass, medical and dental terminology undergoes modifications and changes in meaning. As the dental profession becomes more confident of its members' abilities to carry out techniques in patients' mouths other than purely restorative care, old terminology is lost or new meanings are transferred or

3

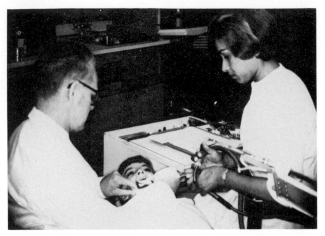

Fig. 1-1. Dentist and assistant examine a child. Dentist and assistant should examine a child in as comfortable a fashion as possible. This dental unit arranged for 4-handed dentistry is ideal for children's dental care. When the occlusion is being checked, however, the child should be in a relaxed position, seated upright in the chair.

substituted. This is quite true in regard to the term *minor tooth movement*.

There was a time when this term implied certain quite circumscribed procedures that would be accomplished almost entirely by the use of one or two simple removable appliances. However, with the acceptance of the reality of new directions in the private practice of dentistry, important changes have occurred in the approach to teaching preventive and interceptive orthodontics within most dental schools during the past few years. In addition, new laboratory equipment and modern technology in stainless steels have made available for the first time to the general dentist and pedodontist finely done and relatively inexpensive custom-made bands, arch wires, attachments, and other appliance components. These technologic advances have eliminated many of the time-consuming methods of fabricating appliances formerly taught in dental school and subsequently used by the dentist in his practice. The new materials offer the general dentist more than just a wider latitude in the selection of minor orthodontic appliances and increased efficiency in accomplishing tooth movement; they offer him

an opportunity to expand his concepts of preventive dentistry into the realm of prevention of many of the minor malocclusions that develop in his younger patients. These expanded concepts include the use of several types of fixed appliances that were not practical for use by the general dentist in the past. With the advent of the many new materials and techniques available to accomplish minor tooth movement, it is hoped that the majority of family dentists will accept this opportunity to diagnose and treat a greater number of the developing minor malocclusions seen among the children in their practices (Fig. 1-1).

Changes in dentists' attitudes

The technologic advances that have brought minor tooth movement procedures within the reach of the family dentist have been accompanied by changes in the dentist's attitude to make him more willing to make minor tooth movement a meaningful part of his practice.

The explicit factors bringing about the tremendously increased interest of the more recently graduated dentist in minor tooth movement procedures that were once deemed separate from his field are not difficult to identify. Pride in his professional ability, better dental school background in diagnosis and treatment of malocclusions, better materials with which to make appliances, simpler techniques of spot-welding and soldering of stainless steel materials, the obvious lowering of caries rates brought about by water fluoridation, the vastly increased interest in preventive dentistry measures, and a better understanding of the physiologic role of the dentition in total body health have all combined to make the newly graduated dentist in general practice ask, "Why shouldn't I accomplish minor orthodontic procedures in my practice?"

In many instances his training in dental school under orthodontic and pedodontic instructors has specifically prepared him to apply many of these preventive orthodontic measures. Dental school teachers are responding to the needs of practitioners and are expanding and clarifying what may be taught in undergraduate orthodontic programs. Yet, commonsense guidelines for interceptive tooth movement in general practice situations still seem ill defined.

Pressures on the family dentist to accept responsibility for the interception of minor malocclusions come from parents and peers alike. Some pressure is generated by dental colleagues exchanging information about tooth movement cases in which they have been successful.

Success must stem from other than casual experimentation, however. To be successful in this area of dentisty, it is necessary that good diagnostic procedures, good treatment methods, and the reasons behind treatment failures be fully explored also. This implies that the dentist must develop a good basic background in the etiology of aberrant occlusions of the growing child. He must know how they develop and why. He must be aware of *normal* growth factors so that he may recognize the *abnormal*. He must select only the *minor* malocclusions to treat, while properly and knowledgeably separating out and referring the difficult malocclusions to orthodontic specialists. Only then will he find that his treatment methods bring success for his individual patients and a renewed sense of fulfillment to him in his practice.

Changing attitudes in the community

Parents' attitudes about orthodontic care for their children are also changing. Information regarding orthodontic care floods parents from many directions. One positive primary force that molds parental opinion regarding children's dentistry emanates from the commercial communication media. Television, radio, women's magazines, family magazines, and newspapers are founts of information and misinformation about dental care. Again and again, from these and other sources, piecemeal information comes to the attention of parents, detailing the transformation that is taking place in medical and dental care for children across the nation. Parents discuss these articles with the dentist to whom they go for family care, and this becomes a social pressure that molds his practice as he allows these changes to come into his office.

The insistence by some parents that their family dentist should handle all of their children's special dental problems is certainly unrealistic. So also is the expectation that all parents will meekly be referred from one dental specialist to another as their children grow up, without occasionally protesting the inconveniences of time and travel.

With excessive referral, responsibility for the child's dental care too often becomes divided and finally lost or neglected by the original family dentist. Parents become unhappy, and the family dentist bears the brunt of parental criticism as well as the loss of patients due to dissatisfaction. Many men have found a new dimension in their family practices by accepting for treatment a limited number of minor tooth movement cases and have ultimately achieved a better balance within themselves of a fuller interest, keener application of their skills, and a deeper understanding of the full spectrum of developing malocclusions. The community image of dentistry is certainly improved by dentists who broaden their practices and continue to grow professionally in such a fashion during their professional lifetimes.

Practice of minor tooth movement by pedodontists

Another source of added interest in minor tooth movement has been an increased flow of information to general practitioners regarding tooth movement techniques due to the burgeoning interest of pedodontists in preventive orthodontic care.

The pedodontist, who once defined himself as "a general practitioner for children 3 to 12 years of age," is gradually being supplanted by the specialist in pediatric dentistry, who is well trained concerning growth and development factors in the healthy child as well as in the ill or handicapped child. Most postgraduate programs now give extensive training in the hospital care of children, and the specialist in pediatric dentistry utilizes in his hospital practice general anesthesia restorative care and in his office practice nitrous oxide analgesia for difficult children.

Partly because of these changes in preparation for his specialty, the pedodontist increasingly has interested himself in the challenge of intercepting minor malocclusions by preventive orthodontic measures, making use of his increased experience in cephalometric analysis of the growth and development problems of children who are passing through the mixed dentition stage. His training in this area usually has been guided by orthodontists or specially trained pedodontists, and his practice reflects this facet of his education. Most pedodontists tend to use a balanced approach to the limited orthodontic care they extend to their young patients. They treat in the primary and mixed dentition almost exclusively. *Most agree that this should never*

include fullmouth corrective orthodontics when the patient has passed the age of mixed dentition. Rather, the pedodontist should carefully limit himself to the younger age group and, in almost all cases, to Class I malocclusions demonstrating dental, not skeletal, arch malformations.

This view is supported by most orthodontic educators, who have repeatedly expressed concern that neither the generalist nor the pedodontist should be involved in full arch orthodontic care. At a recent symposium one educator summed up the consensus of the assembled specialists, broadly based geographically in the United States and Canada, that the expanded recommendations from the teaching conference represented a common approach. The members of the group strongly agreed that they were opposed to the handling of true craniofacial dysplasias by the general dentist and to his use of multibanded techniques for the mass movement of teeth without adequate academic and clinical experience in the physiologic and biomechanical factors involved.[5]

Thus the trained pedodontist often finds himself midway between the family dentist and the orthodontic specialist, from the standpoint of both philosophy and practice in the area of preventive orthodontics.

Obviously, as the years pass, the pedodontist will continue to share a portion of the treatment burden of the less complicated dental malocclusions. Continuing communication among the community of pedodontists and orthodontists by way of shared courses in postgraduate and continuing education and person-to-person discussions concerning patient referrals will do much to lessen the tensions that occasionally arise in their relationships. Members of both specialties recognize the needs of the children with minor malocclusions who may benefit greatly by properly timed treatment performed by the generalist in dentistry.

In some instances the generalist identifies the limited approach that the pedodontist uses as being a more realistic answer to his own needs in general practice. In a sense this stems from the amount of parallel training they have shared as well as the "language barrier" that appears to be present between some orthodontists and generalists.

Future needs of the dental profession

It is fairly obvious that in the coming years the general dentist will accept more responsibility for treating minor orthodontic problems that develop in his child patients. To be able to accomplish this, he must take advantage of more opportunities for continuing dental education in the area. However, some writers express concern not only for this approach but also for the wider problem in dental education pertaining to the teaching of orthodontic techniques to undergraduate dental students and the changing relationships of general practitioners to specialists.

It has been stated that since the general practitioner is unable to cope with the caries problem at hand, he obviously cannot be expected to undertake the very time-consuming preventive orthodontic supervision of even a moderate number of patients. But the argument is put forward that as dental caries is gradually brought under control and increased use of auxiliary personnel helps to make further inroads on the incidence, severity, and time spent in treatment of periodontal disease, more time will become available to the practitioner. On a long-range basis, his energies may be increasingly directed toward care of malocclusions. Even though orthodontic specialists will always be needed to deal with problems truly requiring specialist care, dental educators have the responsibility to see to it that the aims of undergraduate orthodontic education are adapted more closely to the future character of dental practice.[7] One of the needs is for greater in-depth consideration of the multiplicity of factors that function to provide what we call "occlusion."

DIAGNOSING NORMAL AND ABNORMAL OCCLUSION
Defining "normal" occlusion

One of the most difficult judgments the general practitioner will be called on to make in his future practice is: what is a normal occlusion? Children differ considerably from each other even within the same family in regard to growth factors, skeletofacial patterns, and the size, shape, and spacing of their teeth within the arches. As of this moment, there is no diagnostic pattern that, taken in the young child, will outline for the dentist exactly the picture of the matured child. Yet we are often faced with the problem of deciding that a child's occlusion is either normal or not normal.

In one definition, "normal" implies a situation commonly found in the absence of disease, and normal values in a biologic system are given within a physiologic adaptive range. However, it has been stated that normal occlusion should imply more than a range of acceptable values; it should indicate also physiologic adaptability and the absence of recognizable pathologic manifestations. Such a concept of normal occlusion emphasizes the functional aspect of occlusion and the capability of the masticatory system to adapt to, or compensate for, some deviations within the range of tolerance of the system.[3]

A child with normal occlusion, then, will be accepted as one having either no devi-

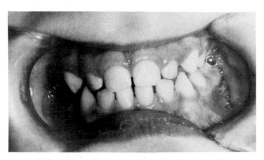

Fig. 1-2. Normal *spaced* occlusion in primary dentition at age 3 years.

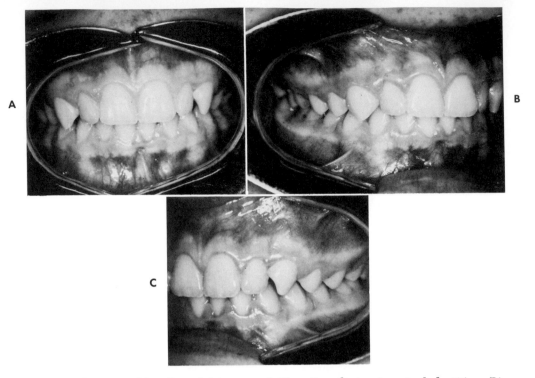

Fig. 1-3. Boy, age 10, who exhibits normal Class I occlusion in mixed dentition. Bicuspids have erupted early. **A,** Front view. **B,** Right view. **C,** Left view.

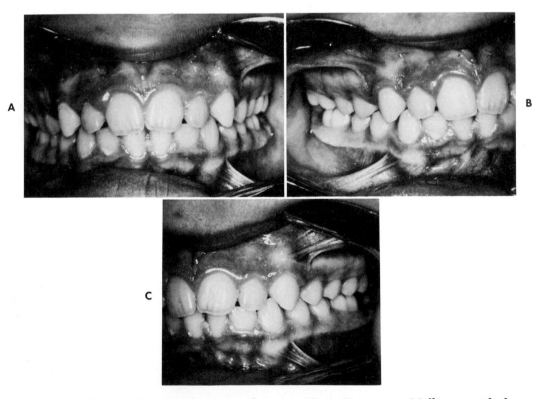

Fig. 1-4. Normal Class I occlusion in a boy, age 12. **A,** Front view. Midlines are ideal. **B,** Right side. Excellent interdigitation of cuspids and bicuspids. **C,** Left side. Excellent intercuspation of cuspids and bicuspids.

ate factors, or extremely minor ones, present in his masticatory system (Figs. 1-2 to 1-4).

Establishing limits of minor malocclusions

Although such cases will be examined in much greater detail in later chapters, parameters establishing what will be termed *minor* malocclusions are listed here so that the general dentist may realize the scope of his responsibilities in this area. Most of these responsibilities have been agreed on and accepted by orthodontists across the nation in educators' meetings and advisory conferences. It is apparent from the following discussion that a satisfying range of interceptive orthodontic treatment can be accomplished by the truly interested general practicing dentist. However, he will be ultimately successful in the treatment of these patients only if he familiarizes himself with certain growth and development factors in children, follows good diagnostic procedures, and assimilates the fundamental essentials of appliance therapy.

1. *Preservation of existing space.* When primary teeth, particularly molars, are prematurely lost by tooth removal, the space occupied by them must be preserved by appliance therapy in many cases. Some orthodontists estimate that 75% of the children they see as referrals suffer from space loss that could have been prevented.

2. *Posterior cross-bites involving primary cuspids, primary molars, and first permanent molars.* When a cross-bite exists on *one* side (i.e., unilaterally), the prevailing opinion is that the condition should be treated early, sometimes even in the primary dentition. The more complicated cases of bilateral cross-bite, involving both primary and permanent molars with an excessively narrowed palate, are usually regarded as a problem for the orthodontist.

3. *Anterior cross-bites involving one or two upper permanent incisors.* These malocclusions may be resolved if care is used to ascertain the etiology of the anterior cross-bite and there is adequate space in the arch to move the tooth or teeth into proper relationship with the other teeth. If this malocclusion appears to be a familial trait with Angle Class III tendencies, almost certainly the orthodontist should be consulted.

4. *Crowding of the lower incisors.* These cases can be treated, provided careful measurements show that space is available in the arch for all the permanent teeth.

5. *Mesial migration of maxillary 6-year molar.* If expectations are not held unreasonably high and space loss has not exceeded 3 mm. in a quadrant, the lost space can often be regained. It should be realized, however, that the treatment difficulties mount with each succeeding millimeter of space lost. In the mandibular arch the story is quite different. As will be seen, regaining lost maxillary space is considered to be much easier than regaining space lost in the mandibular arch.

6. *Mesial migration and tipping of the mandibular 6-year molars.* Orthodontists themselves describe so many difficulties in moving lower molars distally that the red flag of warning should be waved for the general dentist. Again it is a case of the *amount* of tipping or movement that has occurred. Six-year molars can be slightly uprighted posteriorly by simple appliance therapy in many cases if the 12-year molar has not erupted into a position where it can exert a mesially directed force against the distal surface of the 6-year molar. Disappointments, however, can occur far too frequently in these seemingly simple cases. If more than 2 mm. of space have been lost in a lower quadrant, the assistance of an orthodontist may be required.

7. *Closing of diastemas.* These "simple" procedures should be undertaken only after extremely careful diagnosis and study of etiology. Most diastemas existing between upper central incisors at 9 years of age will close spontaneously as the dentition matures. (See Chapter 10 for formula.) Familial history is helpful here.

8. *Flared and spaced upper anterior teeth.* Excessive protrusion of upper incisors can be treated if the molar relationship is Class I and the child is not too resistant to retraining procedures to help him overcome the particular oral habit that has produced the protruding teeth. Often the dentist is faced with the consequences of an early thumb- or finger-sucking habit that has developed into a tongue-thrusting habit.

9. *Anterior open-bite.* Anterior open-bite is nearly always indicative of a long-term oral habit. Commonly there is a problem involving a passive tongue held in position between the upper and lower front teeth or a strong tongue thrust during swallowing. A speech professional may be needed to help diagnose and institute swallowing and tongue therapy, since the possibility of an underlying speech problem exists.

By earnestly applying the few basic principles of diagnosis and a careful study of appliance techniques discussed in this book, the dentist will find the procedures of actual tooth movement can remain reasonably uncomplicated. The fixed and removable appliances described and demonstrated are deceptively simple, and yet their efficacy in general practice situations has often been proved, *provided that each case is diagnosed properly and the etiology of each malocclusion is understood.*

TREATMENT OF MINOR MALOCCLUSIONS
Suggested treatment ages in children

Minor tooth movement, in general, will involve treatment of children whose ages range between 4 and 10 years. In children younger than 4 years proper appliances for the treatment of minor occlusal disorders many times cannot be successfully worn. In children beyond 11 years the prepubertal growth spurt is beginning, and this tends to mask many diagnostic factors that are more easily seen in younger patients. To treat beyond this age is to encroach on the "prime time," so to speak, when full-mouth corrective orthodontics may most favorably be accomplished by the orthodontic specialist.

Essentially, then, minor tooth movement in children probably should be limited to the late years of primary dentition and the early and middle years of the mixed dentition. If this seems a narrow span of ages, perhaps it should be emphasized these are the years in which dentitions give many clear indications of straying from the broad path that may be termed "good occlusion." For the best success in treatment, the diagnostic acumen of each family dentist must be sharpened and his interest in minor tooth movement sustained in his practice. This may effectively avert the necessity of full-arch orthodontic treatment for many children in their teens. Remember that advanced treatment by the orthodontist often becomes necessary because vital arch space has been carelessly lost or poor occlusal relationships have been allowed to persist through the years of mixed dentition. This can occur if the family dentist has not been trained to recognize *beginning* malocclusions. Just as often, improved skill in the recognition of the warnings of poor occlusal relationships will help the family dentist to refer children to the orthodontist at an earlier age if the developing malocclusion appears to be beyond the treatment area he has defined for his practice.

The emphasis in these chapters will again and again point up the value of early diagnosis: *Early recognition of occlusal discrepancies allows the possibility of minimal interceptive treatment.* The diagnostic aids presented here are designed to help every interested dentist check his very young patients for *developing* malocclusions. The chief benefit of minor tooth movement in children is that it allows a child's dentition to be "normalized" so that he has every possible opportunity to attain his best possible dentition in his early adulthood.

It cannot be stated strongly enough that

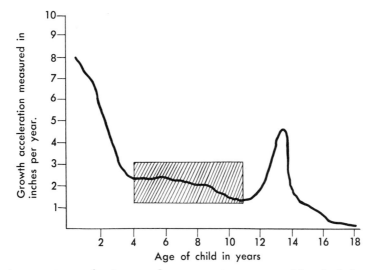

Fig. 1-5. Age spectrum of minor tooth movement, represented by shaded area, should avoid peak growth periods. "Prime time" of pubertal growth spurt should be avoided by the general dentist and reserved for the orthodontist.

the dentist seeking to help his young patients in this fashion must thoroughly review his knowledge of growth and development. Moyers[1], in his recent text, discusses the immense importance of growth factors. He emphasizes that most types of orthodontic appliances will successfully move teeth, but the dentist who fails to do his homework to gain deeper knowledge of the underlying theory necessary for the proper use of these appliances may end up mismanaging even minor malocclusions. Much of this mismanagement is engendered by ignorance of the factors of growth and development (Fig. 1-5).

Types of appliances recommended

Both removable and fixed appliances will be described for use by the family dentist. Among the removable appliances are the upper and lower Hawley appliance with labial bow, the lower clasped space maintainer, the oral screen, and the Kloehn type cervical extraoral force appliance. This last appliance is really both a fixed and removable appliance, since it has bands cemented on the upper 6-year molars.

The fixed appliances to be described are the crown (or band) with soldered loop space maintainer; the cemented lower acrylic inclined plane; the fixed (soldered) lower lingual arch as well as several types of fixed-removable (F-R) lingual arches, and two upper round-wire labial arches, one constructed with heavy wire and one with light wire.

Maintenance of lower arch form as basis of preventive orthodontics

Just as the foundation of a house determines the support of the structures erected above it, so does the form of the lower arch support and maintain the positions of the upper teeth. The ovoid form of the lower arch is the most healthful and natural pattern for these teeth, and this is the form that the dentist seeks to preserve (Fig. 1-6).

It will be seen that the mandibular permanent teeth erupt before the permanent maxillary teeth. Therefore the pattern of occlusion (or malocclusion) is most often seen early by a careful examination of the *lower* arch in the younger child.

The use of the various kinds of mandibular fixed-removable lingual arches will be

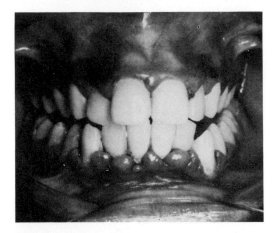

Fig. 1-6. Girl, age 16, front view. Malocclusion present has hastened onset of periodontal disease. Note that lower incisors appear as if they have been depressed lingually and upper anterior teeth appear crowded. Also, upper right lateral incisor is locked in cross-bite. Much of this combination of problems could have been prevented if the family dentist had been able to preserve the proper ovoid form in the lower arch at an earlier age.

heavily emphasized because they best serve as appliances to recover and maintain the natural ovoid form of the lower arch. They are worn as fixed appliances in the patient's mouth and yet can be easily slipped out of their attachments by the dentist at the chairside for periodic adjustments. The term *fixed-removable* lingual arch is a bit awkward, so these will be referred to as F-R lingual arches. They are held in place by horizontal or vertical attachments that have been spot-welded or soldered to the molar bands. Auxiliary springs, or finger springs, may be soldered to the F-R lingual arch wires and then activated so that when pressed against a tooth or teeth (usually the lower central and lateral incisors), the force of the wire, attempting to return to its original shape, will carry the teeth with it.

These appliances are described in more detail in Chapters 5 and 9 in the sections on lingual arches. It is important to remember that the forces built into appliances to move teeth should be light, gentle forces acting over a long period of time. Needless to relate, much damage can be done by activating appliance forces so harsh that they exceed the physiologic capacity of the periodontium. These forces should be adjusted to permit the tooth to move into a new position in the arch and yet maintain its pulpal and periodontal health.

GENERAL PROBLEMS DURING DIAGNOSIS AND TREATMENT PROCEDURES

Preventive orthodontic care must be limited to *minor* malocclusions. Nothing is more embarrassing for the family dentist than to have a seemingly simple problem in tooth position correction suddenly begin to grow more and more difficult to treat. This can occur during therapy when upper 6-year molars erupt ectopically, when lower lateral incisors erupt too far lingual to their normal positions, or when cuspids or bicuspids erupt into unexpected positions after a period of minor tooth movement treatment in the mixed dentition.[6]

Too often, unless the original case presentation to the parents is made extremely specific regarding *which* teeth are involved in the treatment program, the general dentist can find himself out of his depth by the unlooked-for arrival of such problems. In an honest reappraisal of the situation it will nearly always be found that a referral should be made immediately to an orthodontist, complete with a history of the therapy efforts that have been used.

Problems involved when treating too early

There is a strong current of opinion in dentistry which avows that early treatment provides many answers. Occasionally, however, such early treatment creates new problems.

As a specific instance of such a problem of treating too early, let us consider a lower lingual arch placed to support newly erupted mandibular permanent central incisors that have begun to incline lingually under the force of a hyperactive mentalis muscle action present during swallowing. The appliance seems to be successful in preventing the lingual collapse of the central incisors until it suddenly becomes apparent to the dentist that the two lower lateral incisors are erupting *lingual* to the arch wire. The operator is now placed in the position of having *lingually blocked out the lateral incisors,* a most interesting and potentially embarrassing iatrogenic, or dentist-caused, malocclusion.

In most cases a careful look at the periapical radiographs of the lower incisors during the diagnosis would have shown that the roots of the primary lower lateral incisors were not being resorbed in a normal fashion. Since permanent lower lateral incisors almost never erupt labially, the diagnostic conclusion should have been that the lateral incisors were more lingually located than is normal and that placement of the lingual arch wire to prevent lingual tipping of the lower central incisors should have been deferred until the permanent lateral incisors had erupted, despite their lingual positions. Diagnostic factors such as these will be discussed in detail in appropriate chapters.

Problems of retention

After a course of treatment, the dentist must remain alert to the necessity of following his patients to make certain the teeth are being naturally retained in their new positions. In general, fewer problems of retention occur after minor tooth movement accomplished during mixed dentition than is the case subsequent to full-arch orthodontic therapy during and after puberty. Following are several examples of this:

1. Reduction of *posterior* cross-bite. The retention problem is usually solved by tooth intercuspation if the cuspal slopes on the occlusal table of the molars are steep enough; that is, the cuspal slopes on the molars have to be steep enough to cause the molars to "lock" into their new positions reasonably well.

2. Correction of an *anterior* cross-bite. The new incisal relationships tend to be retained quite well, with the arch form of the lower anterior teeth holding the upper incisors in position.

3. Corrective posterior positioning of 6-year molars. The eruption of bicuspids tends to help retain the molars in their new positions.

4. Treatment to align crowded lower incisors into a more normal arch perimeter. The lower permanent cuspids can now erupt and seem to retain quite successfully the incisors' corrected positions in the arch.

5. Retruding (lingual repositioning) of procumbent upper anterior teeth. The existing hypotonicity of the upper lip and the poor swallowing patterns of the child may be changed by training so that more normal lip habits and tongue positions will aid retention. The lips themselves then can serve as muscular retainers to hold the upper anterior teeth in their new positions.

When and how to refer to the orthodontist

When a family dentist is expanding his practice to include the treatment of minor malocclusions in his child patients, he must make certain that his diagnosis is carefully done. If he is in doubt, he may wish to consult with, or refer the child to, an orthodontist. Some general rules regarding situations in which a dentist should refer a child rather than initiate treatment himself are as follows:

1. When the parent of the patient requests this

2. When the problem does not fall within the previously outlined scope of treatment by a general practicing dentist

3. If the patient is older than 10 years

4. If the dentist is informed that an orthodontist has been following the case previous to the present office visit, even though treatment may not have been actually started

Example of a letter of referral to an orthodontist

Dear Doctor Smith:

This is to introduce Jimmy Jones, age 10, son of Mr. and Mrs. Henry Jones, 856 Maple Drive, City. He has been a patient of mine for five years and has cooperated fully with all my toothbrushing and other home preventive care instructions. Jimmy has two younger sisters and two older brothers at home. One of the older brothers received edgewise technique orthodontic care in another city before they moved here five years ago. The results appear to me to be very good.

I would like you to see Jimmy and evaluate his case if you will. He appears to have a Class II, Division 2, malocclusion. His restorative care has been completed, but I WILL BE CHECKING HIM FOR CARIOUS LESIONS, TAKING CAVITY-DISCLOSING X-RAY STUDIES, AND PERFORMING A PROPHYLAXIS AND FLUORIDE TREATMENT EVERY SIX MONTHS. I am sending his recent fullmouth x-ray films in a separate envelope.

Please let me know what you think about Jimmy's case after you have talked with his parents. They will expect a call from your office for an appointment.

Thank you,

(Signed) _____

Copy for Jimmy's file.

---

5. If the dentist has any doubts regarding his ability and training to treat the problem he has diagnosed

Many orthodontists will encourage dentists in their immediate area to telephone regarding patients, even when both realize that this kind of consultative advice leaves much to be desired. Some dentists feel obligated to consult with their orthodontist at least once a month to ask the questions about their patients' malocclusions that puzzle them. It is good practice to keep the channels of communication wide open between the dentist in general practice and the orthodontic specialist. This, of course, applies in equal measure to a pedodontist's relations with these groups.

A referral is usually best arranged if the family dentist writes a letter to the orthodontist (see sample above). He may send a copy to the parents at his option.

The advantages of such a letter of referral are quite obvious. It serves to inform the orthodontist that Jimmy is a good cooperative patient, that his parents know a good bit about orthodontic care already, that there are younger siblings at home, and that you are interested in following Jimmy as his regular dentist. A copy of the letter will remain in your files.

A generalist should not compete with the specialist

As the community in which the dentist practices begins to realize that he will accept minor malocclusion problems for treatment, inevitably he will be asked by some parents to step outside the bounds of his training, skills, and experience to take on a more difficult case for treatment. Tempting as this may be in some instances, he should limit himself only to the minor interceptive orthodontic problems, or he may find himself placed in a competitive position with the orthodontic specialist. To yield to this temptation is extremely unwise. To whom, then, can he refer his orthodontic patients who present difficult malocclusions and for whose care he has not been trained?

Moyers[2] has summed up admirably the attitude of the well-informed general practitioner in this regard. His message is that generalists should realize that all orthodontists are not trained alike and all do not do interceptive orthodontics themselves. Even today, orthodontists do very little treatment in the primary and mixed dentitions, although there has been a stronger tendency toward early treatment in recent years. He should remember that the orthodontist's most difficult job is still the correction of comprehensive problems in the young adult dentition. The orthodontist should never be given the idea that the generalist is planning to do every bit of the interceptive work his training and experience will permit or that he is limiting his practice to this kind of treatment.

Most orthodontists prefer that the family dentist be informed about facial growth, the development of occlusion, and orthodontic care in general. It is fairly obvious that the general practitioner so informed is able to appraise in a better fashion the care that the orthodontist offers to his patients. The skillful orthodontist is not afraid to have his work assessed. On the contrary, he wishes it, since he wants his efforts appreciated. In summary, the well-informed general practitioner can keep many of the minor problems out of the orthodontist's office and is far more likely to get the difficult ones to the orthodontist at the correct time.

SUMMARY

As the dentist utilizes this book to meet his own special needs in the clinical area of minor tooth movement, in either general practice or the field of pedodontics, he will discover that the treatment spectrum outlined here is surprisingly narrow. However, it is to be hoped that he will also recognize the many clinical applications of these ideas to his daily practice. Whether it concerns impression taking and model pouring, fitting and cementing bands to make a lingual arch appliance, or bending arch wire for a fixed light labial arch or whether it is used to train auxiliary personnel to make minor tooth movement appliances in the laboratory, these chapters will open many avenues toward an increased degree of fulfillment for him in his practice.

REFERENCES

1. Moyers, R. E.: Handbook of orthodontics, ed. 2, Chicago, 1963, Year Book Medical Publishers, Inc., p. ix.
2. Ibid., p. 441.
3. Ramfjord, S. P., and Ash, M. M.: Occlusion, Philadelphia, 1966, W. B. Saunders Co., p. 89.
4. Revere, Paul: Dentistry and its victims, New York, 1970, St. Martin's Press, Inc., p. 305.
5. Spengemann, W. G.: Foreword, Dent. Clin. North Am., pp. 267-272, July, 1968.
6. Taylor, G. S., and Hamilton, M. C.: Ectopic eruption of lower lateral incisors, J. Dent. Child. **38:**62-64, July-Aug., 1971.
7. Woodside, D. G.: The present role of the general practitioner in orthodontics, Dent. Clin. North Am., pp. 483-508, July, 1968.

2 | Normal and ectopic eruption of teeth

Before the correction of positions of teeth by minor tooth movement appliances is described in any detail, some normal and abnormal eruption patterns of primary and permanent teeth should be considered. In the traditional views of development of occlusion, the teeth seem to erupt through the gingiva and seek their positions in the dental arch more or less according to a master plan. Certain events, however, which may be observed by the astute dentist, can serve to delay, distort, or even abort this plan.

NORMAL ERUPTION PATTERNS OF TEETH

A careful clinical analysis of forces acting on the teeth as they erupt is extremely revealing. A series of events in the life of each tooth is brought to light, which can give a more dynamic picture of the struggle each tooth undergoes as it responds to the pressures that move it into its arch position.

The final spurt of eruption of permanent teeth and the simultaneous growth of the alveolar crest are interesting phenomena to observe. The illusion is of buds opening and flowering into maturity within a short span of months. After observing many chil-

dren, however, the attentive dentist will see that the following eruption patterns emerge:

1. Teeth tend to erupt along the line of their own axes until they meet resistance, which, for the succedaneous tooth, comes in the form of a primary tooth which must be resorbed.

2. As the primary tooth is resorbed, a channel is created in the alveolar bone through which the permanent tooth moves, pressed on by its own motive force of eruption, a great part of which stems from root formation.

3. If trauma or advanced caries has rendered the primary tooth nonvital, it may act as a shunt, forcing the permanent tooth aside from its normal path of eruption. Lack of arch space can produce a similar shunting aside of an erupting tooth.

4. Genetic factors can cause odd eruption patterns, which often can be seen to be familial in nature.

5. As the tooth erupts, certain forces help guide it into or distort it from its normal arch position. These forces may stem from pressures of adjacent teeth, muscles of the tongue, cheeks, lips, mentalis muscle, and occasionally the thumb, fingers, or other sucked objects.

Because the eruption patterns of teeth are intertwined so inextricably with the subsequent movement and natural migration of these teeth, it is necessary to review these patterns to distinguish between the normal and the abnormal (Fig. 2-1).

Eruption patterns of primary teeth

It is well accepted that fewer malocclusions occur in the deciduous dentition, and yet is it also clear that certain influences can be noted early on, which will be significant and in some cases will permit a prediction of need for treatment later in the permanent dentition.

The sequence of eruption of primary teeth has been well documented by various authors. Finn[2] uses the McCall and Schour modification of the Logan and Kronfeld chart[5] to describe this sequence in his pedodontic text. It is quite normal that by age 3 in the average child the twenty primary teeth have grown into an occlusion that usually exhibits almost no curve of Spee, shallow cuspal interdigitation, very slight overbite and overjet, and very little crowding. Indeed, in many instances they may exhibit generalized interdental spacing, or spaces may occur interdentally in certain specific areas (Fig. 2-2).

Spaced primary dentitions

Baume[1] was the first to name the spaces most commonly found in many deciduous dentitions between the upper lateral incisors and cuspids and between the lower cuspids and primary first molars. Because they so markedly corresponded to the spaces observed in the dentitions of monkeys, he termed them *primate spaces* (Fig. 2-3).

Using this as a guide for naming a deciduous dentition as *spaced* or *unspaced,* Baume also concluded that *no additional spaces appear interdentally as the child gets older if he starts out with an unspaced dentition,* thereby exploding one of the continuing myths of dentistry. It has been observed that the interdental spaces between primary teeth do *not* increase in size after 3 years of age as folklore had insisted; rather it has been found that they tend to disappear during the eruption of the permanent incisors.[7] This is fairly logical when one compares the increased size of the permanent incisors as compared to that of the respective primary teeth.

Having a spaced primary dentition almost certainly gives a child a head start toward having well-spaced permanent teeth. However, this does not always mean that if a child's primary dentition is crowded, he has no chance of having anything but crowded permanent teeth.

Regarding this, Moorrees[7] notes that it is of considerable clinical significance that some of the children studied had a normal occlusion of their permanent dentition in spite of a marked lack of space or a large surplus of space during the transitional period. In part, this is accounted for by the increase in width of the arch during the eruption of the permanent cuspids.

Sequence of normal eruption of permanent teeth
Six-year molars

Most writers agree that the first permanent molar is usually the first permanent tooth to erupt.

Regarding this emergence of the mixed dentition stage, Moyers[10] indicates that with the arrival of the first permanent tooth there begins the hazardous process of transferring from the primary dentition to the permanent. During this period, which normally lasts from ages 6 to 12, the dentition is highly susceptible to environmental changes. Since many malocclusions become evident at this time, it is important to be familiar with the rather complicated process of the normal transfer of dentitions.

Baume emphasized the importance of terminal planes of the second deciduous molars as clues to predicting whether the first permanent molars will erupt into normal, or Class I, occlusion. Even when these

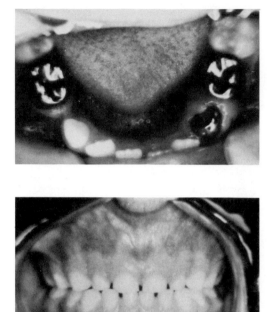

Fig. 2-1. Flattening of the arc of the lower anterior segment in this Class I malocclusion may be seen. It may result in blocking out permanent cuspids labially. Note also distal migration of lower primary cuspids. As this illustration demonstrates, much information can be gained by close observation of the tooth positions in the lower arch.

Fig. 2-2. Girl, age 4½ years. Primary dentition exhibits generalized spacing. With such spacing present, the child usually will have no serious problem erupting her permanent teeth.

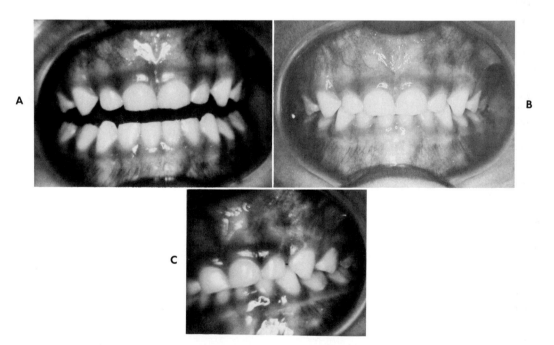

Fig. 2-3. Unspaced primary dentition of girl, age 4 years. **A,** Front view, open. Small primate spaces are evident in this child's teeth. **B,** Front view, closed. **C,** Left view. Note primate space distal to upper lateral incisor.

more obvious clues are used, the dentist must face many problems in making a predictive diagnosis of whether the mature dentition will exhibit a normal occlusion. Nothing can serve as a substitute for careful observation and meticulous measurements of the arch dimensions and the widths of teeth.

However, even if the occlusion of the primary teeth has been observed to be satisfactory in a child younger than 6 years, close attention should be paid to the eruption pattern of the first permanent molars. Careful scrutiny of the positions of primary molars will allow certain predictive assumptions to be made regarding the future occlusion of the 6-year molars, since the terminal planes of the second primary molars guide the erupting 6-year molars into their positions in the dental arch. It is instructive to look at the two desirable ways in which Class I molar occlusion can ultimately develop during the early mixed dentition period.

In observing 60 children during the time of eruption of the permanent first molars, Baume[1] found two chief variations in the mechanism leading to normal (Class I) molar occlusions: (1) a mesial step in the terminal plane of the deciduous second molars permitted the permanent first molars to erupt directly into normal occlusion; (2) a straight terminal plane plus a mandibular primate space that closed up by mesial drifting of the deciduous molars led to a proper occlusion of the permanent first molars.

The second variation has been termed the "late mesial shift" by Moyers.[10] This can occur when there exist a straight terminal plane and an absence of interdental spacing, which has resulted in a temporary end-to-end molar relationship. This may be acceptable but is not considered desirable. Later when the lower second primary molar is lost by normal exfoliation, the lower 6-year molar drifts mesially slightly during the eruption of the second bicuspid, which requires less space than its predeces-

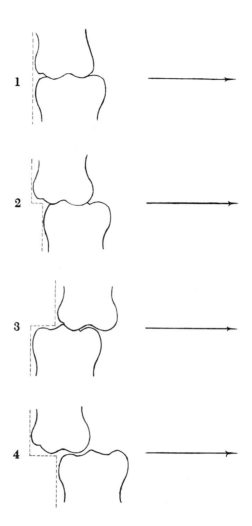

Fig. 2-4. Terminal planes of primary second molars viewed from right side. From careful observation of these terminal planes, certain predictions can be made regarding the future occlusion of 6-year molars. *1,* Flush terminal plane. This will allow first permanent molars to erupt into an end-to-end relationship. Later, when second primary molars are exfoliated, lower 6-year molar shifts mesially more than upper 6-year molar. This is described by Moyers as the "late mesial shift" into normal Class I malocclusion. *2,* Mesial-step terminal plane. This allows 6-year molars to erupt directly into normal Class I malocclusion. *3,* Distal-step terminal plane. This allows 6-year molars to erupt only into Class II malocclusion. *4,* Exaggerated mesial-step terminal plane. This allows 6-year molars to be guided only into Class III malocclusion.

Table 1. Normal ages of eruption of permanent teeth*

Maxillary teeth		6		1	2		4	5	3	7
Age in years	(6)		(7)	(8)		(9)		(10)	(11)	(12)
Mandibular teeth	6	1	2			3	4	5		7

*Palmer method of designating teeth used here. See Table 2.

sor. This results in normal, or Class I, occlusion of the 6-year molars.

Influence of terminal planes of primary molars on 6-year molar eruption. It can be seen that in the prediction of the future positions of the 6-year molars the terminal planes of the second primary molars form an important diagnostic checkpoint. To include Class II and Class III malocclusions* in a broader view, the four types of terminal planes and their influence on the permanent molar occlusion may be diagrammed as in Fig. 2-4. Class II results from an exaggerated *distal* step, whereas Class III results from an exaggerated *mesial* step.

Permanent central and lateral incisors, cuspids, and bicuspids

The eruption of the mandibular central incisors usually follows immediately the eruption of the 6-year molars. Almost without exception the parent will report that the lower central incisors are the first permanent teeth to erupt, since the eruption of the 6-year molars was not noted by the parents or reported by the child. The permanent teeth present in the child's mouth should always be *counted* for the parents both during the examination and case presentation. Rarely are they aware of the presence of the 6-year molars or their significance to the permanent dentition. In case presentations to the parents, these teeth should be referred to as the "corner posts" or "foundations" of a good dentition.

The lower lateral incisors, then the up-

*Angle's three classes of malocclusions and the Dewey-Anderson amplification of Angle's Class I are discussed in Chapter 3.

per central incisors are the next to erupt in a normal sequence. These are followed by the upper lateral incisors, the lower cuspids, the lower second bicuspids, and lastly by the upper cuspids. Diagrammatically, the age of the child and sequence of normal eruption should resemble that shown in Table 1, which employs the Palmer system of notation explained in Table 2.

However, the tooth eruption pattern of some individuals may show considerable variation from this so-called normal sequence. If the eruption sequence of a child differs markedly from the normal, it may be an indication of a developing malocclusion (Fig. 2-5).

Self-correction of malocclusions through growth and development

In the past, many dentists have avoided early treatment of malocclusions because they believed that normal growth and de-

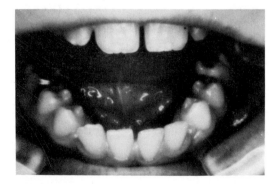

Fig. 2-5. In this 10-year-old child the lower anterior teeth have moved lingually and are flared to the distal due to lack of support from the cuspid area. Main force moving teeth is mentalis muscle. Presence of bicuspids before cuspids indicates this to be a clear case of improper sequence of tooth eruption.

Table 2. Palmer system of identifying teeth

		E	D	C	B	A	A	B	C	D	E			
8	7	6	5	4	3	2	1	1	2	3	4	5	6	7	8
8	7	6	5	4	3	2	1	1	2	3	4	5	6	7	8
		E	D	C	B	A	A	B	C	D	E			

The dentist must have at his disposal a fast, accurate way of designating each tooth in the arch. Because so many orthodontic band kits and some pedodontic stainless steel crown kits use the Palmer system, this is the one chosen for use in this book. It is convenient, widely used, and easily taught to a dental assistant.

Accurate identification of individual teeth present in the arches is of extreme importance in any diagnostic procedure. The use of the Palmer system for identifying missing teeth or those involved in a cross-bite or open-bite relationship permits clear and accurate patient chart notes to be maintained. Since most orthodontists use this system, telephone consultations also become clearer and can be entered as chart notes without the attendant hazards of attempting a translation to another identification code system.

The vertical line is assumed to be the midline of the arches, and the horizontal line is assumed to be the occlusal plane. Deciduous teeth are designated in capital letters. An example would be ⌊E, the upper left second deciduous molar. The permanent teeth are designated by number. 6⌉ is the lower right first permanent molar. This system will be used throughout this book.

velopment of the child would somehow solve the problem. Clinical research has indicated otherwise. Moorrees[8] quotes Silver's (1944) longitudinal survey of 342 children with malocclusions at the Forsyth Dental Infirmary who *did not* receive orthodontic treatment. He showed that either a mesial or a distal relationship of the dental arches has very little chance for improvement under the normal influences of growth and development. Of the Class II type malocclusions, 76% became worse, and of the Class III malocclusions, 89%. Only children with occlusal anomalies belonging to the Class I group showed some self-correction, namely, 47 out of 235 (20%). This means that even with early identification of Class I malocclusions, only one out of five children's arches can be expected to be self-correcting.

ECTOPIC ERUPTION

Ectopic eruption is defined here as the abnormal eruption of a permanent tooth, which is both out of position and causing the resorption of a primary tooth in an abnormal fashion.

Ectopic eruptions of the upper first permanent molar and the lower lateral incisor are the most common positional aberrations that occur during the eruption of permanent teeth. The malposition of the 6-year molar is genetically induced, whereas in the ectopic lower lateral incisor the dentist may be dealing with a muscular force problem. The ectopically erupting maxillary 6-year molar tends to resorb the distobuccal root of the second primary molar, since the former is genetically malposed in a *mesial* direction. The permanent lower lateral incisor, however, is usually forced by crowding to ectopically erupt in a *distal* direction. This causes it to resorb the adjacent root of the lower primary cuspid while erupting. Many times this crowding of the lower incisors results from muscular contractions of the mentalis muscle during swallowing; therefore the genesis of the ectopic eruptions seen in lower lateral incisors may be environmental factors. It is important in a diagnosis to attempt to separate genetic influences from environmental factors when ectopic patterns of eruption are observed; minor tooth movement may correct environmentally caused malpositions, but genetically caused malpositions are much more difficult to correct.

Maxillary first permanent molar

Solving the problem of ectopic eruption of an upper first permanent molar is not easy. In fact, there is a fair amount of disagreement over the proper course to follow in some cases.

A recent article[3] has pointed out the consequences of the ectopic eruption of the maxillary 6-year molar and suggested a remedy. It explains that the ectopic maxillary first permanent molar cannot erupt properly because it is locked on the distal surface of the second primary molar. The second primary molar has become mobile because of the resorption of the distal portions of its roots. The article goes on to suggest that the second primary molar should be extracted when its resultant mobility causes discomfort to the child or when the first permanent molar has moved too far mesially into the space created by its resorption of the roots of the primary molar. It is proposed that an activated space regainer be inserted immediately to reposition the first molar distally, thus attempting to regain the space that was lost as this tooth erupted ectopically. When the space has been regained, a fixed space maintainer may be inserted.[3]

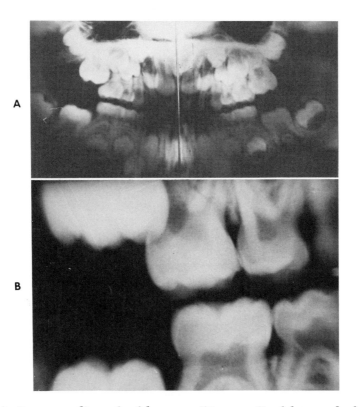

Fig. 2-6. A, Panorex radiograph of boy, age 7½ years. Careful perusal of such radiographs can give the dentist hints concerning eruption paths of teeth. Note ectopically erupting upper right 6-year molar. The adjacent second primary molar has been loosened, and some dentists yield to the temptation to extract these loosened teeth. They may be salvaged, however, by judicious use of the Humphrey appliance. B, Bitewing radiograph of the ectopically erupting 6-year molar seen in A.

It should be noted here that not all clinicians, including myself, agree that the endangered second primary molar should be extracted. Several other methods of treating such cases without resorting to extraction will be offered in Chapter 6. (See Fig. 2-6.)

Mandibular permanent lateral incisors

McDonald[6] notes that in most children the permanent lower lateral incisors erupt essentially normally. However, in some children an excessive amount of tooth material or a genetically inadequate arch length may cause the crown of the lateral incisor to ectopically erupt distal to its normal position and resorb part of the mesial

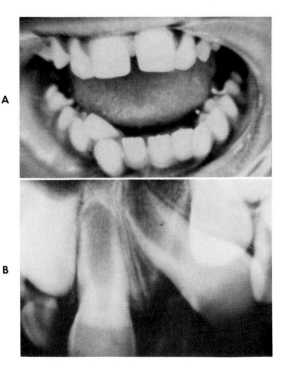

A

B

Fig. 2-7. **A,** Ectopically erupting lower lateral incisor. This is a case beyond the scope of usual minor tooth movement treatment. **B,** X-ray film of upper central incisor erupting ectopically. This occurs much less often than ectopic eruption of the lower lateral incisor seen in **A.** There is a history of trauma to the primary central incisor in many of these cases.

aspect of the root of the primary cuspid. The recognition of this problem should come from x-ray examination of the patterns of resorption of the roots of the primary incisors and cuspids. If only one primary cuspid is lost in this fashion, a measurable drift of the lower dental midline will be seen in the direction of the prematurely lost primary cuspid. Often the dentist may miss this midline change of position because he is not always aware of the seriousness of the too early loss of one or both primary cuspids. Also frequently overlooked are the distorting influences that the muscles of the lower lip can exert on the positions of lower permanent incisors to flatten the arc of the lower anterior teeth. The dental midline between the lower central incisors may drift to the right or left, and the space available in this portion of the arch may be lessened by these muscle forces.

In an unpublished study by Croxton noted by McDonald,[6] it was found that 32 of 400 children had 48 lateral incisors erupting ectopically—17 maxillary and 31 mandibular. It is felt by McDonald that this condition is one indicating a genetic arch length inadequacy. Hyperactivity of the mentalis muscle was apparently not considered in this study, nor was the change of the dental midlines considered. In later chapters much more emphasis will be placed on diagnosing the presence of muscular forces provided by the mentalis and other muscles and their effects in both shaping and distorting the dental arches. The importance of recognizing changes of positions in dental midlines and acting to intercept these changes will also be emphasized. (See Chapter 8 for treatment of this problem of insufficient arch space and Fig. 2-7.)

Shifting of mandibular dental midline in direction of least resistance

Teeth and dental midlines seem to move in the direction of least resistance. Any change in position of the lower dental midline greater than 1 mm. should serve as a warning of a developing malocclusion. Such a shift may result from the ectopic eruption of a lateral incisor and eventual loss of a primary cuspid.

When only a single deciduous cuspid is lost due to ectopic eruption of a lateral incisor, the cuspid is nearly always adjacent to the last lateral incisor to erupt. That

is, the eruption of the first lateral incisor into an arch that is either genetically inadequate or is being muscularly compressed tends to move the lower central incisors slightly to one side, causing the midline to shift from its original position. This usually causes the adjacent primary cuspid to move distally and close the primate space if this is present in the arch. The later-

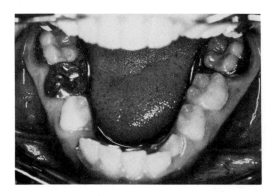

Fig. 2-8. First lower cuspid to erupt in a crowded arch usually is blocked out labially (rarely lingually as shown here), and shifted midline in the lower arch stabilizes in its new position. Note midline shift to the right is in process of being corrected by use of a fixed-removable lingual arch.

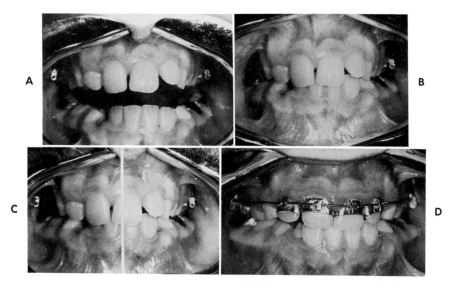

Fig. 2-9. Upper dental midline of a 10-year-old girl has deviated markedly to the right due to the congenital lack of an upper right primary cuspid. **A,** Open view. **B,** Note upper and lower dental midline relationships remain the same as in **A. C,** Dental midlines may be checked and compared with the midsagittal plane by the use of a 15-inch length of dental floss held against the middle of the child's forehead, nose, and chin. **D,** Upper light-wire labial arch appliance (one of the eight basic appliances used in this book) was fitted to begin the recovery of the upper dental midline to normal. Note changes in interdental spacing that have already occurred in upper arch as a result of treatment.

erupting lateral incisor on the opposite side of the arch, however, has been cheated out of a portion of its allotted space, and proceeds to erupt ectopically distal to its usual position, resorbing the primary cuspid root and causing the premature loss of this important stabilizing tooth. The midline is then caused to shift even more in the same direction when the permanent cuspids erupt unevenly in the same sequence. The last permanent cuspid to erupt ends up being blocked out of the arch, usually in a labial position. This is an example of how teeth tend to follow the path of least resistance during their pattern of eruption. Using this rule will aid the dentist in predicting more accurately the position of the fully erupted tooth (Fig. 2-8).

Early recognition that a change in the position of the mandibular dental midline has occurred is best followed by two measures:

1. Careful scrutiny of the x-ray films of the lower anterior region during ages 6 to 8 years to observe abnormal root resorption patterns in the primary anterior teeth
2. Careful observation of the direction of the shift of the dental midline, best done by stretching a piece of dental floss along the forehead-nose-chin line to simulate the midsagittal plane (Fig. 2-9)

The importance of maintaining the positions of the upper and lower dental midlines exactly at the mid-sagittal plane cannot be overemphasized. A dental midline once lost is difficult to regain. It is far better to intercept the beginning malocclusion than it is to correct it once it has fully expressed itself.

The "arrow rule." When a shift in the upper or lower dental midline *has* occurred, the "arrow rule" may help establish the causes of the shift. First, determine in which direction the shift has occurred, using the dental floss as described in the section on arrow rule in Chapter 4. Second, place a mental arrow in that direc-

tion. The cause of the shift will usually be found in the quadrant to which the arrow points (Fig. 2-10). For example, if a lower right primary cuspid has been lost prematurely, the dental midline will move to the right as the incisors drift in the direction of least resistance. These steps in diagnosing and identifying the five types of treatable Class I malocclusions will be examined in much greater detail in the section on the diagnostic quadrangle in Chapter 4.

Importance of environmental factors

Obviously, in space-deficient lower arches an ectopic condition may be present *bilaterally* in the mandibular lateral incisors. This may result in *both* mandibular primary cuspids being resorbed and exfoliated too early by the ectopic eruption patterns of the lateral incisors. If this is the case, environmental pressures acting against the lower incisors may worsen the space problem. Pressures generated by the mentalis muscle during the swallowing act may cause the lower lip to press this immature anterior segment of teeth in a lingual direction, producing a more serious crowding situation. This may occur with

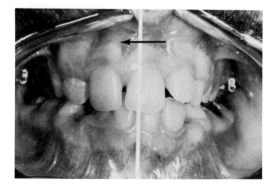

Fig. 2-10. The "arrow" rule: Place an imaginary arrow in the direction of the dental midline deviation. This points to quadrant where the trouble usually lies. This 9½-year-old girl had a congenitally missing upper right primary cuspid, causing the exaggerated midline shift to the right.

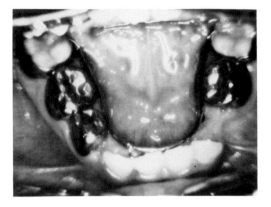

Fig. 2-11. Dentition of girl, age 8½, showing flattening of normal anterior lower arch circumference by the action of a hyperactive mentalis muscle. Note that a fixed-removable lingual arch with a finger spring has been placed to prevent any further lingual tipping of these unsupported lower incisors.

or without a shift of the lower dental midline, but will almost certainly serve to promote two conditions: (1) a flattening of the normally rounded lower anterior arch circumference (Fig. 2-11) and (2) the subsequent blocking out labially of the permanent mandibular cuspids.

Occasionally, in an incipient Class III dentition the lower anterior segment is seen to be flattened, mimicking the condition produced by a hyperactive mentalis muscle action. However, the permanent cuspids in these children usually are seen to be *lingual* to the flared distal surfaces of the lower incisors, not *labial* as in most Class I, Type I, muscular cases (Fig. 2-12).

SUMMARY

The knowledge of how teeth erupt normally in the primary and permanent dentitions offers a firm foundation for detecting early abnormalities in the dentitions of children. Only by constant comparison to the normal patterns can the effects of exaggerated mesial or distal steps in the terminal planes of primary second molars be understood.

So also must the normal positions of permanent lower central and lateral incisors be visualized in order to recognize early that a lateral incisor is undergoing ectopic eruption. This pattern of normalcy should

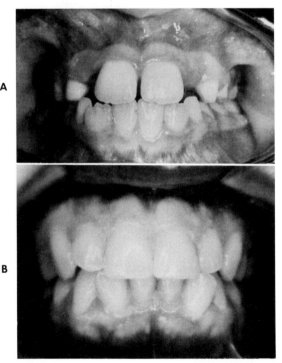

A

B

Fig. 2-12. **A,** Child, age 8 years, developing a crowding and mild Class III tendency in lower anterior teeth. Etiologic factors here are several: hyperactive mentalis muscle, lateral growth in anterior of mandible (particularly evident at this age), and hereditary tooth size/arch space discrepancy. Compare with adult in **B. B,** The 40-year-old mother of girl in **A** who shows genetic similarity in lower anterior region.

include the dental midlines, with the realization that if their position is to right or left of the midsagittal plane (as represented by the dental floss positioned in the middle of the face), this should warn the dentist that teeth are shifting in the direction of least resistance.

REFERENCES

1. Baume, L. J.: Physiological tooth migration and its significance for the development of occlusion. Part I. The biogenetic course of the deciduous dentition, J. Dent. Res. 29:123-132, 1950.
2. Finn, S. B., editor: Clinical pedodontics, ed. 3, Philadelphia, 1967, W. B. Saunders Co., p. 60.
3. Gellin, M. E.: Indications and contradictions for the removal of primary teeth, Dent. Clin. North Am., pp. 899-911, Oct., 1969.
4. Lo, R., and Moyers, R. E.: The sequence of eruption of the permanent dentition, Am. J. Orthod. 39:460-467, 1953.
5. Logan, W. H. G., and Kronfeld, R.: Development of the human jaws and surrounding structures from birth to age fifteen years, J. Am. Dent. Assoc. 20:379-427, 1933.
6. McDonald, R. E.: Pedodontics, St. Louis, 1963, The C. V. Mosby Co., p. 444.
7. Moorrees, C. F. A.: The dentition of the growing child, Cambridge, Mass., 1959, Harvard University Press, p. 122.
8. Ibid., p. 18.
9. Moyers, R. E.: Handbook of orthodontics, ed. 2, Chicago, 1963, Year Book Medical Publishers, Inc., p. 70.
10. Ibid., p. 72.

3 | Recognition of abnormal arch patterns

The ability to recognize that a dental arch pattern is developing into a malocclusion beyond the range considered normal is vital to the dentist contemplating treatment procedures to correct the abnormality. Even though it does not solve treatment problems, the very fact that a malocclusion may be accurately recognized as belonging within a certain category of malocclusions can serve to promote self-confidence in the dentist.

There have been many methods proposed for separating into categories the so-called major malocclusions. It is generally agreed that Edward Angle's method of systematizing these malocclusions has remained preeminent for more than half a century.

One weakness of the Angle system from the general practitioner's point of view is that much attention is paid to identifying the several types of Class II and Class III malocclusion categories and less effort is directed toward clarifying the factors present in commonly recurring kinds of Class I malocclusions. The Dewey-Anderson system of separating Class I malocclusions into five different *types* appears to answer this keenly felt need. Use of this latter system allows simpler methods for recogniz-

ing early arch pattern deviations within the range of Class I malocclusions. Recognition of these factors allows a diagnostic appraisal to take place early in the primary dentition stage, as opposed to the Angle concept that the 6-year molars must be in occlusion before meaningful diagnoses may be made.[5]

In addition to the positions of the molar teeth, the positions of the cuspids, both deciduous and permanent, will be used to "prove" that the positions of the molars are being correctly diagnosed.

REVIEW OF CLASSIFICATION OF MALOCCLUSIONS

Not only individual teeth but the various main categories of malocclusions should also be accurately identified. Although there have been proposed many systems, one of those best accepted, as suggested previously, is the Angle system reviewed in the following section.

Disagreements among dentists over what constitutes "ideal" occlusion have persisted through much of the past century. Even now there are nearly as many definitions of occlusion as there are professors teaching dentistry.

Close study of many hundreds of occlusions in young adults would reveal a broad spectrum of dentition patterns. In general, these patterns can be grouped into several kinds that resemble each other and are found with some predictable consistency within a uniracial population.

To aid in separating these varying kinds of occlusions, Angle and others have proposed using the relative mesiodistal positions of the upper and lower 6-year molars as they mesh together in centric closure. Other men such as Dewey and Anderson have added to Angle's system to describe discrete differences among the Class I malocclusions, dealing mainly with space problems and excessive facial-lingual malpositions of individual or groups of teeth.

Since primarily the treatment of Class I malocclusions are considered here, these are reviewed in some detail in the following section.

Two additional considerations emphasized in this book are methods of identifying muscular forces acting to produce measurable malpositions of teeth within immature arches and the description of a "normal" Class I malocclusion, which has no discernible defects. The concept of a "zero defects" Class I malocclusion can serve as a guide for the dentist as he works to maintain or attain the ideal occlusion for each child in his practice.

ANGLE'S SYSTEMATIZING OF MALOCCLUSIONS

Edward Angle, generally acknowledged to be the father of American orthodontics, felt that there was one malocclusion that had more normal dentofacial relationships than others. This relationship occurred more often than others and was present in persons who were relatively straight featured. He called this a Class I malocclusion.

The next most often seen type of individual, one with a prominent upper lip and a chin less well developed, he called a Class II malocclusion.

He assigned the term Class III malocclu-

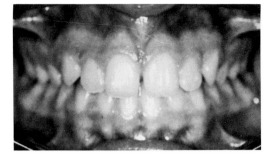

Fig. 3-1. Angle Class I malocclusion in a girl, age 12 years. This case represents nearly ideal occlusion.

sion to the prominent chinned individual whose upper arch and lip appeared to be less well developed.

Even though he divided these occlusions into three groups, one of which was essentially normal, he termed all three dentitions *malo*cclusions. Under his primarily *dental* concept, the intercuspation of the 6-year molars determined into what classification a particular dentition was placed. He viewed the upper 6-year molars as having a fixed, unchanging position and regarded the mandible as being the source of error when a bite other than that of Class I was present. His categories of malocclusions have undergone remarkably few major modifications over the years (Fig. 3-1).

The following list (modified from Hitchcock[5]) presents one of the present views of how the three major malocclusions should be classified, using a system only slightly changed from that originally proposed by Dr. Angle.

Class I As the mandible closes evenly and comfortably into its relationship to the maxilla, the mesiobuccal cusp of the upper permanent molar falls into relationship with the buccal groove of the lower first permanent molar. In the United States Caucasian population 60% to 65% of the children may be grouped under Class I malocclusion.

Class II As the mandible closes evenly and comfortably into its relationship with

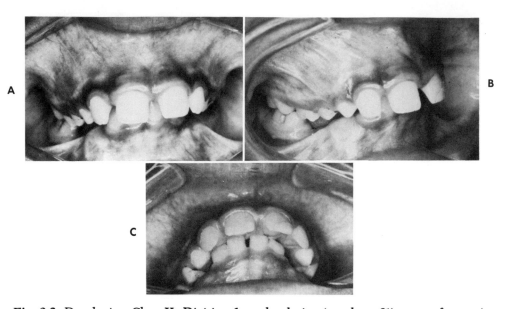

Fig. 3-2. Developing Class II, Division 1, malocclusion in a boy, 8½ years of age. **A,** Front view. Note there has been an early shift of lower dental midline. The prominent feature, however, is the protrusive maxilla. **B,** Right view. Note exaggerated curve of Spee characteristic of this malocclusion. **C,** View of exaggerated overjet common in these cases. Note lower dental midline shift to the right.

the maxilla, the mesiobuccal cusp of the upper first permanent molar is in relation to the embrasure between the lower second bicuspid and the lower first molar. In the United States Caucasian population, 25% to 30% may fall within Class II.

Class III As the mandible closes evenly and comfortably into its closed relationship with the maxilla, the mesiobuccal cusp of the upper first permanent molar falls into relation with the distobuccal grove of the lower first permanent molar. In the United States 3% to 5% of the Caucasian population may fall into Class III.

Divisions of Class II

Angle further divided Class II dentitions into two *divisions.* The divisions are determined by the axial inclination of the upper incisors.

Class II, *Division 1,* indicates that the upper central incisors are protrusive (procumbent) (Fig. 3-2).

Class II, *Division 2,* describes a dentition in which the upper central incisors may

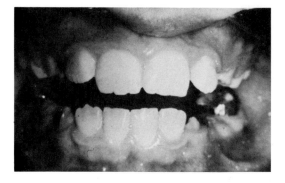

Fig. 3-3. Developing Class II, Division 2, malocclusion of a girl, 9½ years of age. Note upper lateral incisors are beginning to move labially. Flat curve of Spee is evident in lower arch, characteristic of this malocclusion. Note also that the mamelons on the incisors are unworn, indicating inability to incise due to overjet.

vary from a position of approximately vertical to a position more lingually inclined. In this latter division, the upper lateral incisors usually appear to be protruding markedly labial to the position of the central incisors (Fig. 3-3).

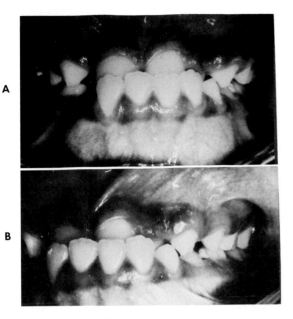

A

B

Fig. 3-4. Developing Class III malocclusion evident in boy, age 9. **A,** Front view. Note shift of upper dental midline to right, which will serve effectively to block out the upper right lateral incisor. **B,** Left view.

Subdivisions of Class II

Each Class II division has a subdivision. A subdivision describes a dentition that has a Class I molar relationship on one side of the arch and a Class II molar relationship on the other. To summarize, an individual exhibiting a Class II malocclusion would be placed in one of the following four categories:

Class II, Division 1
  Class II molar relationship on both sides; procumbent central incisors
Class II, Division 1, Subdivision
  Class II molar relationship on *one* side, Class I molar relationship on the other; procumbent central incisors
Class II, Division 2
  Class II molar relationship on both sides; near-vertical or even lingually inclined central incisors, with protruding lateral incisors
Class II, Division 2, Subdivision
  Class II molar relationship on *one* side, Class I molar relationship on the other; central incisors vertical or lingually inclined, with only one lateral incisor pro-

Table 3. Angle's classification of malocclusions*

Malocclusion	% of United States Caucasian population
Class I	60%–65%
Class II, Division 1,	
Class II, Division 1, Subdivision	
Class II, Division 2	25%–30%
Class II, Division 2, Subdivision	
Class III	
Class III, Subdivision	3%–5%

*This chart serves as an outline description of the seven diagnostic separations in Angle's system of classifying malocclusions. Also included are the approximate population percentages represented (Caucasian).

truding labially, usually on the Class II side.

Class III malocclusions

In describing Class III dentitions, Angle felt that a subdivision was also necessary. A Class III malocclusion is demonstrated when the molar relationship is Class III on both sides of the arches. Class III, Subdivision, describes a dentition in which a Class I molar relationship is present on one side and a Class III molar relationship on the other (Fig. 3-4).

• • •

To review, then, Angle's classification of malocclusions offers seven categories of molar and incisor relationships. Table 3 summarizes the percentage of each malocclusion group that could be expected in a large Caucasian population sample.

DEWEY-ANDERSON MODIFICATION OF ANGLE'S CLASS I

It can readily be seen that there is a large segment of the population (60% to 65%) that would be grouped in Class I. Yet, under Angle's system of classification, this large group was not broken down into diagnostic entities as were Class II and Class

III. It remained for the Dewey-Anderson system to remove this limitation. This system divides Angle's Class I, so that obvious and constantly recurring factors such as *genetically too little arch space, decreased posterior arch space as the result of mesially drifted permanent molars, protrusive incisors, and cross-bites* can be considered specific entities of malocclusion. Each of these Dewey-Anderson diagnostic patterns of Class I malocclusion are called *types.* They are easily recognized and are particularly useful as diagnostic aids during the mixed dentition years, but they become more blurred and therefore diagnostically less important later in the dentition of the young adult.

In the following section is a list of the Dewey-Anderson *types* of Class I, a description of the specific malocclusion they represent, the several etiologies that may help explain the origin of the malocclusion, and a brief explanation of the direction treatment might take. Each type of Class I malocclusion is separated into two general categories, one of which may be treated by the generalist and the other of which is to be referred to the orthodontic

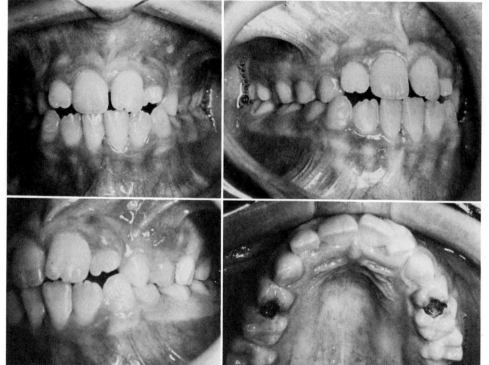

Fig. 3-5. Class I, Type 1, malocclusion in 8½-year-old girl (according to the Dewey-Anderson system of diagnosing *five* types of Class I malocclusions). This system is particularly applicable to primary and mixed dentitions. **A,** Front view. Apparently too much tooth material is present for available arch space. *Etiology: Genetic,* since dentition is crowded in both arches. **B,** Right side. Note slight cross-bite in cuspid area. Chief diagnostic feature is crowding, however. **C,** Left side. **D,** Palatal view. Note *crowded* and rotated upper incisors characteristic of *genetic* case. Some mesial drifting has probably occurred in posterior segments from loss of interproximal tooth structure due to caries. This serves to decrease the existing space in the child's arch length, which is already seen to be inadequate.

specialist. The separation is usually one that is measurable in millimeters by using a Boley gauge.

Class I, Type 1

Class I, Type 1, is characterized by crowded and rotated incisors (Fig. 3-5).

Description of malocclusion

Some children seem to have a genetic expression in their dentitions that can best be described as having too much tooth material present for the available arch space. When the upper and lower permanent incisors erupt, they do not have enough space in the arch to assume normal positions, and so they appear crowded and rotated. Lack of space in the anterior portion of both arches is the criterion, which is not to be confused with a *loss* of space in a *posterior* segment caused by the obvious mesial drifting of one of the first permanent molars. One of the reliable measurements available for the dentist in determining tooth size/arch space relationships is that the crown sizes of the permanent teeth, once formed, do not change appreciably. Yet, although the sum total of the widths of the individual teeth may not change, the size of the arches may be altered by certain growth factors. The widths of teeth may be quite accurately determined, but the measurements of immature arches should be accomplished with extreme caution for these are not nearly so reliable. This is chiefly because the growth of the bony facial complex in the younger child is incomplete. Some young children appear to inherit upper incisors much too large for their faces. It must be realized that the alveolar bone in the maxilla and mandible, the temporomandibular-joint complex, and the whole skeletal-dental bony complex undergo vast growth changes during the childhood growth years. These facial growth changes occur slowly but steadily during the mixed dentition years, then with startling rapidity during the pubertal years. Therefore incisors that seem overlarge in a child whose age is 9 years may appear to be quite normal in the smile of an 18-year-old.[5]

By carefully measuring the total of the widths of the newly erupted incisors and comparing this to the arch space available, one is able to gain a fairly accurate indication of whether there is indeed too little arch space or whether there only *appears* to be too little. If careful measurement indicates there is *more* than 3 mm. too much tooth material when compared with available arch space, then almost certainly the child should be referred to an orthodontist.

A reasonable exception can be made, however, in those rather common cases where space in the *maxillary* arch appears to be adequate but where crowding is present because of too much lingual inclination in the newly erupted lower incisors. Hyperactivity of the mentalis muscle during the swallowing act commonly causes this.

Genetic Class I, Type 1

The child who has *measurably* too much tooth material for his existing arch space is many times mistakenly accepted as a candidate for minor tooth movement procedures. This is the result of poor diagnosis; teeth cannot be compressed magically into an arch space too small to contain them. The first clue that the available arch space is not adequate to allow the unrestricted eruption of the permanent teeth is seen when the lower and upper incisors erupt during ages 6 to 8 years. The diagnostic procedure to determine whether the arch space is adequate is started in the *lower* arch.

First, the width of each permanent central and lateral incisor is accurately measured to the nearest tenth of a millimeter, using the modified Boley gauge described in Fig. 4-9. The second step is to determine the arch space available for these teeth. The most accurate method of doing this is by bending a light arch wire (0.020) around what is estimated to be the anterior perimeter of the arch, using the buccal cusps of the molars as a guide. A mark is made on the wire exactly opposite the mesial surface of each primary cuspid. The arch wire is straightened, then the distance between marks is measured. This measurement is compared to the total measurement representing the widths of the lower incisors. The upper arch space and the widths of the upper incisors are compared in the same fashion. If the total sum of tooth material exceeds the available arch space measurement in either arch by more than 3 mm., it can be assumed that there is a true tooth size/arch space discrepancy.

Because a definite tooth size/arch space discrepancy problem of this kind (*genetic Class I, Type 1*) can be best solved at or around the time of the pubertal growth spurt, these malocclusions (and the planned extraction of bicuspids) will usually be outside the treatment scope of those dentists interested in minor tooth movement in children. Treatment by the orthodontist would follow one of three general pathways in these cases:

1. Expanding the arch anteroposteriorly (increasing arch length)
2. Expanding the arches outward (facially) in an effort to accommodate all the permanent teeth
3. Selective removal of certain of the primary and later certain permanent teeth to provide the space necessary to allow proper occlusion of the remaining teeth (The first or second bicuspids are usually selected for extraction in space discrepancy cases. This method has sometimes been termed "serial extraction" and presents some real difficulties for the generalist. This will be discussed in the following section.)

Fallacy of treating crowding of incisors by serial extractions of deciduous teeth. There exist some well-entrenched fallacies regarding the treatment of crowded arches by extraction of deciduous teeth. For some

years the term *serial extraction* has existed in the dental literature to justify such a procedure. According to most writers, this term describes a therapy program involving the extractions of selected primary teeth to allow for the more normal eruption of crowded permanent incisors. In some instances serial extraction carries the connotation that certain permanent teeth, usually bicuspids, will be removed at a later date. Too often the general dentist has been led to hope that additional arch space in a child diagnosed as genetic Class I, Type 1, would somehow magically appear if selected primary teeth were removed over a period of time in a particular sequence. This is simply not true.

Crowded lower arches resembling Class I, Type 1, malocclusions have been in the past the target of misguided serial extraction therapy. Ultimately space is *lost,* not gained, in the arch by this treatment. To have any chance of success the serial extraction of primary teeth *must* be combined with accurate tooth width/arch length measurements (mixed dentition analysis) and with well-timed lingual arch therapy. The rationale for this combined primary tooth extraction–appliance therapy approach will be more fully examined in Chapter 9. (See Fig. 3-6.)

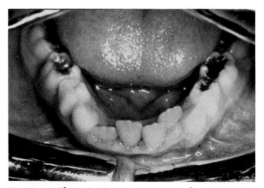

Fig. 3-6. Class I, Type 1, case evidencing *muscular* crowding of lower anterior teeth. Often such cases are treated improperly as serial extraction cases. Although often used, extractions usually fail to solve the problem of crowded teeth due to muscular imbalance.

Extraction of permanent teeth to provide increased arch space. To extract permanent teeth to gain a better balance of arch space is a procedure that can have severe consequences for the child's occlusion. Only rarely is the general dentist justified in deciding this on his own. A good rule for the general dentist to follow is that *whenever a permanent noncarious tooth is chosen for extraction to provide space in the dental arch, an orthodontist should sign the consultation sheet previous to the extraction.* Not only professional ethics but recent decisions rendered by courts of law in the field of forensic dentistry make this rule a wise one in a general dental practice.

• • •

To sum up, there are no easy ways to handle the problem of too little arch space. Diagnosis is the first step. The second is usually a referral to the orthodontist who has the necessary training and experience to deal with *genetically* caused dental problems.

Muscular Class I, Type 1

Crowding of lower anterior teeth caused by pressures generated by muscle of the lower lip is not, however, viewed as a genetic problem but as an environmental one. The mentalis muscle is one that can produce such a malocclusion if its action is too strong (Fig. 3-7). In such instances,

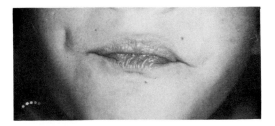

Fig. 3-7. Hyperactive mentalis muscle exhibited by child during swallow. This commonly produces environmental pressures that result in the type of crowding of lower anterior teeth seen in Fig. 3-6.

the malocclusion is termed a *muscular* Class I, Type 1, case. A malocclusion of this type may be treated by the family dentist to correct the lingually directed pressures caused by the mentalis muscle. More will be said concerning the selective diagnosis of cases involving crowded lower teeth in Chapters 8 and 9 on treatment of *muscular* Class I, Type 1, malocclusions.

Hyperactive mentalis muscle pressure and swallowing patterns. A crowding situation involving the lower incisors, which very much resembles the Class I, Type 1, malocclusions previously discussed may occur in some children. This may appear to be a genetic problem, but the diagnostic clues are that the lower lip acts in an acrobatic fashion during the swallow and the measurements of the *upper* arch demonstrate no tooth material/arch space problem. In other words, this crowding of lower incisors is a muscular problem limited to the lower arch only. The mentalis muscle, by contracting excessively during the act of swallowing, can exert enough unbalanced pressure on the newly erupted lower incisors to tip them lingually. Such environmental muscular pressure is of continuing importance in the etiology and subsequent treatment of crowded lower anteriors. To normalize the arc of the lower incisors, this unbalanced force must be counteracted by an appliance such as an activated lingual arch. When hyperactivity of the mentalis muscle is seen in a child, this almost always demonstrates that the child is using an improper swallowing pattern.

Some sort of tongue-thrusting activity will also be present in the child who exhibits a hyperactive mentalis muscle. For the child to correct or inhibit this pattern to aid in reducing the severity of his malocclusion, some form of tongue or swallowing therapy is usually required. Tongue therapy for children exhibiting muscular Class I, Type 1, and other types of malocclusions will be explored in greater detail in Chapter 10.

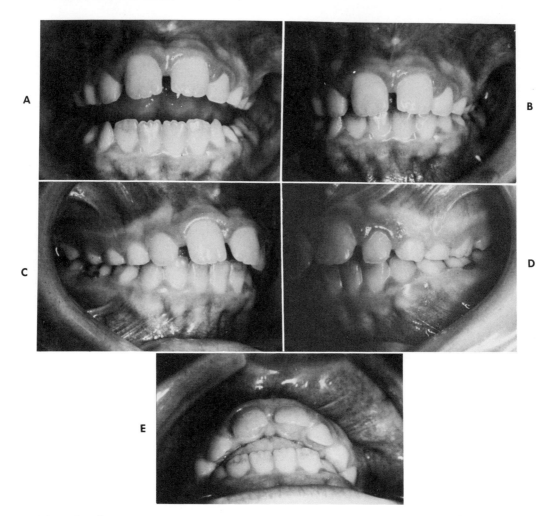

Fig. 3-8. Class I, Type 2, malocclusion in 9-year-old boy (Dewey-Anderson system of diagnosing *five* types of Class I malocclusions). **A**, Front view, open. Note spacing between upper central and lateral incisors. Oral habits are prominent in the etiology of these cases. **B**, Front view, closed. Note upper and lower dental midlines match quite well. **C**, Right view. Note both molar and cuspid relationships are Class I despite "Class II-ish" appearance of upper anteriors. **D**, Left view. Note both molar and cuspid relationships are Class I. **E**, Child's head is tilted back to demonstrate exaggerated overjet although minimal anterior open-bite is present.

Class I, Type 2

Protruded and spaced upper anteriors characterize Class I, Type 2, malocclusions (Fig. 3-8).

Description of malocclusion

At first glance, a Class I, Type 2, malocclusion may seem to resemble the classic Class II, Division 1, malocclusion. The like-

ness is that the upper anterior teeth are protrusive in both instances. However, in Class I, Type 2, the upper incisors are usually well *spaced*, and the molar and cuspid relationship is Class I. In both malocclusions the upper lip appears shorter and acts in a hypoactive (inactive) fashion, so that the lips do not fit together and enclose the teeth during the act of swallowing. The lower lip therefore seems to overact in an inward and upward direction to effect the seal for the swallow. As the overjet increases, the lower lip may effect the seal for the swallow by closing upward and lingual to the upper incisors.

Etiology

The apparent similarities of these two malocclusions should not mask their differences of origin. The Class II, Division I, dentition is the result of a clear pattern of heredity, as a rule. On the other hand, the etiology of Class I, Type 2, is usually a series of protracted oral habits such as early thumb- or finger-sucking, which may give way later to tongue-thrusting or an improper passive tongue posture. Continued for some years, these detrimental oral habits can generate forces that can cause both upper and lower arches to be maligned and perhaps move the upper teeth into quite protrusive positions.

Anterior open-bite

Commonly an *anterior open bite* is present in Class I, Type 2, malocclusions, that is, a distinct opening is seen from the front between the incisal edges of the upper and lower front teeth when the posterior teeth are in occlusion. From the size and shape of this opening the careful dentist can sometimes gain a better understanding of the cause of this malocclusion. For instance, a right-handed thumb-sucker will have a more exaggerated pattern of open-bite to the right side of the dental midline.

Speech articulation problems such as lisping may or may not be present, but a speech test *is* indicated during the diagnostic procedure. This may be administered by the dentist, but it is far more accurately done by a competent speech pathologist. The tongue may thrust through the opening between the front teeth during an abnormal swallowing pattern, tending to maintain the open-bite even after the child has ceased to suck his thumb. During the formation of certain speech sounds such as

s, z, unvoiced *th,* and *zh,* the child may experience difficulty in finding the proper tongue-palate contact. Other sounds made by the lower lip contacting the incisal edges of the upper front teeth, such as *f* and *v,* may also undergo distortion, substitution, or omission.[2]

Diagnosis of oral habit problems

By questioning the patient, examining the calluses caused from sucking on fingers and thumbs, listening to the speech and observing the tongue's actions during speech and the act of swallowing, and by talking with the parents, the dentist may be able to draw a fairly accurate outline of the etiology of the malocclusion. Care must be taken in these cases, however, to avoid excessive zeal in quizzing the youngsters regarding their oral habits. The dentist finds out rather quickly that he has strayed out of his specialty area when problems of a psychic nature are present. It is almost a truism that these Class I, Type 2, children tend to be the unhappy, underachieving, slow to mature children who may present psychological management problems for the dentist. Usually more boys than girls will be found in this category.

In the eagerness to solve the child's dental problems with appliance therapy, it is all too easy to forget or gloss over the deeper-seated personal problems. With care and good judgment, however, many of these potentially disfiguring malocclusions are treatable in the general dentist's office.

It is important to remember that in Class II, Division 2, malocclusions there are usually no interdental spaces between the upper anterior teeth. However, in Class I, Type 2, malocclusions spaces should be available between the teeth to permit the dentist to move the upper anterior teeth back into a more normal relationship with the mandibular teeth. Since an oral habit is nearly always involved, special exercises or counseling should be provided by the dentist to aid in retraining the child to swallow and to avoid mouth-breathing at night and perhaps to aid in regaining correct speech patterns.

Habit retraining

Habit retraining will be found to pose problems for most general dentists, however, and a speech therapist or pathologist, trained in tongue therapy should perhaps be consulted in resistant cases. If none of these professional persons is within a reasonable referral range of the dentist's practice area, he might find it valuable to refer to one of the newer books on retraining therapy that emphasize the dentist's role in such treatment.[4]

The appliance choices are several in these cases, and therefore treatment of Class I, Type 2, malocclusions involving both protruding upper teeth and the problem of anterior open-bite will be covered extensively in Chapter 10.

Class I, Type 3

Class I, Type 3, malocclusions comprise anterior cross-bites involving permanent upper incisors (Fig. 3-9).

Description of malocclusion

Perhaps nothing in the development of an occlusion is as dramatic as the eruption of a maxillary incisor into a lingual cross-bite position. Literally this produces an immediate "locked bite," with all the attendant possibilities of poor lip and facial muscle function, poor masticatory function, and improper incisal and occlusal wear on

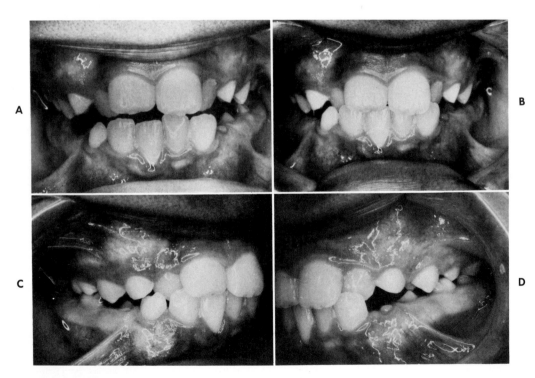

Fig. 3-9. Class I, Type 3, malocclusion exhibited by 8-year-old girl (Dewey-Anderson system of diagnosing *five* types of Class I malocclusions). This patient has an anterior cross-bite, both upper lateral incisors being inlocked. Normal masticatory function cannot take place; instead, the child chews only up and down. **A,** Front view, open. **B,** Front view, closed. Note the mandibular shift on closure as evidenced by comparison to the upper and lower dental midlines in **A. C,** Right view. **D,** Left view.

the occluding surfaces of the teeth and may even produce an odd, truculent look about the face of the child. The parents may spontaneously report that the child chews his food oddly, with up and down chopping motions rather than the normal rotary motions.

An early diagnosis of this condition is important, since these cases should be treated as early as possible. If the dentist sees this malocclusion occurring as the teeth erupt, it is much more easily treated. However, if treatment is delayed until the child is 10 to 12 years of age, many times there is inadequate space into which to move the lingually locked tooth so that it may assume its proper position in the dental arch. Also considerable damage may be caused to the periodontium of a *lower* central or lateral incisor, particularly on the labial aspect, if this condition is *left untreated*. Therefore the more mature child past 10 years of age probably should be referred to the orthodontist, since in most cases the mesial drifting of adjacent teeth has robbed some of the necessary arch space from the tooth that is in cross-bite. Children younger than 10 can usually be treated in the general practitioner's office because there is still adequate room in the arch into which to move the upper tooth in cross-bite. This will normalize the arch shape and "unlock" the bite.

Pseudo-Class III malocclusions

When *two or more* upper permanent incisors are involved in the anterior cross-bite, the prognosis should be less positive that the anterior cross-bite can be successfully reduced. Diagnosis is again of distinct importance because these children may not have simple anterior cross-bites (Class I, Type 3) but indeed may be genetic Class III malocclusion cases. Sometimes diagnosis is clarified during treatment of an anterior cross-bite. Hitchcock[5] notes that if more than 3 weeks of appliance therapy do not succeed in reducing the anterior cross-bite, it should perhaps be regarded as a possible Class III case disguised as a Class I, Type 3. Some writers have called these *pseudo-Class III malocclusions*. In general, it is better to regard Class I, Type 3, cases as being at one end of the spectrum and full Class III malocclusions at the other end. The greater the number of anterior teeth found in cross-bite, the firmer should be the suspicion in the dentist's mind that the child may be developing a Class III malocclusion, which only an orthodontist should treat (Fig. 3-10).

Class I, Type 4

Class I, Type 4, malocclusions are characterized by posterior cross-bites involving primary molars, first permanent molars, or both (Fig. 3-11).

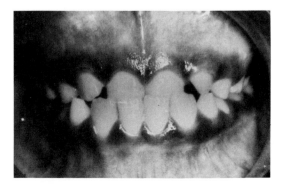

Fig. 3-10. Pseudo–Class III malocclusion. May be confused with Class I, Type 3. After treatment reducing the cross-bite, the incisors may fail to retain their new positions, and the child may continue his development into a Class III malocclusion.

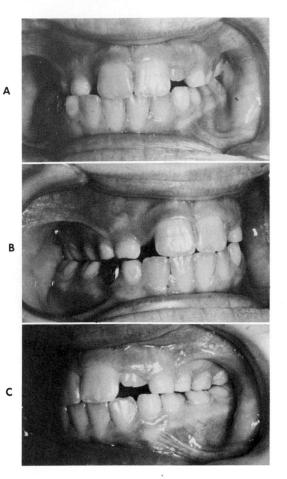

Fig. 3-11. Class I, Type 4, malocclusion (Dewey-Anderson system of diagnosing *five* types of Class I malocclusions). Note marked mandibular shift on closure in this posterior *unilateral* cross-bite. **A,** Front view. **B,** Right view. Posterior cross-bite is evident on the right side. **C,** Left view. Note the relatively normal intercuspation on this side of the arch.

Description of malocclusion

Much confusion exists regarding the terminology for describing posterior cross-bites and the treatment responsibilities in these commonly occurring malocclusions. Perhaps it is time that some of the terminology is modified to aid in clarifying pathways to treatment in the generalist's office.

Most texts in the past have used the terms *functional* and *genetic,* as well as *unilateral* or *bilateral,* to describe the vari-

ous types of posterior cross-bites. A different method using an anatomic orientation is suggested here. With this method it is only necessary to determine how many *maxillary* teeth are in cross-bite relationship and whether the cross-bite is in one of three buccolingual positions in relation to the opposing lower teeth. The three possible positions are *lingual cross-bite, complete lingual cross-bite, and buccal cross-bite.* The differences among these cross-bites are explored in the following sections.

Lingual cross-bite. The diagnosis of a primary molar, first permanent molar, or bicuspid as being in a lingual cross-bite indicates that the buccal cusps of the upper tooth are locked into the occlusal groove of the opposing lower tooth. It also indicates the maxillary tooth is located approximately 3.5 to 5 mm. toward the midpalatal line from its normal position in the upper arch.

With the Palmer system of tooth identification, an entry made on the diagnosis sheet to indicate the upper right 6-year molar was in lingual cross-bite would be as follows:

Class I, Type 4;
6| in lingual X-bite.

If the lingual cross-bite were in the entire upper left posterior segment and involved both primary molars as well as the 6-year molar, the malocclusion would be charted:

Class I, Type 4;
|D E 6 in lingual X-bite.

Complete lingual cross-bite. If an upper bicuspid or molar erupts fully to the lingual of the corresponding lower tooth, so that the *buccal* surface of the maxillary tooth in cross-bite occludes with the lingual surface of the opposing mandibular tooth, the upper tooth is said to be in complete lingual *cross-bite.* Such a cross-bite would be charted:

Class I, Type 4;
|6 in complete lingual X-bite.

Buccal cross-bites. Occasionally a posterior tooth or the whole posterior segment of an arch will erupt in *buccal cross-bite.* This term describes a condition in which the whole crown of the upper tooth in cross-bite is entirely buccal to the opposing lower tooth. Therefore the *lingual surface* of the maxillary tooth occludes against the *buccal surface* of the mandibular tooth. If a child exhibited a buccal cross-bite involving the upper right first and second bicuspids, such a cross-bite would be charted:

Class I, Type 4;
5 4| in buccal X-bite.

• • •

In addition, it should be indicated that all three of these types of posterior cross-bites may be expressed by the child in his occlusion as either unilateral or bilateral.

Arch distortions in cross-bite cases

Lingual cross-bites comprise by far the most common type seen in children. Three to five per cent of the children in some populations exhibit these malocclusions. When a typical lingual cross-bite occurs in posterior permanent teeth, usually it is the maxillary tooth that shows the most deviation to the lingual from its normal position in the arch. The mandibular tooth usually tends to maintain its position, so that little alveolar bone distortion occurs toward the buccal in the mandibular arch of the younger child.

This is clearly not the case when either a buccal or a complete lingual cross-bite occurs. In each of these the tremendous forces generated by closure into biting relation are dissipated against the buccal and lingual surfaces of the opposing teeth, as if two inclined planes move pressed together. Each tooth and the alveolar ridge area enclosing it move in response to this vector of forces, but the greatest movement occurs in the maxillary arch. The relatively harder and more dense mandibular bone acts to resist

the movement of teeth through it and thus minimizes mandibular arch distortion in most younger cross-bite cases.

Etiology

Although it may not be possible to prove the etiology of posterior cross-bites in all cases, some educated guesses should be attempted. The most common cross-bites seen in children during the primary dentition stage are lingual cross-bites involving the maxillary deciduous cuspid and both of the maxillary primary molars on one side. Almost always these give the clinical appearance of being *unilateral cross-bites,* whereas on the other side of the jaw the bite appears normal.

Functional vs. genetic considerations in cross-bites. Other writers dealing with these occlusal dysfunctions called cross-bites have separated them into *functional* and *genetic* types. Usually it is implied that functional posterior cross-bites may be treated in the general dentist's office, whereas the genetic cross-bites should be referred out. It is usually explained that when a child opens his mouth and closes *slowly* into a comfortable bite, his cross-bite is a functional one if his mandible is seen to deviate *toward* the cross-bite side to accommodate the cuspal interference during the last 2 or 3 mm. of closure. However, if no deviation of the mandible is observed during closure, then the cross-bite is said to be of genetic origin.

This diagnostic separation does not appear to be always a valid distinction in practice. Particularly this is true when a functional cross-bite can assume the "no shift" characteristics of the genetic cross-bite as the child gets older and the upper *and* lower alveolar bone can distort in response to the odd pressures of this occlusion.

First permanent molar. Usually the first permanent molar can be expected to erupt into cross-bite when a primary molar cross-bite has persisted from the early age when the deciduous molar occlusion was originally established. Treatment can be accomplished by maxillary arch expansion using several appliance methods (Chapter 12), in addition to the disking described below, but the timing of treatment is more important than the method.

The ectopic eruption of 6-year molars can also develop a cross-bite relationship, since many of these molars erupting *mesially* from their normal arch positions also may be found rotating in a lingual direction. This may produce a lingual cross-bite.

Primary cuspids as "culprits." The primary cuspids may be the culprits in many posterior cross-bite cases. Erupting as they do before the posterior occlusion is well established in the deciduous molars and meeting each other as round, pointed teeth, there appears to be ample opportunity for the occluding cuspids to slide down the wrong slope, causing a "locked" bite to occur. It is interesting to note that if the unilateral cross-bite is diagnosed early, at age 2 or 3, the dentist should attempt first to disk the cuspids on the offending side and the cross-bite may resolve itself. Other authors have indicated that the cusps of primary molars should be disked even if the age of the child indicates the cross-bite has persisted for 5 or 6 years. Before such a course is embarked on, it should be remembered that although the primary molar cuspal discrepancies would be freed and the normal lateral excursions of the mandible made possible after disking, the distorted maxillary alveolar ridges have not changed their configuration. Therefore when the 6-year molar and the bicuspids erupt in this area they may well be in cross-bite also. Ideally, treatment to reduce cross-bites involves moving the affected teeth out of cross-bite as well as changing the configuration of the upper alveolar ridge to one of "normality."

Other causative factors in unilateral cross-bite. Explanations in the past have attempted to imply that a local etiology may produce posterior cross-bites. Some of the causes suggested are as follows:

1. The child wads a pillow against his face and sleeps on the same side each night.
2. Cheek sucking as an oral habit.
3. Trauma to one of the posterior segments at an early age.
4. Formocresol pulpotomized or abscessed primary molars do not exfoliate normally and may cause the bicuspids to erupt buccal or lingual to their normal positions in the arch.

No one has yet successfully documented that these suggested etiologies are indeed true causes of malocclusions.

Early treatment of posterior cross-bites advised

Because a posterior cross-bite in the primary dentition may not be confirmed until after age 3, the maturity of the child would dictate that treatment methods should wait until at least age 4. This is indeed the case with most children. If treatment is initiated at age 4, *with great care,* the posterior segment that is in cross-bite can be corrected over a period of 2 or 3 months. The child then has 2 years or so of normal masticatory function to stimulate and guide the 6-year molars into a more normal pattern of eruption within the alveolus. Many times after early treatment of the primary dentition, the 6-year molar on the side of the former cross-bite will erupt in a normal fashion. When treatment has not been initiated early, and the cross-bite is left to "self-correct," it is common to find that the distortion of the alveolar ridge has caused the 6-year molars to erupt in cross-bite, following the pattern of the primary molars.

Bilateral posterior cross-bites

Occasionally a child is seen with a cross-bite present on both sides of the arch. As in the unilateral case, the bilateral cross-bite usually involves the narrowing or deformation of the maxilla, not an increase in the width of the mandible. The measurable narrowing of the maxilla in such cases may vary from 8 to 20 mm. Long-term allergic

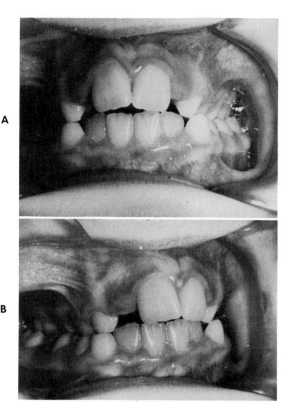

Fig. 3-12. Class I, Type 4, *bilateral* posterior cross-bite in a 9-year-old girl. A marked narrowing of the maxillary arch and crowding of the upper front teeth are evident in these cases. Etiology is *both* genetic and muscular. **A,** Front view. **B,** Right view.

rhinitis, mouth-breathing, and perhaps persistent tongue and cheek habits may be causative or harmful influences in these cases. The palatal vault commonly appears constricted and heightened in these children. Certain speech sounds, mainly sibilants, may be defective. Referral to speech professionals may be indicated in some instances. These types of cases will be examined in more detail in Chapter 12. (See Fig. 3-12.)

Treatment of cross-bites in general

Most unilateral posterior cross-bites involving primary molars and 6-year molars are amenable to treatment by the family dentist. The oral habit cross-bites are per-

haps the most difficult to treat, involving as they do the suggested course of appliance treatment and tongue or habit therapy at the same time.

As in the case of the Class I, Type 2, malocclusion (protruding, spaced upper anterior teeth), the counsel of the speech pathologist and the orthodontist should be sought to help sort out the etiologic factors that have produced and are helping to sustain the malocclusion. If a speech professional is not available for consultation, the orthodontist should be consulted.

A good rule to remember seems to be that in reducing any cross-bite, anterior or posterior, there must be adequate space in the arch so that the inlocked tooth or teeth can be brought into correct alignment without significant changes in the positions of the adjacent teeth.

Class I, Type 5

Class I, Type 5, malocclusion involves loss of space in the posterior segment (Fig. 3-13).

Description of malocclusion

This malocclusion resembles Class I, Type 1, in that the *lack of arch space* available for the permanent teeth is able to be clearly ascertained. Although it may superficially resemble Class I, Type 1 (genetic lack of space), Type 5 involves an *arch space loss,* not a *genetic lack* of space. Also, the arch space loss is in the *posterior* (buccal) segment, not the anterior segment as in Class I, Type 1.

The usual dental arch discrepancy in Type 5 is caused by the mesial drifting of the 6-year molar. If it happens in the upper arch, the drift tends to be a bodily one, with not too much tilting of the axis as the 6-year molar moves mesially. This is particularly true if the second primary molars have been lost as early as 3 or 4 years of age. Lower arch x-ray films, however, will commonly show that tilting *and* mesial bodily movement of the molar occurs. When the 6-year molar has drifted mesially

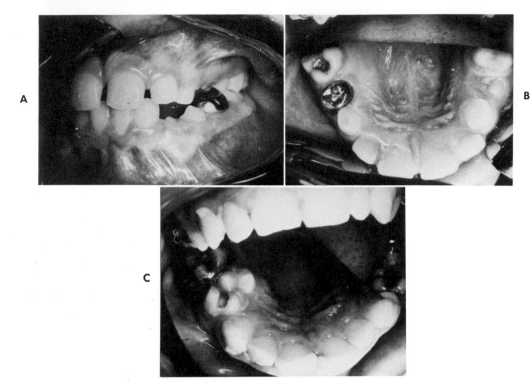

Fig. 3-13. Class I, Type 5, malocclusion. **A,** Left view. Upper left molar appears in good Class I relationship. **B,** Palatal view of case shown in **A** demonstrates almost complete closure of space formerly occupied by the primary second molar. Space-regaining would almost certainly prove unsuccessful here. Upper right 6-year molar exhibits a false Class II position until it is "mentally" repositioned to its former Class I relation. **C,** Palatal view of another Class I, Type 5, case in which the upper right second bicuspid has been blocked out lingually as well as rotated 180 degrees! This is not an unusual consequence in the upper arch.

in the typical case, the total arch length is dramatically lessened. When this occurs, almost inevitably the last bicuspid to erupt in the quadrant where space has been lost is "blocked out" of the normal arch. The second bicuspid may be forced lingually or impacted in what appears to be an otherwise normal arch, since it is commonly the last bicuspid to erupt. In the rare event that the first bicuspid is last to erupt, it will be forced buccally most of the time. The upper cuspids also may be blocked out labially or lingually. When maxillary cuspids are blocked out labially they present one of the most dramatic demonstrations of the sequelae of loss of critical arch space in the posterior segment.

Etiology of posterior space loss

In general, any of three causes may be assigned to the mesial drifting of 6-year molars: caries, extraction (iatrogenic), and genetic factors (ectopic eruption). Loss of arch space due to interproximal caries is the fault of the child's parents, but space loss as the result of early primary molar extractions should, in most cases, be considered iatrogenic space loss. This is particularly true if the dentist makes no attempt to place a space maintainer to prevent the almost certain loss of space after the extraction of a primary molar.

Ectopic eruption of the first permanent molar is a mesially oriented eruption pattern found in maxillary molars. Barber[1]

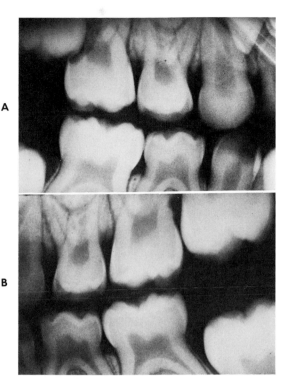

Fig. 3-14. X-ray films of child, age 7. A, Ectopic eruption of upper right first permanent molar. Upper molars have a greater tendency to erupt ectopically than do lower molars. In doing so, they can dramatically decrease the arch length. B, Opposite side of child's arch shows normal molar eruption pattern.

states that mandibular first permanent molars erupt ectopically very rarely. (See Fig. 3-14.) When, less commonly, ankylosis or palatal impaction of the upper cuspid occurs, it is well to observe the rest of the family carefully and inquire into the familial history regarding "missing" or impacted teeth. Usually it will be found that a genetic factor is involved in these impaction cases.

Loss of primary molar space can also be present due to long-term neglect of carious lesions in these teeth.

Treatment of Class I, Type 5, malocclusion

Perhaps it is best to assume that in all Class I occlusions except Type 1, there was once sufficient arch space available to allow normal eruption of the first and second bicuspid and the permanent cuspid. By measuring the spaces occupied by teeth on each side of the arch on the models and in the radiographs and comparing measurements, a close scrutiny will reveal the discrepancy in millimeters. Then by measuring the widths of the permanent teeth in the area, a determination regarding treatment or referral may be made.

It must be emphasized that treatment by minor tooth movement in Class I, Type 5, cases does not involve the distal repositioning of a drifted 6-year molar over a great distance. Perhaps no more than 3 mm. in the maxilla and 2 mm. regained space in the mandibular arch would be all that could be reasonably hoped for in minor tooth movement treatment procedures.

Referral to the orthodontist would be indicated in those cases where diagnostic measurements showed the space loss due to the mesial drift of the 6-year molar exceeded these dimensions. Bear in mind that these arbitrary dimensions are used as a guide, not as a rule. Knowledge and confidence in diagnosis and experience in the use of appliance therapy compiled over the years ultimately serve as the best guides for which cases to refer and which to treat. (See Table 4.)

Class I, Type 0—perfect occlusion

Although admittedly the incidence is low in most sections of the United States, still another type of Class I malocclusion should be discussed. This involves the child in whom all the teeth interdigitate normally into a good Class I relationship and the upper and lower dental midlines match each other and the facial midline. In other words, this is the case where no apparent occlusal discrepancy is present in the dental arches *at this age*. It is proposed that this normal dental arch be designated Class I, Type 0 (for zero defects). (See Fig. 3-15.) To designate such cases merely as "Class I" on the dental chart is to deny the depth

Table 4. Review of diagnostic considerations in Dewey-Anderson modification of Angle Class I malocclusions*

Classification	Etiology	Suggested: refer or treat
Class I, Type 1	Crowded, rotated upper and lower anterior teeth *Cause:* Usually genetic	Refer
	Crowded lower anterior teeth, normally spaced upper teeth *Cause:* Hyperactive mentalis muscle	Treat
Class I, Type 2	Protruding, spaced upper anterior teeth *Cause:* Mild tongue thrusting and lip habits	Treat
	Protruding, spaced upper anteriors pronounced open-bite *Cause:* Oral habits present, poor swallowing pattern, and poor tongue position at rest	*Treat* with extreme care if in conjunction with tongue therapy
Class I, Type 3	Anterior cross-bite involving 1 or 2 upper incisors *Cause:* Trauma to upper primary teeth	Treat
	Anterior cross-bite involving 3 or 4 upper incisors *Cause:* Commonly genetic	Treat with care, may be Class III malocclusion
Class I, Type 4	Posterior cross-bite, unilateral *Cause:* Primary cuspids interdigitating improperly	Treat early
	Posterior cross-bite, bilateral *Cause:* Genetic, or possibly allergic rhinitis or cheek-sucking habits	Refer
Class I, Type 5	Posterior loss of space due to mesial drifting of 6-year molar; space loss 2-3 mm. in one quadrant *Cause:* Early extraction or carious destruction of primary molars	Treat
	Posterior loss of space due to mesial drifting of 6-year molar; space loss greater than 3 mm. in one quadrant *Cause:* Early loss of primary molars, ectopic eruption of the 6-year molars, carious destruction of primary molars	Refer

*This summation of the ideas in this chapter should provide the family dentist with a "check-list" to help him to decide whether to treat or refer a child patient who has a minor malocclusion.

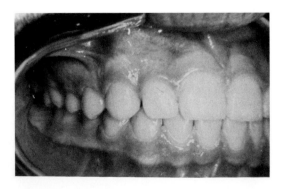

Fig. 3-15. This young lady has ideal occlusion. Not every child has the potential for an ideal dentition, but future efforts by family dentists can normalize many more malocclusions than is now being accomplished. In the system suggested here this child would be classified as Class I, Type 0, since there are zero defects in her occlusion.

of diagnostic skills of the dentist who classifies the case by excluding all other possibilities.

In all the other malocclusions discussed there has been a specific diagnostic entity present that makes the dental arch abnormal. It may have been a genetic pattern of aberrant dentoalveolar growth, a mesial drifting of 6-year molars, a protrusion of upper anterior teeth, a cross-bite relationship, or a crowded anterior segment. Therefore to allow the proper designation of *all* types of malocclusions, it is proposed that Class I, Type 0, be used for those Class I malocclusions that include no apparent occlusal discrepancies or abnormal positions of teeth.

Hopefully, in the near future, the children in our practices will reap the full benefits of preventive dentistry, including dentist-applied topical fluorides, community water fluoridation, the daily use of fluoride toothpastes and fluoride mouthwashes, and the routine use of dental floss. Therefore a quarter of a century from now the dentist may be able to assign to this new classification many more children in the mixed dentition years and even in the permanent dentition years than is now possible.

SUMMARY

The Angle system of diagnosing malocclusions has been reviewed and the Dewey-Anderson modification by separating Angle Class I malocclusions into five types has been described. Each type of Class I has specific characteristics such as genetic lack of space in the arch, protrusive upper incisors, anterior or posterior cross-bites, or space loss in the posterior segments. Etiologies and directions for treatment are discussed for each of the five types of Class I malocclusions. A new type, Class I, Type 0, is proposed for those young arches that show no abnormalities of tooth position or arch alignment.

REFERENCES

1. Anderson, G. M.: Practical orthodontics, ed. 9, St. Louis, 1960, The C. V. Mosby Co., p. 144.
2. Coleman, R. O., and Gullikson, J. S.: Speech problems in children, J. Dent. Child. 38(6):17-20, Nov.-Dec., 1971.
3. Ehrlich, A. B.: Training therapists for tongue thrust correction, Springfield, Ill., 1971, Charles C Thomas, Publisher.
4. Graber, T. M.: Orthodontics: principles and practice, ed. 2, Philadelphia, 1966, W. B. Saunders Co.
5. Hitchcock, H. P.: In Finn, S. B., editor: Clinical pedodontics, ed. 3, Philadelphia, 1967, W. B. Saunders Co., pp. 240-306.

4 | Using the diagnostic quadrangle

The family dentist who wishes to increase the dimension of his practice to include the treatment of minor malocclusions usually expresses a need for a confidence-building series of steps leading to a good diagnosis, which will then suggest a pathway of treatment. If treatment is being considered in the primary and mixed dentition stages, there should be a series of trustworthy and practical diagnostic steps. These, when completed, will furnish the dentist with all the necessary information to allow him confidently to decide to treat the child or refer him to an orthodontist. Unfortunately, in this area no fool-proof diagnostic processes are known, but certain precautionary steps, if followed with reasonable care, can yield a surprising amount of directional diagnostic information. The findings from such a diagnosis should lead fairly directly to considerations for the method of treatment the dentist will best pursue, should he make the decision to treat the child.[4]

CHOOSING THE BEST DIAGNOSTIC METHODS

Diagnostic methods that are suitable and necessary for an orthodontist may not be compatible with the procedures used in the office of a generalist. The generalist is usually more concerned with the successful management of arch space while maintaining the full complement of permanent teeth.[1] As a rule, he views the extraction of two or four bicuspids to provide arch space as being beyond his level of expertise. Although there are really remarkably few shortcuts to a good diagnosis, it certainly behooves the general dentist to be able to eliminate all except the essential elements he needs in the material he gathers for diagnosing a minor malocclusion.

STEPS IN DIAGNOSIS OF MALOCCLUSIONS

Basically the dentist should perform the following checks:

1. Examine the soft tissue facial profile of the child to see whether the profile is in agreement with the arch relationships.

2. *Count the teeth,* both in the mouth of the child and in the fullmouth radiographs or panographic film.

3. Determine the terminal plane relationship of second primary molars (if the child is younger than 6 years). See Fig. 2-4.

4. Examine the first permanent molar relationships (if child is older than 6) and

48

note them to be Angle's Class I, Class II, or Class III.

5. Examine the cuspid relationships on both sides of the arches (primary cuspids are usually the ones present in the younger age group). The permanent lower cuspids appear between ages 8 and 10. The upper cuspids are commonly the last of the replacement permanent teeth to erupt.

6. Establish the relationships of the upper and lower dental midlines to the midsagittal plane. The position of the lower dental midline must be compared to the midsagittal plane in both the *bite-open* (2 to 4 mm.) and *bite-closed* positions.

7. Note any oral habits of the child that are creating malpositions of teeth. These may include digital sucking habits, tongue-thrusting, hyperactive mentalis muscle patterns during swallowing, and others.

8. Examine the overbite relationships of the upper to the lower incisors. If an anterior open-bite exists, this is measured as a *negative overbite*.

9. Check the overjet relationship of the upper to the lower incisors. In the case of an anterior cross-bite or a Class III malocclusion this may be measured as a *negative overjet*.

10. Note the approximate angle of the longitudinal axes of the lower central incisors to the mandibular plane (lower border of the mandible). In most cases this angle will be within a range of 90 degrees.

11. Ascertain the proper arch perimeter of the lower arch so as to be able to estimate closely where the incisal edges of the permanent lower incisors will best be located.

12. Do a space analysis, which includes checking the *existing space* in the posterior segments of all four quadrants to ascertain whether there is room to allow the unhindered eruption of the permanent cuspids and the first and second bicuspids. This analysis can be accomplished accurately only if the four 6-year molars and the lower four incisors have erupted.

PREPARING GOOD DIAGNOSTIC RECORDS FOR EACH CASE

Without good diagnostic records of a child who is suspected of having a malocclusion, the dentist is crippled in his approach to excellence either in diagnosis or treatment. Good, clear periapical radiographs of all the teeth or a clear panographic film allows the dentist to view

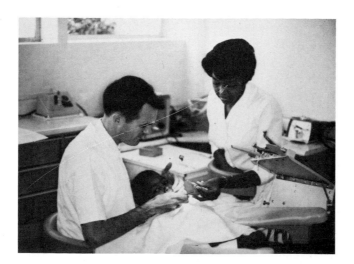

Fig. 4-1. Orthodontic impressions can be taken (utilizing 4-handed dentistry procedures) while the child is in a reclining or semireclining chair position.

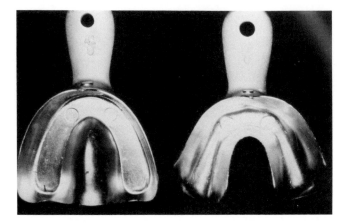

Fig. 4-2. Use of a set of solid aluminum trays aids considerably in impression taking. The dental assistant will appreciate the ease with which they may be cleaned and sterilized.

unerupted permanent teeth to ascertain their positions as well as count them to check for the possibility of missing or supernumerary teeth.

Alginate impressions, properly taken, can ensure good quality plaster casts for measuring arch length and checking arch perimeter (Fig. 4-1). The appearance during a case presentation of a set of orthodontic casts that are nicely finished, bubble free, and smudge free is one demonstration of the dentist's skills that should not be taken lightly.

Taking impressions and finishing orthodontic casts

Within this section are incorporated many "pearls" of information passed on by pedodontists and orthodontists. Particular thanks should go to Dr. John R. Rogers, Bellevue, Washington, whose innovative approach to many of these procedures helped stimulate the writing of this book.[9]

The following are the steps for taking impressions:

1. Select an upper and lower *solid aluminum* tray (see components list, Chapter 14) of proper size, usually one size larger than might otherwise be chosen (Fig. 4-2).

2. Contour soft beeswax or boxing wax around the whole perimeter of each tray.

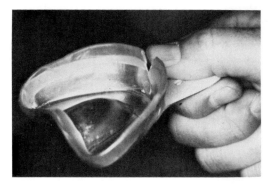

Fig. 4-3. Soft beeswax sheets are cut into strips. These strips are warmed and used to line the solid aluminum trays so that the impression may be extended into the alveolar sulcus without trauma to the child's soft tissue.

The wax should be warmed slightly over a flame first if flat beeswax strips are used. The wax is contoured highest in the labial area, slightly lower on the buccal areas. Leave an open area for the upper and lower labial frenums.

3. Pinch the wax upward in the distal palate area (corresponds to postdam area). This serves to cut off the alginate that normally flows back to the "gag" area at the juncture of the hard and soft palate (Fig. 4-3).

4. Mix a *regular* alginate, but use 15% to 20% *less* room-temperature water than

the directions call for. This makes a "heavy" mix that tremendously increases the hydrostatic pressure during the seating of the impression, presses soft labial and buccal tissue away from the alveolar ridges, and at the same time gives better detail. In addition, the heavy mix cuts the alginate setting time in the mouth to a minute or less. For younger children this is a real advantage.

5. Loading the lower tray is done in two quick strokes, using one full spatula of alginate. Then the spatula is used to *smooth* each posterior molar area and *add* material to excess in the anterior part of the tray.

6. The child's lower lip is held out away from the anterior teeth with one hand. *The lower tray is seated in the anterior of the arch first and then is rocked into position posteriorly,* using finger pressure first on the right side then on the left.

7. Loading the upper tray is also accomplished in two quick strokes of a spatula full of the thick alginate mix. The spatula is then used to remove most of the alginate in the molar areas, adding this alginate to the anterior portion of the tray.

8. *The upper tray is seated in the anterior part of the arch first, then rocked posteriorly,* using alternate finger pressures as with the lower. If this is done slowly, the dentist can control the amount of alginate material that escapes past the wax ridge at the distal end of the tray. Children do not appreciate having their gag reflex tested, and this method of taking impressions lowers the gagging rate considerably.

9. Take two single-thickness beeswax or pink baseplate wax registration bites. Each wax wafer should be warmed before the bite registration is taken. One wax bite is used to ensure accuracy of the bite during trimming of casts, and the other remains in the model box. It may be used to cushion the casts during the case presentation.

Trimming orthodontic casts

Whether the vacuum method or the "shake" method is used to mix the plaster,

the casts should be poured so they are almost free of bubbles.

The steps used in trimming casts are as follows:

1. Separate the casts from the rubber bases and wet them with cold water.

2. Grind the heel of the *upper* cast at 90 degrees to the midpalatal line.

3. Grind the sides at 60 degrees to the heel line, using as a reference the flat aluminum template (Fig. 4-4). Then place the top of the cast against the wheel and grind until the occlusal plane of the upper teeth is approximately parallel to the top of the cast.

4. Recheck each side at 60 degrees by setting the cast on the aluminum template, then grind the anterior faces of the upper cast at 25 degrees to a perpendicular drawn to the mid-palatal line, with the point making an extension of the midline of the palate.

5. Grind the heel of the lower cast, and grind each side at 60 degrees to the heel.

6. Place one of the wax-bite wafers between the casts to orient the bite and cushion the teeth. Then turn the casts upside down and using the *top* of the upper cast as a reference, grind the heels of both casts so that they are flush.

7. Now grind the sides of the models as they are occluded upside down.

8. Then using the flush heels as an index, grind the *bottom* of the lower cast so that it parallels the *top* of the upper cast. Then grind heel bevels at 60 degrees to the heel.

9. Remove the lower cast from the wax bite and grind a rounded toe on the lower cast from lower cuspid to cuspid.

10. Smooth all ground edges with a medium-fine flat Arkansas stone kept wet with cold water (Fig. 4-5).

11. Remove all bubbled bits of plaster, then fill in any hollow bubbles with wet plaster on the wetted casts. Smooth all buccal and labial tissue areas, using wet-or-dry black sandpaper, grit 280 or 400.

12. After the models have dried for 24

hours, soak them for 20 minutes in a covered plastic container half-filled with
Model Gloss.

13. Remove, rinse with cool water, and
dry all surfaces with a rubbing motion
using a soft cotton cloth.

It should take an experienced dental assistant 20 to 45 minutes to fiinsh one set of
casts if she is doing several sets at a time.
The dentist will save much time by teaching his auxiliaries to perform these time-
consuming procedures using the aluminum

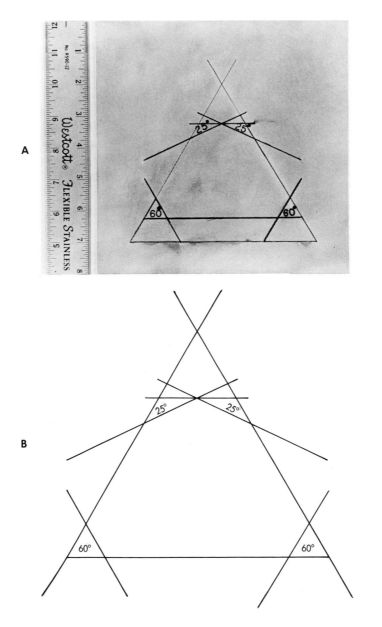

Fig. 4-4. A, A 60-degree guide scribed into an aluminum sheet will help the dental
assistant when she grinds the dentist's models for case records and demonstrations. **B,**
Drawing here may act as a template for making the aluminum plate, **A,** used as a
guide to check angles on plaster models.

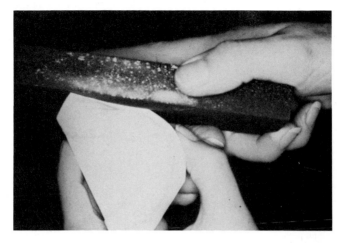

Fig. 4-5. Dental assistant smoothing model base with wetted Arkansas stone.

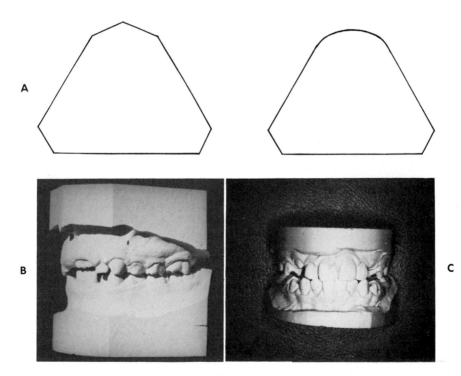

Fig. 4-6. A, Convenient outlines of model bases. Used properly, the metal guide form will help the dentist's assistant trim models with correct angles. **B,** Finished models of a 7-year-old child. Well-finished models allow a dentist to take justifiable pride in his case presentations. Poorly finished study casts, **C,** do little to enhance the dentist's reputation for excellence in his practice.

Date:_____

Name:_____ Age:_____ B.D._____
Parent:_____ Address:_____
                                                Phone:_____

Diagnostic Quadrangle

Molars   Cuspids

R__   1   2   R__
L__   L__
Type__

        |- - - - - -|

        3   4

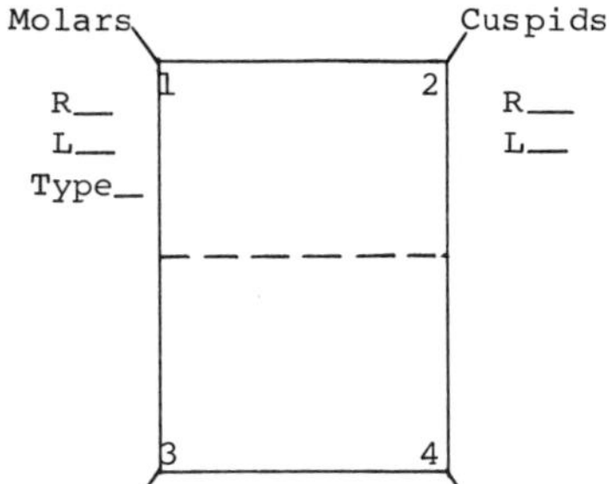

Mid-Lines

1. U. Dental__mm.
2. L. Dental__mm.
3. Mand. Shift__mm.

Oral Habits

1. Over-jet__mm.
2. Over-bite__mm.
3. Angle 1|1__°

Space Analysis

Space existing__mm	Space existing__mm
Space needed__mm	Space needed__mm
Difference__mm	Difference__mm

R _____ L

Space existing__mm	Space existing__mm
Space needed__mm	Space needed__mm
Difference__mm	Difference__mm

RESULTS OF MOYERS' ANALYSIS:

RESULTS OF COMBINATION ANALYSIS:

Check following:

Soft tissue profile	Yes	No		Yes	No
Normal	__	__	Occlusal table normal	__	__
Convex	__	__	Occlusal table shallow	__	__
Concave	__	__	Curve of Spee excessive	__	__
Deviate swallowing pattern	__	__	Child emotionally stable	__	__
Hyperactive mentalis muscle	__	__	History of allergies	__	__
Tongue positional problem	__	__	Study models taken	__	__
Lip competency normal	__	__	Full mouth x-rays taken	__	__
Palatal vault normal	__	__	Panographic x-ray taken	__	__
Excessively high	__	__	Headfilm taken	__	__
			Cephalometric tracing	__	__
			Color slides taken	__	__

TREATMENT DECISION:

    Suggest no treatment at this time_____
    Suggest minor tooth movement_____
    Suggest referral to orthodontist, Doctor_____Tel._____
Statement of MTM problem:_____
_____
_____
Estimated length of MTM treatment time:_____

Date initiated treatment:
    Completed treatment:
        Retention removed:
            Check-ups: 6 months_____ One year_____

Fig. 4-7. Malocclusion analysis chart. As the dentist completes the steps in diagnostic quadrangle (upper left portion of chart), he has already been able to enter the decision-making process that will lead him to an accurate diagnosis of the child's malocclusion. The space analysis section (upper right portion of chart) will give him the information he needs to decide whether the existing arch space in all four quadrants is adequate to allow permanent teeth 3 4 5 to erupt properly. Remainder of the chart is a check list to make certain nothing is overlooked.

template and the steps as outlined here. It has been demonstrated that with only a 1-hour instruction period the office auxiliaries can learn this method.[2]

Often an additional "pour" can be made of each alginate impression to serve as the working model for appliance fabrication.

The test of a good set of diagnostic casts is whether they can be set on their heels with the teeth in occlusion and the bite, as judged by the pink wax wafer, does not change (Fig. 4-6).

Composition of the orthodontic plaster can be altered to make harder casts. This is done by adding white Hydrocal (white stone) to the plaster. Hydrocal is available through dental supply dealers (who usually stock the traditional buff-colored stone), but it is also available at one third the cost in large amounts from hardware and lumber dealers. It must be noted that the harder the cast, the harder it is to grind on the model trimmer.

DIAGNOSTIC QUADRANGLE

The diagnostic quadrangle was formulated to provide a framework for organizing the twelve steps outlined earlier in the chapter for gathering diagnostic information from each child. After having taught this to students for five years, I realized that such an organization aids the diagnostician by being a mnemonic device. In addition, it serves as a definite diagnostic pathway that can both elicit the needed information and provide the organization of information needed during a case presentation to parents.

Of the twelve steps discussed, only steps 1, 2, 11, and 12 are not represented in the diagnostic quadrangle. They are, however, present on the diagnostic examination sheet. (See Figs. 4-7 and 4-8.)

Separation of tooth-to-tooth from tooth-to-skeleton relationships

The *upper* half of the diagnostic quadrangle is concerned with the relationships of lower teeth to upper teeth. These relationships are strictly tooth to tooth, with no skeletal components intruding. The terminal planes of the second primary molars and the relations of the upper and lower 6-year molars and cuspids to each

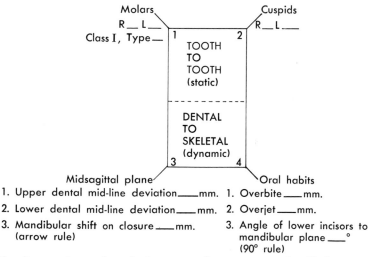

Fig. 4-8. The diagnostic quadrangle is presented as a mnemonic aid that may be used to begin the diagnosis of any case. This must be accomplished with the child at the chair, since steps 3 and 4 require an examination of dynamic relationships not available from the study casts.

other comprise the tooth-to-tooth aspect of the quadrangle.

In the *lower* half of the diagnostic quadrangle, however, the positions of teeth are related to two skeletal landmarks, the midsagittal and mandibular planes. These may be seen in the child as well as in the frontal and lateral positions of the cephalographs. First, the positions of the upper and lower dental midlines are compared with the midsagittal plane of the child. To accomplish this accurately, a 15-inch length of dental floss is held against the child's forehead, nose, and chin to represent the midsagittal plane of the child's face and skull. The positions of the dental midlines are compared to this plane. Second, a hypothetical line is drawn through the longitudinal axis of the lower central incisors, and the approximate angle of its juncture with the mandibular plane is noted. According to Tweed's rule, this angle should be about 90 degrees in most Angle's Class I children. A fairly accurate estimate of this angle may be made using two tongue blades or the dentist's hand.

· · ·

The use of the diagnostic quadrangle itself is divided into four main steps, each with several substeps. Each of the four main steps involves a decision the dentist must make in order to proceed logically to the next step in the diagnosis. The element of decision making is considered one of the chief reasons why a dentist should use a logical step-by-step routine to arrive at his diagnostic destination.

With the completion of steps 1 and 2, the evaluation of *tooth-to-tooth* relationships have been considered. This is called a *static* evaluation because the same evaluation may be made on upper and lower plaster casts related together with a wax-bite wafer.

In steps 3 and 4 a *dynamic* relationship is established, which involves consideration of opening and closing the jaws to test mandibular shifts on closure and looking for the functional causes of protrusion of upper incisors and the lingual tipping of lower incisors.

Each of the steps can be accomplished in the child's mouth at the chair; however, some of them are better done with the diagnostic casts at hand. This is particularly true where actual measurements with a Boley gauge are concerned (Fig. 4-9).

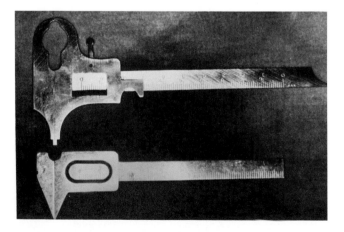

Fig. 4-9. Boley gauge must be modified considerably to be useful in measuring children's dental arches for space requirements as well as for overjet, overbite, and midline changes. When compared with the unmodified instrument, note the ruler end has been cut off at the zero mark in the modified instrument.

Step 1: Determine the molar relationships and the type of Class I malocclusion

If the 6-year molars have not yet erupted in the child undergoing diagnosis, the terminal planes of the second primary molars may be used to establish the probable Angle classification. (See terminal planes, Chapter 2.)

If the child is older than 6 years and the first permanent molars have erupted, the dentist examines the molars on the right and left sides of each arch and classifies them as Angle Class I, Class II, or Class III. If the molars appear to be in Class I relation on each side of the arch, then the dentist assigns a Dewey-Anderson *type* to the child. These types of Class I malocclusions are discussed in detail in Chapter 3.

If there is any uncertainty on the part of the dentist in assigning a Dewey-Anderson *type* to the child, he may wait until step 4 has been completed. In some cases, *two types* may be assigned to the same child. In such cases, the *predominant type* should be listed first.

• • •

A short summary of each of the Dewey-Anderson types of Class I malocclusions is included here.

TYPE 1 Too little arch space available in the anterior areas of the arches, resulting in crowded and rotated permanent incisors. Etiology: genetic; mentalis muscle hyperactivity.

TYPE 2 Protruded and spaced upper incisors. Etiology: oral habit such as digital sucking or tongue-thrusting.

TYPE 3 Anterior cross-bite involving one, two, three, or four upper incisors. Etiology: genetic, or early trauma to primary incisors.

TYPE 4 Posterior cross-bite involving one or both upper primary molars and perhaps including the upper deciduous cuspid and the 6-year molar as well. The cross-bite may be lingual, complete lingual, or buccal and also unilateral or bilateral. Eti-

ology: genetic, complicated by local environmental factors.

TYPE 5 Mesial drifting of one or more 6-year molars or ectopic eruption of the 6-year molar. Etiology: iatrogenic, caries, or genetic.

TYPE 0 A case where, by the best judgment of the dentist, there are no malposed teeth present and the arches are in a good Class I relation. Type 0 stands for zero defects.

Step 2: Determine the cuspid relationships to "prove" the molar positions

The relation of the upper and lower cuspids is examined on each side of the child's arches, and a decision is made to classify each side as Class I, Class II, or Class III. Because they do not have a tendency to drift out of position as much as the 6-year molars, the relative positions of the cuspids on each side of the arch are used as proof that the molar relation was judged correctly on that side of the arch.

The cuspid proof method should be used especially when molars on one side read Class I and on the other side a Class II relation appears. If an upper primary molar has been lost prematurely on the Class II side, the 6-year molar may have drifted mesially from a normal Class I to a Class II relation. The cuspid relationship allows the dentist to see that the upper molar erupted in Class I but has drifted forward and is now giving a false Class II reading.

Step 3: Determine the midsagittal relation of upper and lower incisors

To achieve an accurate simulation of the midsagittal plane without resorting to a frontal cephalograph, a length of dental floss may be used. The length of floss, 15 inches long, may be held to the child's face, centered on his forehead, nose, and chin. With the child's jaws slightly apart, the upper and lower dental midlines are noted in relation to the dental floss. If either is to the right or left of the floss (midsagittal plane), the dental midline is presumed to have moved from its normal midsagittal position, and the distance the midline has moved may be measured accurately with the sharpened tips of a Boley gauge (Fig. 4-9).

After the positions of the upper and lower dental midlines in relation to the midsagittal plane have been checked, the child is asked to close his lower jaw slowly into occlusion. If a deviation or shift of the mandible is noted during the last 3 mm. of closure, then the *amount* and *direction* of mandibular shift is carefully noted.

The substeps in carrying out these measurements are the following.

Upper dental midline relation. Any change noted to the right or left of the simulated midsagittal plane is measured in millimeters, and the direction is entered on the chart. If a change of more than 3 mm. is noted in the upper dental midline, the upper teeth will exhibit a pronounced tilting in the direction of the change. The primary cuspid will usually be lost on the side of the arch toward which the midline has deviated.

Lower dental midline relation. As was stated previously, it is very important to check the relation of the lower dental midline to the midsagittal plane while the child has his teeth 3 to 4 mm. apart. The muscles of mastication act to balance the mandible's position, and the relation of the lower dental midline to midsagittal plane can then be judged accurately.

Just as with the upper arch, if a deviation of more than 3 mm. has occurred, the teeth will appear slanted in relation to the occlusal plane of the lower teeth. Also the lower cuspid on the side of the deviation will usually have been lost due to ectopic eruption of the lateral incisor.

The direction and the exact amount of deviation are noted on the chart in the lower left corner of the diagnostic quadrangle.

Mandibular shift on closure. The mandibular shift on closure is the change (in millimeters) in the position of the lower dental midline from the open-jaw position to the closed-jaw position. Although prematurities in cusps of teeth may cause minor shifts on closure up to 1 mm., a large shift of 2 to 4 mm. on closure almost certainly indicates the presence of a cross-bite. Anterior cross-bites cause less shift, and posterior cross-bites cause greater shift.

In most cases the shift of the mandible is *toward* the side of the upper arch that contains the malposed teeth contributing to the cross-bite relationship. This leads us to the arrow rule, described next.

Arrow rule. The arrow rule emphasizes two important considerations regarding the etiology of midline changes and mandibular shifts. The arrow rule states that if a dental midline deviates to the left, the reason for the deviation will be found in the quadrant to the left. A corollary to this rule is that if a significant mandibular shift to the left is noted during the last 3 mm. of closure, then the cross-bite causing

Fig. 4-10. Use of the arrow rule: If a dental midline deviates to the left, the etiology of the deviation will be found in the left quadrant. A corollary is: If the mandible shifts perceptibly on closure, the reason for the shift will be found in the direction of the shift. Many posterior cross-bites that might escape notice may be detected by noting such a mandibular shift.

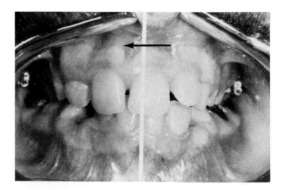

the shift is also located on the left side of the arch. (See Fig. 4-10.) The exception to the arrow rule is noted when a supernumerary tooth is present on one side of an arch.

Application of the arrow rule. If either an *upper* or *lower* dental midline is seen to be deviated to the right or left, place an imaginary arrow above the teeth pointing in the direction of the deviation. The arrow will point to the quadrant where the trouble originated to cause the midline shift.

Step 4: Determine the presence of oral habits

An oral habit of long standing in a child almost certainly is an indication that changed oral environmental factors have contributed to malpositions of teeth. Many of these malpositions of teeth are not lasting if the child outgrows his habit before age 4 or 5. However, the following three common habits, which appear with a high frequency among children beyond age 6, can act to distort the genetic potential toward well-shaped arches and normally arranged dentition in Class I children:

    a. Digital sucking, which may cause spaced, protruding upper anterior teeth and also an anterior open-bite

    b. Tongue-thrusting during swallowing or a passive tongue position where it is held between the teeth, both of which promote an anterior open-bite

    c. Hyperactivity of the mentalis muscle during the swallowing act, which causes excessive, unbalanced pressures against the lower incisors and may act to tip them lingually so that they appear crowded when the space may indeed be adequate if the mentalis muscle action were not so strong

The best available tests to determine the presence of oral habits are to measure the overbite and the overjet and to check how close to 90 degrees to the mandibular plane is a line drawn through the lower central incisors. These tests work best in children exhibiting Class I malocclusion.

Measuring overbite. Overbite is the distance in millimeters by which the incisal edges of the lower incisors close past the incisal edges of the upper incisors. In a normal bite the overbite is 1 to 2 mm. If the upper and lower incisal edges touch together in full bite closure, the overbite is considered to be zero, or end-to-end. It is proposed here that if the incisal edges are apart when the teeth are in full occlusion (anterior open-bite), the condition be regarded as *negative* overbite (Fig. 4-11).

Overbite is accurately determined by having the child close his teeth together and then marking with a sharp lead pencil on the labial surfaces of the lower incisors

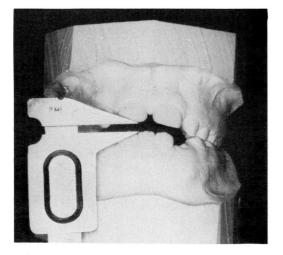

Fig. 4-11. Anterior open-bite (negative overbite) is being measured with a modified Boley gauge. Overbite is measured by having the child close his bite and marking on lower central incisors the level of the incisal edges of the cupped central incisors.

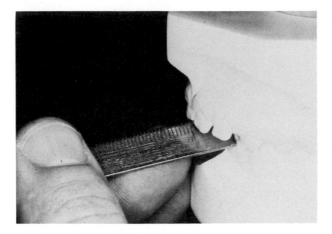

Fig. 4-12. Overjet of a child may be measured either directly in the mouth or on the record models as demonstrated here, using the rule end of the modified Boley gauge, which has been cut off at the zero mark.

the level of the incisal edges of the upper incisors. The overlap of the teeth can then be measured in millimeters with the sharpened tips of the Boley gauge.

A good working rule is that if a child has an anterior open-bite *before* the loss of the primary incisors at age 6, the chances are excellent that it is being caused by a digital sucking problem. However, if the child has an anterior open-bite *after* age 8, a good hypothesis might be that it is caused by a tongue thrust. The reason is that most children have dropped the original sucking habit by age 8 due to social pressures from their peers. However, the tongue thrust continues because the established open-bite acts as an avenue of convenience for the tongue to enter and seal the opening during the swallowing act.

Measuring overjet. Overjet is the distance in millimeters from the incisal edges of the lower incisors to the incisal edges of the upper incisors measured anteriorly on a flat plane. The normal overjet is considered to be 1 to 2 mm. in adult dentition, but it may vary from zero (edge-to-edge incisors) to 3 mm. in children and still be in the range of normality. Excessive overjet beyond 5 mm. is usually indicative of a digital sucking habit in a Class I child.

Measuring overjet is made simpler if the

Boley gauge is cut off at the zero mark at the end distal from the jaws. This allows the dentist to slide the Boley gauge, end in, against the labial surfaces of the lower incisors and read directly the overjet of the upper incisal edges from a position looking down over the child's nose (Fig. 4-12).

Determining the angle of lower incisors to the mandibular plane. The normal range of angles of the lower incisor axes to the mandibular plane is 90 degrees, plus or minus 5 degrees. This is called Tweed's rule.[10] A fairly accurate estimate may be made of this angle in a child's mouth by either of two methods: (1) a pair of tongue blades may be used, one of which is oriented to the lower border of the mandible and the other is held parallel to the axis of the most labial lower central incisor, or (2) the dentist's hand with thumb extended at 90 degrees may be placed so the thumb rests parallel to the underside of the jaw and the edge of the index finger acts as the plane to compare the axis of the most labially inclined lower central incisor (Fig. 4-13).

As a rule, if the lower central incisors are perceptibly inclined lingually, the hyperactive mentalis muscle during the swallowing act is at fault. If the problem is severe, the child may need to undergo

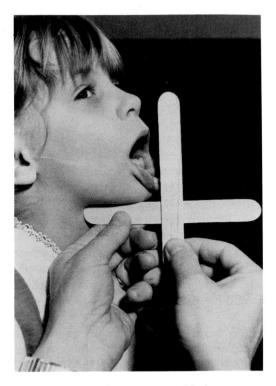

Fig. 4-13. Use of two tongue blades to measure angulation of a child's lower central incisors to the mandibular plane. Tweed's rule states that the angle should approximate 90 degrees, ± 5 degrees. As a rule, the tongue blade would be placed flat against the lower border of the mandible. It was placed on edge here to provide clarity in the illustration.

swallowing therapy or exercises to balance the forces acting against the lower anterior teeth so that the tongue forces equal the forces generated by the lower lip.

• • •

It can be seen that the four steps just described, which comprise the diagnostic quadrangle, may assist the dentist to identify the arch segments in which a molocclusion exists. Furthermore, they are designed logically to help him to decide what course he should take in the treatment of the child's malocclusion. The diagnostic quadrangle organization is easily learned, and the steps can be followed from memory

after practicing a few times with child patients.

ARCH SPACE ANALYSIS

After the recording of data acquired by the dentist from the diagnostic quadrangle, a space analysis must be done in each quadrant if a space problem appears to exist. Of the five types of Class I malocclusion, it will be noted that only Type 1 and Type 5 present problems of lack of space. Type 1 demonstrates lack of *anterior* space and Type 5 demonstrates lack of *posterior* space.

It is unusual that a problem involving lack of space will exist in the primary dentition when all of the deciduous teeth are in good health. The stages of early and middle mixed dentition (ages 6 to 10) present the dentist with spacing puzzles most often.[7]

To gain information that will tell him whether the erupting permanent teeth have a good chance to take their places in the dental arches unhampered by lack of space, the dentist should consider doing a mixed dentition space analysis for each child who appears to have an arch space problem (Fig. 4-14).

In general, three methods of space analysis may be used. Two of these are fairly popular and have been used for some time with excellent results. The third is new with this book, so far as the author is aware, and provides a different approach to estimate quickly and fairly accurately the space needed in each quadrant.

Moyers method of space analysis[6]

Moyers's predictive analysis of space in the child's arches during the mixed dentition helps the dentist decide whether or not the permanent teeth have proper room to erupt and align themselves normally in the existing arch space. By accomplishing this during the mixed dentition years the dentist may act early to solve some of the problems he sees by such interceptive procedures as space maintenance, space re-

Table 5. Probability chart for predicting sum of the widths of 3 4 5 (mandibular cuspid and first and second bicuspids) from the total widths of 2 1 | 1 2 (mandibular central and lateral incisors)*

2 1	1 2 =	19.5	20.0	20.5	21.0	21.5	22.0	22.5	23.0	23.5	24.0	24.5	25.0	25.5	26.0	26.5	27.0	27.5	28.0	28.5	29.0
95%	21.1	21.4	21.7	22.0	22.3	22.6	22.9	23.2	23.5	23.8	24.1	24.4	24.7	25.0	25.3	25.6	25.8	26.1	26.4	26.7
85%	20.5	20.8	21.1	21.4	21.7	22.0	22.3	22.6	22.9	23.2	23.5	23.8	24.0	24.3	24.6	24.9	25.2	25.5	25.8	26.1
75%	20.1	20.4	20.7	21.0	21.3	21.6	21.9	22.2*	22.5	22.8	23.1	23.4	23.7	24.0	24.3	24.6	24.8	25.1	25.4	25.7
65%	19.8	20.1	20.4	20.7	21.0	21.3	21.6	21.9	22.2	22.5	22.8	23.1	23.4	23.7	24.0	24.3	24.6	24.8	25.1	25.4
50%	19.4	19.7	20.0	20.3	20.6	20.9	21.2	21.5	21.8	22.1	22.4	22.7	23.0	23.3	23.6	23.9	24.2	24.5	24.7	25.0
35%	19.0	19.3	19.6	19.9	20.2	20.5	20.8	21.1	21.4	21.7	22.0	22.3	22.6	22.9	23.2	23.5	23.8	24.0	24.3	24.6
25%	18.7	19.0	19.3	19.6	19.9	20.2	20.5	20.8	21.1	21.4	21.7	22.0	22.3	22.6	22.9	23.2	23.5	23.8	24.1	24.4
15%	18.4	18.7	19.0	19.3	19.6	19.8	20.1	20.4	20.7	21.0	21.3	21.6	21.9	22.2	22.5	22.8	23.1	23.4	23.7	24.0
5%	17.7	18.0	18.3	18.6	18.9	19.2	19.5	19.8	20.1	20.4	20.7	21.0	21.3	21.6	21.9	22.2	22.5	22.8	23.1	23.5

*From Handbook of orthodontics by Dr. Robert E. Moyers. Copyright 1958, Yearbook Medical Publishers. Used by permission.

Table 6. Probability chart for predicting sum of the widths of 3 4 5 (maxillary cuspid and first and second bicuspids) from the total widths of 2 1 | 1 2 (mandibular central and lateral incisors)*

2 1	1 2 =	19.5	20.0	20.5	21.0	21.5	22.0	22.5	23.0	23.5	24.0	24.5	25.0	25.5	26.0	26.5	27.0	27.5	28.0	28.5	29.0
95%	21.6	21.8	22.1	22.4	22.7	22.9	23.2	23.5	23.8	24.0	24.3	24.6	24.9	25.1	25.4	25.7	26.0	26.2	26.5	26.7
85%	21.0	21.3	21.5	21.8	22.1	22.4	22.6	22.9	23.2	23.5	23.7	24.0	24.3	24.6	24.8	25.1	25.4	25.7	25.9	26.2
75%	20.6	20.9	21.2	21.5	21.8	22.0	22.3	22.6	22.9	23.1	23.4	23.7	24.0	24.2	24.5	24.8	25.0	25.3	25.6	25.9
65%	20.4	20.6	20.9	21.2	21.5	21.8	22.0	22.3	22.6	22.8	23.1	23.4	23.7	24.0	24.2	24.5	24.8	25.1	25.3	25.6
50%	20.0	20.3	20.6	20.8	21.1	21.4	21.7	21.9	22.2	22.5	22.8	23.0	23.3	23.6	23.9	24.1	24.4	24.7	25.0	25.3
35%	19.6	19.9	20.2	20.5	20.8	21.0	21.3	21.6	21.9	22.1	22.4	22.7	23.0	23.2	23.5	23.8	24.1	24.3	24.6	24.9
25%	19.4	19.7	19.9	20.2	20.5	20.8	21.0	21.3	21.6	21.9	22.1	22.4	22.7	23.0	23.2	23.5	23.8	24.1	24.3	24.6
15%	19.0	19.3	19.6	19.9	20.0	20.4	20.7	21.0	21.3	21.5	21.8	22.1	22.4	22.6	22.9	23.2	23.4	23.7	24.0	24.3
5%	18.5	18.8	19.0	19.3	19.6	19.9	20.1	20.4	20.7	21.0	21.2	21.5	21.8	22.1	22.3	22.6	22.9	23.2	23.4	23.7

*From Handbook of orthodontics by Dr. Robert E. Moyers. Copyright 1958, Yearbook Medical Publishers. Used by permission.

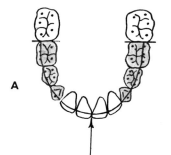

A

Fig. 4-15. **A,** More practical method of measuring arch length (formerly termed arch circumference). **B,** Method of measuring arch length occupied by the primary teeth (sometimes termed the *prime arch*). The instrument is made of two flattened bands and a length of resilient arch wire. In the case presented here, eruption of the four lower permanent incisors has not changed appreciably the length of the prime arch.

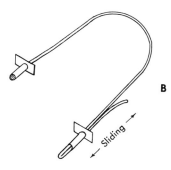

B

Table 7. Mesiodistal crown diameters of deciduous teeth*

Tooth	Sex	Mean (mm.)		S.E.$_M$ (mm.)	S.D. (mm.)	C.V. (%)	Range (mm.)	Number
Maxilla								
di$_1$	♂	6.55		0.05	0.36	5.53	5.8–7.2	64
	♀		6.44	0.05	0.43	6.65	5.4–7.5	69
di$_2$	♂	5.32		0.05	0.39	7.39	4.5–6.6	64
	♀		5.23	0.04	0.33	6.37	4.5–6.2	69
dc	♂	6.88		0.04	0.36	5.16	6.1–7.9	65
	♀		6.67	0.04	0.35	5.29	5.9–7.6	69
dm$_1$	♂	7.12		0.05	0.38	5.33	6.3–8.3	64
	♀		6.95	0.04	0.36	5.14	6.3–7.9	68
dm$_2$	♂	9.08		0.06	0.46	5.07	8.0–10.4	63
	♀		8.84	0.07	0.55	6.21	7.5–10.0	68
Mandible								
di$_1$	♂	4.08		0.04	0.30	7.23	3.0–4.7	64
	♀		3.98	0.04	0.30	7.42	3.2–4.7	68
di$_2$	♂	4.74		0.04	0.35	7.43	4.1–6.0	65
	♀		4.63	0.05	0.39	8.48	3.9–5.7	69
dc	♂	5.92		0.04	0.32	5.39	5.1–6.7	65
	♀		5.74	0.04	0.35	6.06	5.0–6.6	68
dm$_1$	♂	7.80		0.05	0.42	5.38	7.0–8.9	65
	♀		7.65	0.04	0.35	4.55	6.7–8.5	69
dm$_2$	♂	9.83		0.07	0.52	5.32	8.5–11.0	63
	♀		9.64	0.06	0.49	5.07	8.6–10.9	69

*From Moorrees, C. F. A.: The dentition of the growing child, Cambridge, Mass., 1959, Harvard University Press.

perament, the degree of his cooperativeness, and the amount of cooperation from the parents are all factors that enter into the dentist's decision to select a specific fixed or removable appliance to accomplish treatment.

Choice must be made to use either a fixed or removable appliance

Almost always for the treatment of each type of Class I malocclusion described in this book two different kinds of appliance will be available. One of these is the fixed appliance, which can be removed and adjusted only by the dentist. The other is a removable appliance, which is worn by the child at times suggested by the dentist but which the child is able to remove from his teeth during specified intervals such as mealtimes or active play times.

Should the appliance be active or passive?

Most of the types of appliances considered here are *active*. They are capable of being adjusted to exert the necessary amounts of pressure against one or more teeth to cause them to move into the more desirable position in the dental arch envisioned by the dentist during his diagnosis. The only appliances that are not adjusted to accomplish active movement of teeth are the space maintainers, designed only to hold space in the arch, and the retention appliances, used to retain the teeth in their new positions in the arches after active appliance therapy. These last two generally are called *passive appliances*.

Continued use of gentle forces is important

Perhaps one of the greatest errors the dentist can fall into is to attempt to hurry the movement of teeth by using greater pressure when it appears that the gentle biomechanical forces are not producing results. By making careful Boley gauge measurements in the mouth of the child and comparing these to the measurements ob-

tained from the original study casts, the dentist will usually find that continuing movement is indeed occurring.

If it is not, one of two things may be happening: the adjustments of the fixed appliance to maintain light pressures against the teeth have not been made properly, or the child is not wearing his removable appliance.

Appliances must be comfortable to wear

This raises the point of the last appliance objective—comfort for the child. The appliance must be comfortable for the greatest part of each 2-week adjustment period. Children do not care to be heroes and have to withstand constant and unnecessary discomfort. Although it is true that a new adjustment of pressures, particularly in a fixed appliance, can cause some slight discomfort for as long as 24 hours after the adjustment appointment, most of this should not be actually painful. A child who is hurting constantly during the course of appliance therapy rapidly becomes a whining, morose child at home. This scarcely enhances the image of the dentist as the fabricator of comfortable appliances. Until one of your own children has undergone such a treatment program, these ideas may not be fully appreciated.

Children should never have to endure intense discomfort during minor tooth movement procedures. If this is occurring, the appliance design should be immediately changed. Too much discomfort is a good warning to the dentist that there is an error in pressures built into his appliance and the child's tolerance is being exceeded.

APPLIANCES USED TO TREAT CLASS I, TYPE 1, MALOCCLUSIONS

The two different etiologies involved in Class I, Type 1, malocclusions were described in Chapter 3. In the first, the lack of space in the arches results from an inherited imbalance of oral structures. The child's teeth are *measurably* too large to fit into the space provided by nature in his arches. In the second, the upper arch appears to have adequate space for the permanent teeth, but the lower arch appears to be crowded by being depressed lingually in the lower incisor region. Here the lower front teeth are not being allowed to assume their proper alignment in the arch. The cause of this is often the swallowing patterns of the child who demonstrates a hyperactive mentalis muscle. These patterns have been called "the acrobatic lower lip" or "the visible swallow." Such muscle forces can act to crowd lower incisors and fold them lingually or may flatten the entire anterior portion of the lower arch.

The treatment approach is distinctively different in each of these two kinds of Class I, Type 1, malocclusions. So, too, are the appliance choices for children who exhibit these problems.

Genetic lack of space cases

The only time that malocclusions caused by genetic lack of space should be treated by the generalist is when the measured arch length deficiency is minimal. Usually this means that the observed lack of space is less than 3 mm. in the upper arch and less than 2 mm. in the lower arch. To gain this space, careful arch expansion therapy may be used in a child 8 to 10 years of age.

It must be noted that excessively expanded arches do not retain their new positions well and tend to relapse to the former configuration. Relapse after treatment of the lower arch is most prevalent, so of the two arches, expansion therapy in the maxillary arch enjoys the most success.

Split-palate expansion appliances. Two kinds of split-palate expansion appliances may be used to expand upper arches and gain needed space for permanent teeth: the jackscrew and the narrow U wire spring. The use of each during treatment procedures is described in Chapter 12. The buccal expansion to gain arch space is of a smaller dimension than that needed to reduce posterior cross-bites.

The jackscrew appliance (Fig. 5-1) is removable and may be adjusted with a small lever arm either by the dentist or by the child's parent. As a rule the amount of maxillary expansion possible by adjusting the jackscrew is 4 mm. If more maxillary arch expansion is necessary, the appliance may be remade, incorporating the same jackscrew.

When a narrow U wire spring is used (Fig. 5-2) instead of the jackscrew to activate a split-palate appliance, the dimension of possible arch expansion is greater, per-

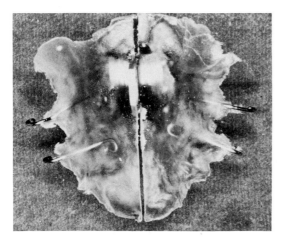

Fig. 5-1. Split-palate expansion appliance, a removable device used to expand upper arches in children who need to gain a minimal amount of additional arch length to allow eruption of all permanent teeth. This appliance has been split to separate the jackscrew elements. A thin separating disk is used in most instances. Same appliance may be used to increase palatal dimension by 4 to 6 mm. in posterior cross-bite cases discussed later. Appliance shown here has been removed from laboratory model but not trimmed and polished.

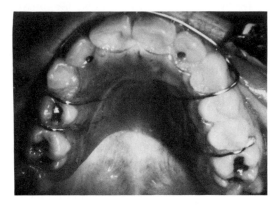

Fig. 5-5. Upper Hawley appliance, one of the most versatile appliances the general dentist will use. Here a Class I, Type 2, case (protruding upper incisors) is being treated. After the protrusion has been reduced, the appliance may be used as a retainer appliance for a period of 3 to 6 months. Note that upper right second bicuspid is congenitally missing.

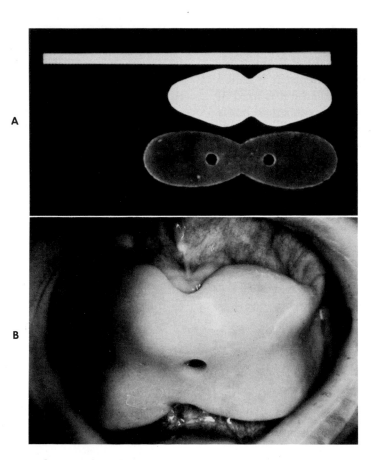

Fig. 5-6. A, Rabinowitch oral habit appliance made of soft gum rubber is one of the simplest appliances to use in cases of protruding anterior teeth and also anterior open-bite cases. Here it is pictured in relation to a 3½-inch paper pattern for making acrylic oral screens. (See Fig. 15-11, C.) It works best in anterior open-bite cases. This requires no laboratory work to fabricate and yet can be worn comfortably by the child. B, Acrylic oral screen in position in a child's mouth.

Retention for the appliance is provided by C (circumferential) clasps, Adams clasps or modified Crozat clasps on the upper 6-year molars. The labial bow wire should be shaped to have an "indent" over the lateral incisors so that the incisors do not have a "denture" appearance when they reach their desired positions.

The dentist is reminded that there is usually a sucking habit in the background of the child in such cases, and he is urged to make certain the child no longer practices the habit.

Anterior open-bite cases

Children who exhibit anterior open-bite also usually have a history of a prolonged sucking habit. In many cases the original habit has been dropped, but a mild to moderate tongue thrust persists, maintaining the open-bite. It will be recalled that in Chapter 3 it was made plain that only *spaced* open-bites should be treated and among these only the open-bites in which the cuspids still have incisal contact. In other words, only the upper and lower incisors are involved in the labial protrusion and exhibit an open-bite.

There are two general methods of treatment for children exhibiting these malocclusions. One is the use of a removable oral screen that the child holds in place by lip pressure, and the other is the use of appliances that exert wire forces against the labial surfaces of the incisors to move them back into proper alignment.

Oral screen. An oral screen (Fig. 5-6, A) is a device made of latex rubber, Plexiglas, and soft or hard plastic materials. It is usually shaped by the dentist to fit the individual child, who wears it held against his front teeth inside his lips only at night during treatment.[3] It acts to increase the pressures exerted by the lips, particularly against the upper anterior teeth, and at the same time changes the swallowing pattern to reduce the tongue-thrusting habit (Fig. 5-6, B). The tendency of the child to

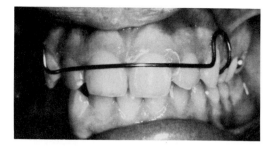

Fig. 5-7. Upper Hawley appliance serving as a retainer after tooth movement procedures.

mouth-breathe at night is also reduced considerably.

Upper Hawley appliance. The upper Hawley appliance used to treat anterior open-bites may be utilized better as a finishing appliance after treatment has been initiated with an oral screen. The labial bow wire is adjusted so that gentle forces are exerted against the labial surfaces of the upper incisors to move them back into a more upright position. It may also be used as a retainer when the teeth have been moved to the more acceptable alignment (Fig. 5-7).

Lower Hawley appliance. Although the lower Hawley appliance is more complicated to make than the oral screen, it can apply more selective pressures by the labial bow wire against individual lower incisors. It is also effective as a retainer after treatment by other methods.

APPLIANCES USED TO TREAT CLASS I, TYPE 3, MALOCCLUSIONS

Four of the eight basic appliances discussed in this book may be used to treat children with anterior cross-bites. They include the inclined plane, the upper Hawley appliance with bite plane, the upper heavy labial arch, and the upper light labial arch. The inclined plane may be a lower acrylic inclined plane cemented over all six anterior teeth or one of the two variations of the inclined plane, which are particularly effective in their application to one-tooth

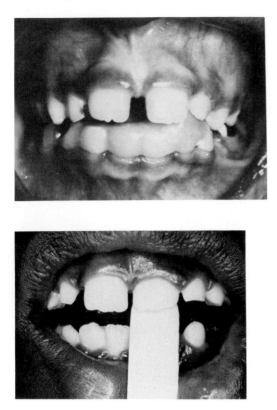

Fig. 5-8. Lower acrylic inclined plane, which may be worn as removable or fixed. It is more reliable as a fixed appliance cemented to place over the lower six anterior teeth.

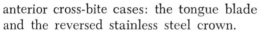

Fig. 5-9. A 9-year-old child is holding a tongue blade in place to guide the inlocked upper central incisor into a more labial position so that the anterior cross-bite will be reduced to normal bite.

anterior cross-bite cases: the tongue blade and the reversed stainless steel crown.

Inclined plane

Lower acrylic inclined plane. The lower acrylic inclined plane can be used to treat anterior cross-bite cases. It is a plastic covering cemented over all six lower anterior teeth with an inclined plane sloped to the labial, which is only as wide as the upper teeth that are in cross-bite. When the inclined plane is at 45 degrees to the axes of the upper teeth, the force exerted by the child in closing his mouth to chew or swallow is directed against the teeth in cross-bite by the sloping plane and moves these upper teeth labially.[3] A more detailed explanation of this is found in Chapter 11. (See Fig. 5-8.)

Tongue blade. The tongue blade held in his own mouth by the child (Fig. 5-9) is one of the variations of the inclined plane used by many dentists to treat a one-tooth

anterior cross-bite. It works best with a central incisor that has only recently erupted into cross-bite because there is minimal overbite and minimal disturbance in the periodontium of the opposing lower central incisor, which is usually forced labially as the teeth close in their "locked" bite. Such a cross-bite has been termed an *inlocked* incisor, which accurately describes the condition.[4] If the tongue blade is held properly by the child, the force of biting on the inclined plane of wood can cause the cross-bite to be reduced in less than an hour. This method is described in detail in Chapter 11. Follow the cardinal rule: Always be certain enough arch space is available for the tooth in cross-bite to fit into the arch in normal relation.

Reversed stainless steel crown. The treatment of a one-tooth cross-bite by the reversed stainless steel crown (Fig. 5-10) is another variation of the use of an inclined

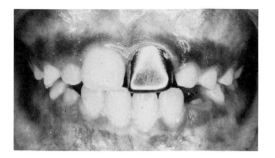

Fig. 5-10. Reversed stainless steel crown acts as an inclined plane to force the upper central incisor labially to create a normal bite in the incisor region.

plane to move a tooth in cross-bite into normal arch relation. Cemented on a child's upper central incisor, the reversed stainless steel crown can reduce the cross-bite in 2 to 4 weeks, as a rule. The tooth must have room in the arch into which to move, however, and a deep overbite should not be in existence when this method is used.

Upper Hawley appliance with bite plane. The upper Hawley appliance used to treat children who have anterior cross-bites is essentially the same appliance described previously in this chapter. How-

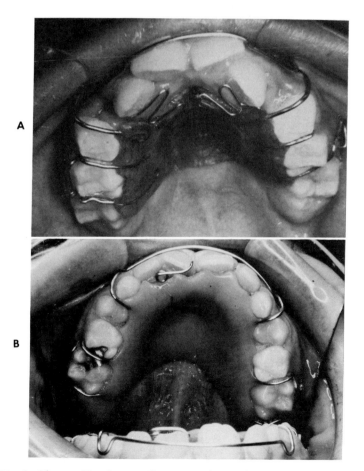

Fig. 5-11. **A,** Upper Hawley appliance used in Class I, Type 3, case. The dentist has not chosen well in this child's appliance. He has used the weaker W springs to attempt to move the two lateral incisors out of their anterior cross-bite positions. A heavy fixed labial arch wire might have been a better choice here. **B,** Upper Hawley appliance utilizing helical spring. A single central or lateral incisor in cross-bite may be moved into normal arch position quite efficiently with this appliance.

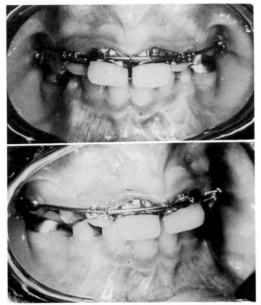

Fig. 5-12. Heavy labial arch with anterior bands being worn by child under treatment for anterior cross-bite. The cross-bite has been reduced, and the lateral incisors are being rotated into position. **A,** Front view. **B,** Right view.

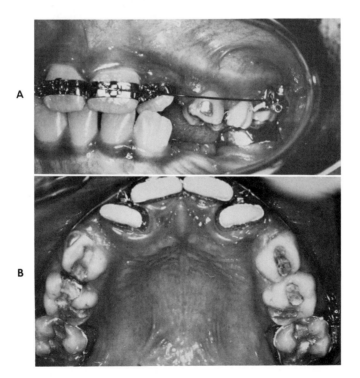

Fig. 5-13. **A,** Left view of light-wire labial arch appliance being worn by 8½-year-old child to reduce anterior cross-bite involving both upper lateral incisors. This permits controlled movement of teeth over period of several months. Teeth are moved out of cross-bite, then rotated using same appliance. Labially directed forces are generated by opening slightly the U-loops immediately mesial to where the arch wires insert into the molar buccal tubes. **B,** Same light-wire labial arch, palatal view. Note deformation of wire from ligature ties.

ever, in the anterior portion an S, W, or helical spring is embedded in the acrylic so that spring action will move the tooth or teeth in cross-bite in a labial direction. Overlaying the spring(s) is a shelf of acrylic that is contacted by the lower anteriors as the child closes into his bite (Fig. 5-11).

Such a bite plane prevents the teeth in cross-bite from inlocking as the child closes his bite and allows the labial movement of the upper teeth under the impetus of the springs to occur with no incisal interference. Oldenburg[6] and McDonald[4] have expressed doubt that a bite plane is necessary in most cases.

Upper heavy labial arch. The upper heavy labial arch (Fig. 5-12) is used to treat anterior cross-bites involving the upper lateral incisors. In the fabrication of the appliance, the upper 6-year molars and the four upper incisors are banded. Buccal tubes spot-welded on the molar bands serve as the insertion areas for the 0.036 arch wire, and the anterior bands have single edgewise brackets spot-welded to their labial surfaces to act as tie-points for the arch wire. By the careful ligation of the arch wire to these brackets, the teeth in cross-bite are gently moved labially into the normal arch relation with the other incisors. Such movement may take 2 to 4 months to complete. The labial directed force is generated by soldered U-loop springs of 0.020 wire placed immediately mesial to the insertion of the 0.036 arch wire into the molar buccal tubes. The heavy labial arch may also serve as a retainer when the desired movement has been accomplished.

Upper light labial arch. The upper light labial arch is constructed exactly as is the heavy arch just described. The difference lies in the size of the arch wire (0.020), which is small enough to fit into the anterior brackets and permit a degree of resiliency in the wire that gives the dentist better control of tooth movement. Fitting the bands, adjusting the bracket levels in a proper fashion, and contouring the con-

figuration of this light wire requires a certain degree of skill in this area. The light-wire arch can be a quite sophisticated appliance when used in experienced hands to treat anterior cross-bites. (See Fig. 5-13.)

APPLIANCES USED TO TREAT CLASS I, TYPE 4, MALOCCLUSIONS

Three of the eight basic appliances discussed in this book are used to treat posterior cross-bites in children. These common malocclusions among children may be treated with either fixed or removable appliances, the former having fewer advantages. All these appliances are discussed in greater detail in Chapter 12.

Bands, hooks, and cross-elastics. An auxiliary appliance to correct one-tooth posterior cross-bites may be fabricated of two cemented bands with soldered hooks, to which are attached cross-elastics (Fig. 5-14). The combination serves as a fixed appliance with removable elastics. It is easily worn by the child and can reduce a one-tooth cross-bite during a treatment period of 2 to 4 months.

Palatal expansion appliances. Both types of upper split-palate appliances used to treat posterior cross-bites have been pre-

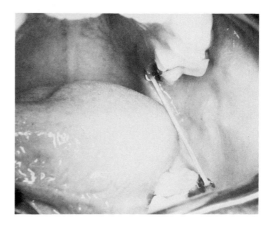

Fig. 5-14. Cemented bands with hooks and cross-elastics will act to reduce a posterior cross-bite involving one upper molar within a period of 5 to 6 weeks. The elastics must be replaced each day by the child and worn faithfully to produce good results.

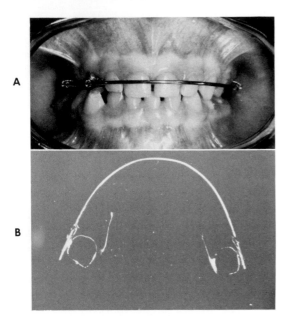

Fig. 5-15. A, Heavy round wire labial arch worn by 4½-year-old child. Lingual arms are soldered to the band. A soldered hoop just anterior to each round buccal tube serves both as a tie point for the ligature wire and as a stop. **B,** Heavy round wire labial arch removed from mouth. Note ligature wires may be attached around distal of buccal tubes and twisted into pigtail at hook stops. Appliance is designed to reduce a unilateral posterior cross-bite.

Fig. 5-16. Porter, or **W,** appliance is used to reduce a posterior cross-bite by expanding the upper alveolar ridge in a buccal direction. Unless appliance is made as a fixed-removable one, it is very difficult to adjust in the mouth.

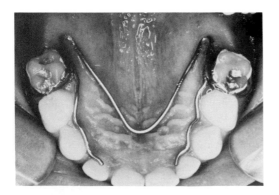

viously described in this chapter in the discussion of genetic lack of space cases. The methods of treatment to reduce a posterior cross-bite and to expand an upper arch to gain arch length are remarkably similar. The differences between the two methods are clarified in Chapter 12.

It is important to note, however, that these appliances have the advantage of expanding the alveolar ridges in a buccal direction and not just the posterior teeth alone. This advantage has caused this appliance to be one of the most widely used in the offices of generalists and pedodontists.

Upper heavy labial arch. The upper heavy labial arch appliance used to treat posterior cross-bites has an added configuration when compared to the same appliance described earlier in this chapter to treat anterior cross-bites. Soldered to the lingual surfaces of the maxillary 6-year molar bands are two 0.036 wires contoured against the lingual surfaces of the teeth forward to the mesial surface of the cuspids. Therefore as the main heavy arch wire is expanded to reduce the cross-bite, the lingual arms act to carry the teeth they touch outward in a buccal direction. (See Fig. 5-15.) The wearing of the heavy labial arch appliance is difficult for the child the first few days and may cause a severe chapping of the lips. Use of a lip ice or other lip emollient helps solve this problem.

Porter, or **W,** *appliance.* The Porter, or W, appliance is used as a fixed appliance to reduce posterior cross-bites in the primary dentition. It is essentially an upper lingual arch combined with lingual arms such as were described above. The Porter appliance may be fabricated as a fixed soldered appliance or may be made more versatile by the addition of vertical tubes on the molars bands to allow the appliance to be used as a fixed-removable one. This greatly facilitates the adjustments made every 2 or 3 weeks in the dentist's office. (See Fig. 5-16.)

APPLIANCES USED TO TREAT
CLASS I, TYPE 5, MALOCCLUSIONS

Loss of space in the posterior segments of the arch may be due to a variety of factors such as interproximal caries, affecting the primary molars, premature extraction of the deciduous molars, or the ectopic eruption of a 6-year molar. This change of molar position can act to block out the normal eruption of the bicuspids, particularly the second bicuspid. The two objectives in treatment of posterior space loss are maintaining adequate space (described in more detail in Chapter 8) and procedures that may cause the lost space to be regained by moving the mesially drifted 6-year molar distally to a position that matches its antimere on the opposite side of the arch.

Fixed and removable space maintainers. Several kinds of fixed and removable space maintainers are used to prevent the loss of posterior space caused by mesial drifting of the six-year molar. Among the fixed space maintainers recommended here are the band and loop, crown and loop, and fixed soldered lingual arch (Fig. 5-17).

Removable space maintainers resemble the lower Hawley appliances described previously in the section of this chapter on genetic lack of space cases. The difference is that a small acrylic saddle is formed over the space on the alveolar crest formerly occupied by the natural tooth, since extracted.

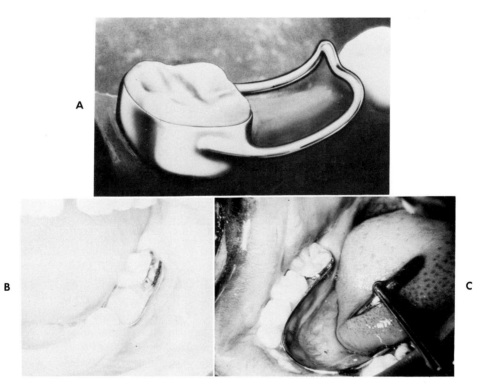

Fig. 5-17. **A,** Band and loop space maintainer. The solder joints should be made on the buccal and lingual surfaces of the band and polished to a high finish. **B,** Soldered band and loop space maintainer. To see a bicuspid erupting within the loop of a properly constructed space maintainer should be a rewarding experience for the dentist. **C,** Soldered (fixed) lower lingual arch. This type of arch has limited use in tooth movement procedures and is most useful as a bilateral space maintainer in the lower arch. (**A** courtesy Rocky Mountain Dental Products Co., Denver, Colo.)

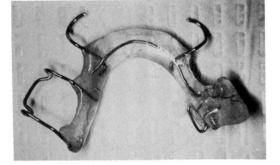

Fig. 5-18. Acrylic removable space maintainer. This type of space maintainer may utilize clasps and even springs to reposition teeth slightly.

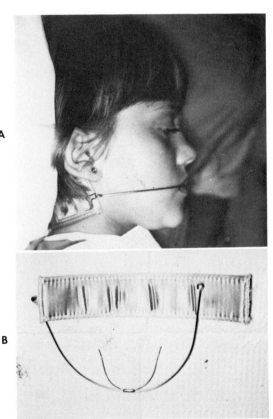

Fig. 5-19. A, This girl is wearing a cervical extraoral force appliance. Outer bow is contoured close to her cheeks. Solder joint in front of her upper incisors should be 3 mm. away from their labial surfaces to allow distal movement of the molars to occur without having the appliance touch the teeth in the anterior area. B, Same cervical extraoral appliance is shown removed from the girl. Note the stops in the inner arch about 6 mm. from the rounded tips of the wire.

Clasps may also be fitted to the primary cuspids as well as the molars, and the usual labial bow wire may be omitted (Fig. 5-18).

Upper Hawley space-regaining appliance. As a rule, the upper Hawley space-regaining appliance is made in much the same fashion as other upper Hawley appliances previously described. The difference is that a helical spring device is fabricated and placed against the mesially drifted molar to enable it to be moved distally during treatment so that it will closely match the position of its antimere in the opposite arch. Two types of wire spring configurations are suggested to achieve distalization of the 6-year molar: (1) a helical spring shaped to provide a force directed to the distal against the molar and (2) a dumbbell-shaped wire spring embedded in acrylic that is split much as in the split-palate appliances. The ends of the dumbbell-shaped wire are not embedded and serve as adjustment areas to allow the split in the appliance to be widened and so exert pressure against the molar to move it distally.[6]

Both of these appliances are easily made and are comfortable for the child to wear. However, they suffer the disadvantage of being removable and therefore are liable to loss or damage by the child. The appliance is also worn at the child's option, not at the dentist's as with a fixed appliance.

Extraoral force cervical appliance. The extraoral force cervical appliance (Fig. 5-19) is in reality a combination appliance. Parts of it, the upper molar bands to which are welded buccal tubes, are fixed by being cemented in place. The face bow and neck strap are removable by the child, and it is worn only at night for about 12 hours each day.

With proper angulation of the inner and outer bows and adjustments of pressure of the elastic neck band, the cervical appliance can move one or both upper molars distally over a period of 6 months or so. It is, however, one of the more sophisticated appliances among the basic eight to use and requires a higher degree of skill in wire contouring on the part of the dentist. Two of its chief advantages are its invisibility during the day (the molar bands do not show) and the fact that only the upper 6-year molars need be banded.

Lower Hawley space-regaining appliance. The lower Hawley space-regaining appliance is fabricated in much the same fashion as the upper Hawley appliance discussed previously. The difference is that a distalizing force is generated by the incorporation of a helical spring or a dumbbell wire split-acrylic device against one or both lower 6-year molars. Adjustment of these springs can act to move the molar(s) distally to their original positions in the lower arch over a period of 4 to 6 months.

F-R lower lingual arch. The fixed-removable lower lingual arch may be worn comfortably by the child patient and may be contoured to provide distalizing force against either one or both of the lower 6-year molars. The tubes attaching the appliance to the 6-year molars may be horizontal or vertical; the horizontal ones occupy less occlusogingival space and are more comfortable for the younger child of 7 to 10 years of age. (See Figs. 5-11, *A*, and 5-3.)

The springs used to generate the distalizing force are of two types: (1) U-loops placed in the main lingual arch wire in the bicuspid areas, which may be opened to provide additional force, and (2) a helical spring added as an auxiliary to one side and contoured to provide a distal force against one 6-year molar. In the latter, a stop wire is soldered at a right angle to the lingual arch wire and contoured against the distal surface of the tooth adjacent to the space being opened. The helical spring is soldered at a right angle to the lingual arch wire distal to the stop wire. Adjustments over a period of 4 to 6 months will allow one or both molars to be moved by such appliances.

A precaution to note is that a buccal tube is soldered on the *lingual* surface of the molar band on the side where space is to be regained. This allows a free-sliding action of the lingual arch wire within the round tube.

SUMMARY

A series of eight basic appliances have been described, which may be used to treat the following five types of Class I malocclusions: genetic or muscularly induced lack of arch space, protrusion of upper incisors and anterior open-bite, anterior cross-bites, posterior cross-bites, and posterior space problems caused by mesial drifting of upper or lower 6-year molars. With each type of malocclusion have been described the several choices of appliances that might be made by the dentist in selecting the route to treatment, including the advantages, disadvantages, and necessary precautionary measures for each appliance.

REFERENCES

1. Adams, C. P.: The design and construction of removable orthodontic appliances, ed. 4, Bristol, 1971, John Wright & Sons.
2. Graber, T. M.: Orthodontics: principles and practice, ed. 2, Philadelphia, 1966, W. B. Saunders Co., p. 167.
3. Hitchcock, H. P.: Preventive orthodontics. In Finn, S. B., editor: Clinical pedodontics, ed. 3, Philadelphia, 1967, W. B. Saunders Co., p. 298.
4. McDonald, R. E.: Dentistry for the child and the adolescent, St. Louis, 1969, The C. V. Mosby Co., p. 361.
5. Mayne, W. R.: Serial extraction—orthodontics at the crossroads, Dent. Clin. North Am., pp. 341-362, July, 1968.
6. Oldenburg, T. R.: Personal communication, 1970.

6 | The case presentation to parents

When a dentist has invested a great deal of time and effort in acquiring new skills in diagnosis of children who have primary or mixed dentition malocclusions, he may feel a high degree of satisfaction. As he puts these skills to use in selecting and fabricating minor tooth movement appliances, his satisfaction will grow.

However, there exists a barrier that most dentists must cross before they achieve the feeling that they are accomplishing minor tooth movement procedures as efficiently as their other practice efforts. The barrier has been called "lack of communication" between the parents of the child and the dentist who is suggesting treatment. A better term might be "poor translation" on the part of the dentist.

If he has found it difficult to translate other facets of dental care into the lexicon of his patients, the descriptions of malocclusions and proposals of options for treatment may be quite baffling to the dentist whose training did not include case presentations.

CASE PRESENTATION

Perhaps the goal of a case presentation should be that *what the dentist says and what the child's parents understand him to say should be as similar as possible.* In this chapter and in Chapter 20 are presented both techniques and language that should make the translation of these ideas to the parents flow more smoothly during case presentations.

Each dentist will, of course, present his cases and treatment plans for minor tooth movement in his own individual manner. However, the procedures discussed in this chapter, which were gathered from the combined experiences of many practicing pedodontists and general dentists, will serve as aids for the less experienced dentist as well as reminders for those who have had wide experience with this important communication problem. *There is no one thing in a dental practice that enhances a dentist's reputation quite so much as his ability to communicate to the parents of his young patients his ideas regarding the problem of a malocclusion as he sees it and the treatment solution.*

Where to hold the case presentation

The dentist who attempts to explain all the details of a malocclusion to a parent at the chairside in a busy office is doomed to failure. He must arrange a special appointment with both parents for a case presentation. The best place for this is his private office.

Ideally he will have a case presentation area at one side of his private office where he and the parents can be seated. Although all the following items may not be necessary in each case, this list of equipment can serve as a goal to work toward in planning case presentations:

1. A table or shelf to display the models of the child's dentition
2. Child's study models and wax bite
3. Example models of other children's teeth, preferably showing both pretreatment and posttreatment occlusions
4. Dental chart with malocclusion analysis chart included (Fig. 4-7)
5. X-ray viewer with mounted x-ray films
6. Custom-prepared Boley gauge
7. Small tensor light for good illumination

Enhancing parents' understanding of malocclusions

One of the stumbling blocks that may prevent the dentist from accomplishing the type of minor tooth movement procedure he may wish to do is the parents' lack of understanding of the serious consequences of the child's malocclusion. It is extremely important for the dentist to remember during a case presentation how little he knew about malocclusions, and indeed the whole dentition, *before he went to dental school.* Quite probably the parents understand even less than this.

Use of the "second language" of dentistry (discussing the problem in lay terms) with the aid of sources such as the booklets *So Your Child Needs Orthodontics* and *Your Child's Teeth** is very helpful. These booklets are published by the American Dental Association, the former with ap-

proval of the American Association of Orthodontists. In clear language using lay terms they explain the difficulties presented by childhood malocclusions and the methods for correcting them.

It is better to proceed one step at a time with parents in a case presentation, showing the problem of the "meshing" of the teeth together, noting which teeth are out of position, demonstrating the loss of space in any of the quadrants, and describing the probable future growth so the parent can visualize what the final development of the malocclusion will be.

It is helpful to point out in a friendly fashion that no one ever becomes ill from a malocclusion. It is not a disease. Yet poor appearance of their teeth becomes an unhappy emotional burden for many individuals. If the dentist feels that preventive orthodontic care during the mixed dentition years will be helpful, this is the time to indicate it to the parents. If he feels that the child's malocclusion presents so difficult a treatment problem that it is out of his area of training and experience, then he should discuss the referral of the child to an orthodontist.

Many time-consuming explanations will be saved if the dentist requires both parents to read "For the Parents," which is the last chapter in this book. Use by the dentist of language and terms similar to those in the chapter will be helpful as he makes his case presentations.

Steps in the case presentation

Hollander[1] offers in his excellent book a series of interesting and productive steps to follow in any case presentation. In general, they include determining the awareness of the parents of the child's problem, description of the normal as compared with the child in question, explanation of treatment procedures and the benefits of treatment, arrival at a decision with the parents regarding treatment, description of fees and methods of payment, explanation of frequency and number of visits,

*Both booklets are available through the American Dental Association, 211 E. Chicago Ave., Chicago, Ill.

and, finally, the arrangement of appointments.

Methods for demonstrating need for treatment

The dentist who treats developing malocclusions in his practice should never be placed in the position of having to persuade the parents of his child patients to initiate minor tooth movement procedures for their children. Indeed, the very opposite situation may occur. Too often the parents may try to urge the general practicing dentist to try to do more with appliances than he is properly trained to do. Rather than the persuasion of parents, the central force behind the dentist's watchfulness where occlusion is concerned should be his own deep interest in the child's growth and development. The child's facial structures and dentition are not divorced from the rest of him. It is careful observation of the *whole* child on the part of the family dentist that more than any other one factor acts to gain the attention of the parents when the dentist notes that there appears to be a discrepancy in the occlusion.

Once the parents have been alerted to the possibility of a malocclusion problem, the following are several items to be presented as evidence of how serious the case is:

1. Nothing the dentist may do is quite so impressive for the parents as when he measures the existing space in each quadrant in the child's mouth with specially prepared calipers. This certainly can be one of the first clear indications that there is a developing malocclusion in many instances. (See Fig. 4-9.)

2. Full mouth x-ray films should be presented, although these demonstrate the relationships of the teeth much better to the dentist than to the parents.

The following observations should be pointed out and explained:
   a. The number of teeth, primary and permanent
   b. Root relationships and resorption patterns of primary teeth
   c. Relative level of crown positions of erupting permanent teeth
   d. Carious lesions that may have been overlooked

3. Panographic type x-ray film should be presented. This will show the parents more clearly the relationships of the teeth in the dental arch than any other type of film. Particularly it shows crowding, poor angulation of roots, and the positions of unerupted teeth.

4. Upper and lower plaster study models of the child's dentition should be available. These show the parent the failure of the teeth to interdigitate properly. Also, mixed dentition analysis measurements may be taken off the casts to demonstrate to the parent the child's space needs in each quadrant. The arch length instrument is valuable for this. (See Fig. 4-15.)

Parental consent for treatment necessary

When the evaluation of the malocclusion has been accomplished and it has been established firmly as a treatable Class I malocclusion (Table 9), the parents must give their consent for treatment at the case presentation. *Both parents must be present at this time if it is at all possible.* Dentists report that most unsatisfactory situations arise from the misinformation concerning the child's need for treatment carried home by the one parent to the other. Consent must not be implied but must be verbally given or signed on a treatment form. A parent must not be allowed to be given the chance to say later, "I was never really given a chance to give or withhold my consent for treatment by the dentist."

Goals of treatment

At this time the dentist outlines his goals of treatment so that there will be no possible misunderstanding. The summing up by the dentist might go as follows.

Now, Mr. and Mrs. Peterson, let me review this treatment plan I have worked out for Debbie so that we may see that we all agree. As I have explained, Debbie's 6-year molars on her right side are in a cross-bite type of malocclusion. It is clear from the x-rays and models that nothing else is amiss at this time with the rest of her occlusion, and I can see no other teeth out of line in the x-rays at this time. However, on this score, only in time can we be really certain whether any other teeth will erupt in malocclusion.

By placing orthodontic bands with hooks on the upper and lower 6-year molars on her right side she will be able to wear cross-bite elastics. These tiny rubber bands will act to move the teeth gently into the correct occlusal positions over a period of the next 3 or 4 months.

Debbie will find it is a bit of a chore to take the elastics out while she eats her meals and then replace them, but they should not be uncomfortable for her beyond the first two or three nights when the teeth may be a bit sore.

You are aware that you are to call me immediately should one of the bands come loose or in any other way begin to bother her. She will keep her own supply of elastics in her purse. Later we may have her wear two elastics at a time on the hooks.

As I explained, we charge an initial fee to begin Debbie's case and then a fee for each visit. I will plan to see Debbie twice a month during treatment until I am certain her teeth are holding in the correct occlusion. I have explained my "clean teeth" program to Debbie very carefully, and she understands the importance of brushing and flossing after each meal. And I have given her an appliance schedule she is to fill in all by herself.

Do you have any further questions about Debbie's treatment program?

Very well. Now please remember—I want you to call me if she has any problem at all while she is wearing her appliance.

Debbie's parents should leave the dental office with the feeling that they know what the problem is concerning their daughter's malocclusion, that the treatment is not terribly complicated, and that the malocclusion should be reduced within a period of 3 or 4 months. After this, there will be an observation period to make sure the malocclusion does not relapse after treatment. Such a careful approach will increase the level of confidence within Debbie's parents and will build a dentist's practice in minor tooth movement in his community.

Prime emphasis in the presentation should be on health service rendered

Several authors emphasize: *Fees should never be discussed until the entire case presentation or explanation is finished. If the patient (parent) has any objection to the necessary treatment other than the fee, this is the opportune time to bring out these objections.*[1]

All contingencies and potential problems that may arise in the treatment should be explained thoroughly.

The greatest emphasis must be placed upon the health service rendered, not upon appliances and materials.[3]

Closing case presentation

There appear to be many dentists who feel quite confident during the presentation of a case to a child's parents until it comes to the nitty-gritty of talking about fees. As soon as money is mentioned, the acute discomfort of the dentist is transmitted to the parents, and suddenly the previously professional atmosphere can become embarrassingly uncomfortable. This situation need never arise if certain pitfalls are avoided.

For the dentist who has ever floundered into one of these pitfalls and who desires a better method of presenting fees and closing his case presentations more successfully, the following five steps are presented. Each will be familiar to the practicing dentist, although he may never have used them together in this fashion.

1. *Describe the child's malocclusion thoroughly, using terms the parents understand,* but remember that some parents reject the idea that their child can be "abnormal" in any way. It is better to emphasize what must be done to move the teeth to *a more acceptable relationship.*

2. *Maintain eye contact with the dominant parent* as the initial fee or the appli-

ance fee is quoted. Explain that a fee will be charged for each visit twice a month, and state the visit fee. You are not trying to stare the parent down, but rather trying to emphasize the confidence you feel in your ability to accomplish the treatment being explained.

Maintaining eye contact is difficult for most dentists, and it takes practice to do it skillfully, but it is the most important factor in the entire case presentation!

3. *Do not stop talking after the fee has been presented.* This is like dropping a wet blob on the table and having everyone stand around looking at it.

4. Without losing eye contact, move easily into an explanation of approximately how many visits to the dental office will be necessary and over what period of time the active treatment will take place. Then ask the dominant parent if he (she) feels that these visits can be arranged, emphasizing that some of them will require absence from school for short periods of time.

If eye contact has been maintained comfortably and the dentist's explanation has been unhurried and thorough, the answer regarding the visits will usually be "yes." In most instances the parent is saying "yes" to the fee as well as indicating agreement that the schedule of office visits can be met by the family.

5. Now is the appropriate time to ask both parents if they have any questions concerning any part of the case presentation. Maintain eye contact as these questions are answered in an easy manner. Good rapport and a high level of confidence should be apparent in the relationships between the parents and the dentist at this point.

• • •

This method of case presentation has been successfully taught to, and used by, many practicing generalists and pedodontists. It appears to overcome what for many men is a barrier to closing successfully a case presentation to parents.

REFERRAL FOR CONSULTATION

More than occasionally, the dentist who treats the developing malocclusions of children during the mixed dentition stage will hear the question from parents, "Shouldn't these braces you are suggesting be done by an orthodontist?" Echoing Moyers's philosophy,[2] the answer should be straightforward and truthful and should put the parents at ease, perhaps as follows.

Whenever possible, during the time of the child's development when deciduous teeth are coming out and the permanent teeth growing in, I prefer to guide the simpler cases of malocclusion myself. My consultant in these matters is Dr. Smith, who is an orthodontist and has a practice here in our area. If you wish, we can arrange that your child has a consultation in his office. He is excellent in these matters and he and I discuss most of the appliance patients whom I decide to treat.

TIMING OF TREATMENT AND REFERRAL

Perhaps no one facet of minor tooth movement is misunderstood so often by parents as the timing of actual treatment of a child's malocclusion or referral to the orthodontist. Regarding the latter, one writer notes, "Referral should be made when an abnormal condition is noted *regardless of age.*"[4] The parents should thoroughly understand the reasons why the dentist has decided on a course of treatment. Likewise they should understand exactly why their child is being referred, if this is the dentist's choice.

Such a positive statement is not possible concerning the age of treatment of the various Class I malocclusions, however. Rather than list ages of children, perhaps a better method is to use the maturity of the child's dentition as a guide. The treatment timing charted in Table 9 appears to be agreeable to many experienced pedodontists and general practitioners in their practices. (See also Chapter 2, Table 4.)

Table 9. Treatment timing chart

Types of Class I	Preferred dental age for beginning treatment or for referral
Type 1	
Genetic crowding of anteriors	*Refer* to orthodontist during early mixed dentition so that he may advise should serial extractions become necessary
Crowding of lower anteriors caused by hyperactive mentalis muscle	*Treat* crowded lower anteriors during early-to-middle mixed dentition
Type 2	
Protruding and spaced upper anteriors caused by thumb-sucking or tongue-thrusting	*Treat* during middle or late mixed dentition with both appliance therapy and habit retraining procedures
Gross anterior open-bite caused by tongue positional habit or tongue-thrusting	*Refer* during middle mixed dentition
Type 3	
Anterior cross-bite, 1 or 2 teeth, caused by genetic influences or trauma	*Treat* during early mixed dentition
Anterior cross-bite, 3 or 4 teeth involved, possible pseudo-Class III	*Refer* during middle mixed dentition
Type 4	
Unilateral posterior cross-bite	*Treat* during primary dentition or early mixed dentition; treat as early as recognized
Bilateral cross-bite, high narrow palate	*Refer* from late primary to middle mixed-dentition stages
Type 5	
Posterior space loss, minimal, caused by slight mesial drift of molar(s)	*Treat* as soon as recognized in mixed dentition with space-regaining appliance
Posterior space loss, maximal, caused by early extraction of deciduous molars (iatrogenic space loss)	*Refer* in middle mixed dentition so that planned extraction of bicuspids may be begun

DIVISION OF RESPONSIBILITIES

After the case presentation has demonstrated the need for treatment to the parents and the dentist has decided to undertake treatment, he must make absolutely sure that the division of responsibilities during treatment of the case is clearly spelled out.

The dentist's responsibilities

The dentist has taken on the task of moving one or more teeth in the arch from an abnormal position to one more nearly normal. He has agreed to accomplish this with appliances that are effective, comfortable to wear, and not harmful to the teeth in any way. This is not a case of *caveat emptor,* or "let the buyer beware." He has

promised to put forth the best of his professional ability to accomplish a goal, but he must also leave room for possible failure on his part! His patients do not expect him to be God. All they expect is good care and the intelligent use of appliances. If the case is started and goes poorly or appears to be beyond his skill, the dentist should arrange an immediate consultation with an orthodontist to discuss the refractory case with him.

During active treatment most patients should be seen for appliances adjustments twice a month. Less than this usually does not indicate good treatment supervision. Remember that this means only ten adjustments are available to the dentist after the first month if he expects to accomplish his treatment goals during a 6-month period, which is usually suggested as the time goal the dentist should set for himself in most minor tooth treatment cases.

The parents' responsibilities

There is no doubt that during the treatment of each case of minor tooth movement some troubled moments will occur in the parents' minds along the way. Problems may stem from the child's not wearing his appliance, a gingival inflammation due to the fit of the appliance or lack of a good tooth-brushing regimen, or sore teeth at the start of a period when new pressures are exerted on the teeth with the adjustment of the appliance. Difficulties may arise over simply transporting the child to the office twice a month for adjustment appointments. The parents may not be aware of the progress that dentist sees in the case and may feel their time and money are being poorly spent. All these problems and a dozen others may occur during the course of treatment.

After a while, even the most patient dentist can become a bit short in his answers to parents asking what can be a series of interminable questions regarding their child's progress.

It would seem best in most treatment plans to have a "progress report" arranged by the dentist for the parents at the end of the first 3 months of appliance treatment and again every 6 months thereafter until the case is treated out.

Reassuring the parents and the child takes real skill in words and demeanor on the part of even the experienced dentist. Most men experienced in these skills would agree that if the dentist carefully outlines what he expects of the parents and child, the in-treatment problems are usually seen to be minimal. Careful presentation of the goals of the dentist and emphasis on the home procedures that must be accomplished to make the treatment successful will help a great deal to eliminate undue friction between the par-

ents and dentist during appliance therapy.

There are several important but more general considerations that promote understanding on the part of parents. The dentist should make certain that these are discussed with the parents if they appear to be pertinent to the child's treatment course.

Some specific actions the dentist might request of his patients' parents are as follows:

1. All restorative procedures on both primary and permanent teeth must be accomplished for the child *before* treatment is begun.

2. Supervised tooth brushing at home is essential, particularly if several of the teeth are to be banded to utilize a fixed appliance.

3. All appointments at the dental office are to be scrupulously kept. The parents must understand that cancellations without cause can upset a busy office routine and make a chaos of good schedules.

4. Any broken or loose appliances must be reported promptly to the dentist so that he may arrange for repair at the earliest possible opportunity.

5. Primary teeth that loosen and are near exfoliation should be reported to the dentist, not because of their long-term importance but because of the possibility that the parents may not have understood that the loss of these teeth was a part of the original planning.

6. Above all, the schedule of wearing of appliances as assigned by the dentist must be rigidly adhered to. To expect good results of treatment with intermittent or haphazard wearing of the appliances is obviously far from realistic.

Some parents will require only praise of their efforts to keep them in a cooperative mood. Others will not cooperate fully until a mild scolding from the dentist brings home the seriousness of their lack of discipline at home. Reminding them that the success of the treatment depends on them and that they are prolonging it unnecessarily and making it more costly by allowing the child to neglect his appliance can serve effectively to obtain the cooperation the dentist must expect and receive.

The child's responsibilities

The age of the child is important to consider when his responsibilities are outlined by the dentist. In general, children younger than 6 years of age should be treated with fixed appliances whenever possible, for the following reasons:

1. The younger child does not always have the necessary maturity to maintain a schedule of wearing removable appliances.

2. Fixed appliances do not become lost or misplaced as often as removable devices.

3. Treatment time in many children is substantially lessened when fixed appliances are utilized. (See Fig. 6-1.)

The younger child and his appliance. The younger child must have a good overall idea of *why* the minor tooth movement procedure is being done. His pride and his maturity must be praised by the den-

---

Appliance schedule for _____, starting _____:
                                    (Name)   (date)

You are to wear this interceptive orthodontic appliance each day according to the instructions Dr. _____ has given to you. To help you do this the following calendar of days will be carefully filled in by you by <u>checking</u> the <u>day</u> <u>in</u> <u>red</u> after you have worn the appliance. Please remind your dentist when you need another calendar.

Month <u>September</u>

1	2	3	4	5	6	7	8	9	10	
11	12	13	14	15	16	17	18	19	20	
21	22	23	24	25	26	27	28	29	30	

Month <u>October</u>

1	2	3	4	5	6	7	8	9	10	
11	12	13	14	15	16	17	18	19	20	
21	22	23	24	25	26	27	28	29	30	31

Month <u>November</u>

1	2	3	4	5	6	7	8	9	10	
11	12	13	14	15	16	17	18	19	20	
21	22	23	24	25	26	27	28	29	30	

Please bring your calendar in to the dentist each time you have an appointment.
Thank you.

Fig. 6-1. Home appliance schedule.

tist so that he becomes eager to help in every way to accomplish the dentist's and his parent's goals.

During the taking of radiographs and fullmouth impressions the dentist will have an excellent opportunity to assess the child's attitude of helpfulness. If these two steps are accomplished only after some difficulty, then perhaps the dentist should think about delaying for a time before beginning treatment. The fitting of bands on primary molars for a fixed appliance such as a Porter appliance or a heavy labial arch to reduce a posterior cross-bite may provide another test to learn whether the child is wholeheartedly accepting the procedures. If, after these three steps, no difficulty is encountered, then almost certainly the child will be able to wear his fixed appliance.

By substituting words such as "pressure" for *hurt,* "cough" for *gag,* and "tight" for *interproximal pressures,* the dentist can guide the child psychologically over the uncomfortable impression-taking moments and the little hurts encountered when he is fitting bands and ligating wires. Also, a child at this age seems to understand the term "glue" better than *cement* when speaking of bands being attached to his teeth. To emphasize good tooth-brushing habits, it is helpful to speak of keeping the bands and wires "silvery" or "shiny" rather than merely *clean.*

Preparing the child for some postfitting discomfort is only fair play on the part of the dentist. Children's aspirin taken before bedtime for one or two nights will help relieve the initial discomfort after new pressures have been added to the appliance during adjustment procedures.

Nothing is more essential than the proper home care of his appliance by the child. This means more than simply good tooth brushing. It means *no* candy or gum should be eaten and heavy, chewy foods should be avoided. Also, curious fingers should stay away from his mouth so that improper pressures are not added to the wires.

To sum up, there really is no problem for the younger child in wearing a fixed appliance as long as he is not *forced* into wearing it. His level of maturity and cooperation must be tested by the x-ray, impression, and band-fitting procedures before the dentist can be sure of his full cooperation. *With the younger child the dentist must be prepared to go slowly enough in his treatment procedures that he does not out-pace the child's level of tolerance of discomfort.*

· · ·

The essence of the problem of obtaining patient and parent cooperation lies in aiming for the ideal relationship: child and dentist working together, with the parents standing by for help only when needed. Such a confident understanding gives the child status and a feeling of responsibility, which serves to enhance the respect he has for the dentist who has placed such confidence with him.[3]

WHAT IS A FAIR FEE?

The fee question remains an obstacle in some dentist's minds when they consider all the aspects of minor tooth movement.

"What is a fair fee?" is a question commonly asked.

The often stated guide to dental fees— "Whatever you feel your services are worth"—is in this case not a very useful approach. Charging fees in the general practitioner's office for a special procedure such as preventive orthodontics requires more than passing thought. In general, there are three approaches to follow:

1. Quoting a total fee for the case at the beginning
2. Charging an initial fee as a down payment, then additional fees during treatment to be paid at each visit, as was suggested in the section on closing the case presentation
3. Charging an appliance fee each time a new appliance is inserted in the child's mouth and, in addition, a monthly or quarterly fee for each period the child remains in treatment

```
                                        Models #

   Name_____Age_____B.D._____Date_____

   Parent_____Address_____

   Tel._____Fee Estimate and Payment Program_____

      Treatment:



   Started_____         Satisfactory_____

   Completed_____         Unsatisfactory_____

   Check 6 mos._____12 mos._____18 mos._____24 mos._____

      Remarks:
```

Fig. 6-2. File card for active minor tooth movement cases.

Of these choices, the appliance fee plus monthly payments is the most popular among general practitioners and pedodontists. This method has been widely criticized because it seems to place emphasis on the mechanical aspects of the treatment program and not on the overall physiologic changes in the dentition that are brought about by the actions of the dentist. Also, there may be questions asked by the parents concerning whether a second or third change of appliances is necessary.

It would seem that the second choice might avoid this problem in most instances, but this is for each practitioner to decide for himself. It must be emphasized, however, that if a *firm* financial commitment is not made at the start of the case, misunderstandings on the part of the parents almost certainly will occur.

FILE CARD SYSTEM FOR ACTIVE MINOR TOOTH MOVEMENT CASES

It is essential that the dentist keep a close check on his active tooth movement cases. There are many ways of doing this, but one of the simplest is to have a card file holding 3 × 5 lined cards. The dental assistant can copy on them the headings in the example (Fig. 6-2), or the dentist can have some printed up. Only the essentials of the case are entered on the file card.

These file cards may be color-tabbed to indicate the type of treatment and type of appliance being used or to indicate that the child is finished with the active treatment phase and is in the retention phase.

SUMMARY

An attempt has been made in this chapter to clarify various approaches to making successful case presentations of minor tooth movement procedures to parents. For the dentist who has experienced pitfalls in the past in quoting fees, closing the case presentation, making clear the parents' and the child's responsibilities during treatment, and explaining the many general considerations that may arise during active treatment procedures, the methods presented here may give new language to enable him better to "translate" his ideas to the parents of his child patients.

REFERENCES

1. Hollander, L. N.: Modern dental practice, concepts and procedure, Philadelphia, 1967, W. B. Saunders Co., pp. 165-184.
2. Moyers, R. E.: Handbook of orthodontics, Chicago, 1963, Year Book Medical Publishers, Inc., pp. 188-195.
3. Ibid., p. 436.
4. Rehak, J. R.: Corrective orthodontics, Dent. Clin. North Am., pp. 437-450, April, 1969.

7 | Tissue response to natural and biomechanical forces

Because there are several excellent orthodontic texts that offer abundant and detailed descriptions of the responses of hard and soft alveolar tissues to the application of both natural and biomechanical forces,[5-7] only a rather sketchy review of these important factors will be attempted here.

The dentist almost certainly absorbed the essential peculiarities of these tissue changes from his training in dental school, continuing dental education courses, or his professional reading. It *is* necessary, however, to have in his mind's eye an accurate view of what occurs when natural forces are in action as well as when biomechanical forces (artificially induced pressures generated by appliances) are brought to bear against teeth in a child's mouth. He must have an idea of the amount and the direction of forces that will best move teeth. He should know whether he should plan to move teeth through bone in a particular case or whether he may move both bone and teeth to accomplish his objectives. He should also have a basic understanding of anchorage.[1,6]

The short review that follows will aid him in understanding how natural forces may act to aid or hinder him as he utilizes the eight basic appliances described in this book to apply biomechanical forces to malposed teeth so that they will be moved into more acceptable relationships.

NATURAL FORCES

The natural forces that act to change the positions of teeth may be thought of as being generated mostly by the muscles of the lips, cheeks, and tongue. These muscles act as a functional matrix of soft tissue, a sort of envelope of pressures surrounding the bones of the jaws and the dental arches. Some of the natural forces may act in a balanced fashion that might be described as normal, whereas others may seem to act in an unbalanced fashion and are then referred to as abnormal.

Normal forces that affect tooth position

A host of natural forces may act to affect a tooth's position in the alveolus. In some cases these forces may act in concert to cause movement of a tooth at a rate rivaling that produced by biomechanical forces generated by appliances.

Residual eruption force

Although the primary motive force for the eruption of a tooth may be expended once the tooth reaches occlusion, what might be called a residual force of eruption remains during an individual's lifetime. This force serves to keep teeth in normal alignment and allows occlusal wear and abrasion to occur. In some cases this may result in a tendency toward supraeruption, or an eruption beyond the plane of occlusion.

Supraeruption. Supraeruption is the phenomenon noted when opposing occlusal contact is removed from primary or permanent teeth. This occurs most often when opposing teeth are extracted. Teeth tend to continue to erupt until they meet occlusal pressure from other teeth in the opposing arch. An example is seen when a primary molar is lost by too early extraction and the succeeding bicuspid continues its eruption beyond the occlusal plane into the space in the opposing arch where the opposing primary molar may also have been lost. In the Class II malocclusion cases, the lower anterior teeth can erupt until a deep overbite results. Perhaps the lower anterior teeth may even bite into the palatal tissue behind the upper anterior teeth. Supraeruption, in this case, acts to increase the curve of Spee.

Muscle forces

As teeth thrust themselves through the alveolar crest to a height at which they can be acted on by facial and lip muscle pressures, they may have not reached a level where they are stabilized by touching opposing teeth or by adjacent teeth. Slender-rooted lower anterior teeth are particularly vulnerable to these muscular forces because the lower lip presses inward at almost 90 degrees to their labial surfaces. The development of their root structure is incomplete, and arch stability at this stage is lacking. Many arches can be distorted by muscle forces.

Tongue forces

The normal action of the tongue on newly erupted anterior teeth is to press them labially. The tongue acts most strongly in this regard during the act of swallowing, which is accomplished during the waking hours of children between six and thirty times a minute. During sleep the salivary flow is almost shut off, so the swallowing process is much less important. Of less concern, but still an effective force, is tongue pressure against the teeth during speech. A repetitive habit of licking the lips can also serve as a disruptive force against the lower anterior teeth.

In addition, the position the tongue assumes at rest is extremely important. If the tongue at rest is habitually held between the front teeth for long periods of time, the process of eruption of the lower and upper anterior teeth may be distorted or inhibited. The teeth will not meet incisally, and alveolar growth in the anterior regions may be affected markedly. The result of this forward passive tongue position may be an anterior open-bite. Posterior open-bites may occur in those children who hold the *lateral* edges of the tongue between the teeth as a habitual passive tongue position.

It is the belief of many who have studied the problems of constant and abnormal tongue thrusting during swallowing that these types of deviate muscular patterns can be retrained to a more normal and balanced pattern with the help of competent speech pathologists and therapists.[9] Therapy is usually better timed if it is given *during* the course of minor tooth movement treatment while the child is wearing appliances. In this way the deviate habit patterns can be effectively retrained to produce more acceptable muscle actions that *assist* the formation of proper arches instead of disfiguring them. (See Chapter 10.)

Distal drifting of the permanent lower lateral incisors

In some children whose tongue pressure is overbalanced by excessive and unbalanced pressure of the lower lip (mentalis muscle) the lower incisors are crowded lingually. As a consequence, the lower lateral incisors erupt ectopically against the primary cuspid roots, causing the primary cuspids to be lost by early resorption. This poses a serious problem. Without the primary cuspids, there is no confining pressure or arch stability to prevent the distal drifting of the lateral incisors. If only a single cuspid is lost, a shift in the dental midline toward the area of least pressure is to be expected. A shift in the lower dental midline is serious because it complicates appliance therapy to recover lost midlines.

These factors can make the unguided arch positioning of the upper and lower central and lateral incisors appear to be more a product of chance than of planning. In actuality, the influence of heredity is very powerful. Constant checking to determine variations in the upper and lower midlines will be extremely helpful. As was explained in Chapter 4, the maintenance of a good dental midline is one of the four important "legs" of the minor tooth movement diagnostic quadrangle.

Mesial vector of force

The pronounced tendency toward mesial drifting of teeth in both arches is spoken of as the *mesial vector (component) of force.* It is best seen in how the first permanent molars seem to compel any teeth they touch to move in a mesial direction. This vector of force is not completely understood, and Moyers[7] separates it into two kinds of force. However, here are some rules it seems to follow:

1. The mesial vector of force is not strongly present until after the 6-year molars erupt. Probably the establishment of the curve of Spee is a factor here.

2. Mesial vector is present only if *all* the teeth in the arch are *in contact* with one another mesial to the first permanent molar (Fig. 7-1, *A*).

3. If the interproximal contact of teeth is lost (as by an early extraction of a second primary molar), the vector only acts mesially through the area of the second bicuspid. In the area of the first bicuspid and cuspid the vector of force may well act distally (Fig. 7-1, *B*).

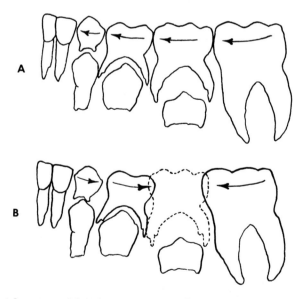

Fig. 7-1. A, Mesial vector of force as it acts in a lower quadrant when all teeth are in contact. **B,** Mesial and distal vectors of force acting in the same lower quadrant when a second primary molar has been lost prematurely.

When analyzed, the mesial vector of force seems to be a function of several factors: the angle of the axes of the upper and lower 6-year molars as they occlude, the cuspal slopes of these molars, the curve of Spee, and the pressure generated from the distal side by the maturing 12-year molars.

Depths of occlusal tables in primary and permanent molars

The shallower the occlusal table on a molar, the more likely is the possibility of a change in its cuspal relationship. Conversely, the deeper the occlusal table, the more likely the teeth will remain in the same "locked" position as they bite together. The cuspal slopes on the occlusal surfaces of molars are genetically controlled and therefore difficult to change. However, if molars are moved out of crossbite by appliance therapy, it should be no surprise to find that steep-cusped molars retain their new positions better than shallow-cusped molars.

Alveolar growth factors when teeth are congenitally missing

Alveolar growth can be affected if there is no succeeding tooth to replace a primary molar. The mandibular second bicuspid is congenitally missing more often than any other except the upper lateral incisor. In the former case a decision must be made whether to hold the space by retaining the primary tooth or to remove the primary molar and control the space closure and the undesirable changes in the axial inclination of the 6-year molar which might result.

A tooth should not be maintained in the arch if it is becoming totally submerged by the growth of alveolar tissue mesial and distal to it.

Ankylosis of primary molars. Commonly when a second bicuspid is hereditarily missing, the portion of the alveolar ridge in which the primary second molar is present fails to grow properly, and the primary molar seemingly becomes depressed or ankylosed (Fig. 7-2, *A*). Somewhat less commonly ankylosis of the first primary molar occurs. In a recent study in which 1100 complete radiographic examinations of children ranging in age from 2 to 13 years were evaluated, it was found that the incidence of ankylosis of the primary molars was 5.8% for the second and 4.3% for the first.[3] Interestingly enough, the same

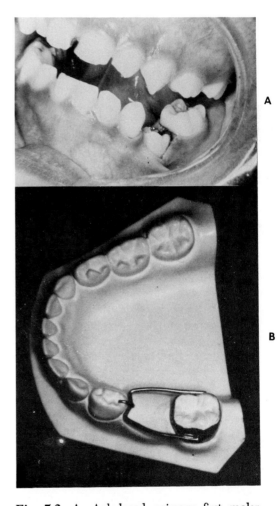

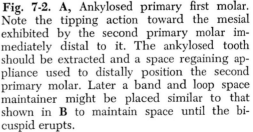

Fig. 7-2. **A,** Ankylosed primary first molar. Note the tipping action toward the mesial exhibited by the second primary molar immediately distal to it. The ankylosed tooth should be extracted and a space regaining appliance used to distally position the second primary molar. Later a band and loop space maintainer might be placed similar to that shown in **B** to maintain space until the bicuspid erupts.

study showed that there were more congenitally missing second premolars than congenitally missing permanent maxillary lateral incisors, which is contrary to the findings of most other studies.

It is extremely important that a second bicuspid not be judged missing even though calcification in the area of the tooth bud is not visible in the radiographs at 5 or 6 years of age. Fass[3] showed that these teeth may not begin to visibly calcify until as late as the sixth to ninth year.

Treatment should be initiated to maintain the space until the ankylosed primary molars may be crowned (Fig. 7-2, *B*) or if extraction is indicated, until the child is old enough to have a fixed bridge made. This prevents the mesial drifting or, in some cases, the mesial tipping of the permanent molars onto the distoocclusal portion of the infraerupted primary second molar.

Abnormal habit forces that can move teeth

In addition to the normal forces that can affect the positions of teeth, there are also many abnormal forces that may cause or sustain malocclusion. Many of these forces result from acquired oral habits or the retention of infantile muscle patterns of mastication and swallowing. Prominent among these abnormal forces are excessive tongue-thrusting, thumb- and finger-sucking, lip habits (hyperactive mentalis muscle action), and oral play.

Tongue thrust

As mentioned previously in this chapter, the effect of a deviate swallowing pattern (also termed aberrant swallow, tongue thrust, and retained infantile swallow) can have a pronounced effect on the newly erupted anterior teeth, which have little arch or root support. Tongue thrust can cause or perpetuate an anterior open-bite in some cases, or it can make worse a developing Class II malocclusion, especially if it is Class II, Division 1. (For a discussion on

tongue or swallowing therapy for such children see Chapter 10.)

Retraining children away from such muscular patterns and into more acceptable swallowing patterns usually calls for the services of a speech pathologist or therapist who has been trained in tongue therapy. Interestingly enough, many speech professionals believe that a child who thrusts his tongue during swallowing also exhibits tongue-thrusting during speech, resulting in an anterior lisping.

Thumb- and finger-sucking

In the past too many dentists have attempted to intervene at too early ages to prevent damage to the dental arches in younger children who exhibit thumb- and finger-sucking habits. This intervention has often taken the form of fixed devices fabricated by the dentist, such as tongue traps, rakes, screens, or removable palatal appliances with tines, knobs, or wire loops. (See Chapter 10 for treatment of these children.)

Relationship of sucking habits and tongue thrusting to malocclusion

To properly understand the relationship between sucking habits, tongue thrusting, and malocclusion in children whose ages range through the years of mixed dentition, it may be pertinent to review what several authorities have concluded from their studies. This is an area of dentistry in which the speech pathologist is most helpful. It has been confirmed by speech investigators that an infant's normal swallowing pattern is much like a tongue thrust, with the tip of the tongue extending between the gum pads to contact the lower lip to effect the seal for the swallow. Only with maturation and the eruption of the primary teeth does a slow change toward the normal adult pattern emerge. Even so, a study has shown that the infantile swallowing pattern still persists in a high percentage of 4- to 6-year-old children.[9]

However, in children who have digital

sucking habits, the open-bite that results in the anterior region provides a perfect pathway of convenience through which the tongue may thrust. The longer sucking habits persist, the more difficult it will be for the swallowing pattern to mature to normal.

It is important to realize that malpositions of the young permanent anterior teeth, which have been caused by the sucking habits, may be retained or even worsened by the continuing aberrant swallowing habit.

Norton and Gellin[9] have reviewed these relationships recently in an excellent article. These authors also present some practical suggestions for the interested dentist to follow in his office treatment of these common problems. (See Chapter 10.)

As long as the sucking habits (of the finger, thumb, etc.) continue, the tongue-thrusting swallowing pattern is usually retained. As the habit pattern becomes more firmly established with age, the tongue-thrusting during swallowing may persist even when the sucking habits are outgrown. Ordinarily it is expected that in the general population a sharp natural decline in tongue thrusting should occur at about age nine.

Lip habits and the mentalis muscle

The orbicularis oris muscle fibers, decussating as they do near the corners of the lip, act to close the mouth much as a purse string would draw a purse closed when pulled in opposite directions. These labial muscles seem to become mature in their actions about the age of puberty. The pursing action of the lower lip appears to differ considerably, however, from the upper. The mentalis muscle, which originates in the incisive fossa of the mandible and inserts into the integument of the chin, complicates the musculature of the lower lip region. The mentalis, in fact, has been indicted as the villain in many analyses of muscle action where the unprotected lower central and lateral incisors are pressed in

a lingual direction during deviate swallowing patterns. This occurs because the tongue thrusting in most cases appears to coincide with a marked *hyperactivity* of the mentalis muscle and a lessening in the activity of the temporalis muscle. (See Chapter 9.)

Oral play

Other oral habits found in children may be lumped together as "oral play." These may be cases of constant tongue-biting, lateral (toward the checks) tongue-thrusting, cheek-biting, frenum-thrusting (usually occurring when a diastema is present between the upper centrals), and clenching or sucking some object. At one time or another all these oral habits have been condemned as culprits causing abnormal movement or positioning of the teeth. Careful questioning of the child and his parents will usually elicit the reasons for the positions of oddly posed teeth. The dentist should feel that there is *always* a reason for malposed teeth. Writing "etiology unknown" on a malocclusion chart should be considered a *last* resort.

Scalloping of tongue from lateral pressures. The thrusting action of the tongue is not confined to forces directed anteriorly.

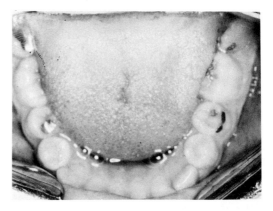

Fig. 7-3. Note scalloping along margins of tongue. This indicates a considerable lateral pressure directed outward against the buccal segments of both upper and lower arches.

Laterally directed forces are present also. In general, the tissue response to forces acting on the teeth are thought of as occurring in the periodontal membrane and alveolar bone. Changes in the margins of the child's tongue may be seen occasionally, however, when lateral tongue pressures against the enclosing teeth cause the edges of the tongue to assume a scalloped appearance (Fig. 7-3). The incidence of this is probably wider than is generally supposed. In oral examinations of 150 freshman dental and medical students at the University of Alabama, it was found that more than 50% of the students exhibited definite scalloping along the borders of the tongue due to lateral tongue pressures.[11]

BIOMECHANICAL FORCE APPLICATION

With the use of carefully controlled biomechanical forces generated by fixed or removable appliances, the dentist can tip or bodily move teeth into more desirable positions in the dental arches. Just as he must understand the natural forces acting against teeth, so too should he be knowledgeable concerning the responses of soft and hard tissue to adjustments of pressures in appliances.

When a force is incorporated into an appliance to move a tooth, it must be realized that the distance over which the force can act effectively cannot be more than the thickness of the periodontal membrane. If too heavy a force is used, a localized crushing and subsequent necrosis of the periodontal membrane can occur, and *the movement of the tooth ceases until the force is lessened.* In other words, good physiologic tooth movement occurs only when the forces against the teeth are light enough to maintain the health of the periodontal membrane, yet heavy enough to obtain the desired response of *osteoclastic action* on the pressure side of the tooth, and *osteoblastic action* on the tension side. Individual differences in physiology prevents a "formula" approach to forces used in appliance therapy, however. This is one of the areas of minor tooth movement that must be understood through experience and cannot be summarized simply.

Continuous, interrupted, and intermittent forces

The pattern of orthodontic force as it is applied may be described as *continuous, interrupted,* or *intermittent.* From the preceding discussion, it is seen that *continuous forces* on a tooth must be the lightest of all forces, since the rapidity with which bone can undergo restructuring is necessarily limited. With the use of the recently developed light, highly resilient Australian wire, for instance, continuous light forces may be applied to teeth. *Interrupted forces* act over a short distance, then are stabilized for a period. An example is a helical spring on a Hawley appliance being adjusted at 3-week intervals to move an upper lateral incisor out of cross-bite. *Intermittent forces* are usually applied for a short time, then released, as in the use of the Kloehn cervical extraoral force appliance. This is worn for 12 hours each night, with no appliance being worn during the day, allowing the teeth and tissues a recovery period.[7]

Use of anchorage during tooth movement procedures

A fixed appliance can be made of bands fitted and cemented, with wires ligated to attachments, and a force can be applied by this appliance to attempt to move *one* tooth. In a reciprocal fashion, it must be understood that the same force that seeks to move the tooth in one direction is directed equally and oppositely against all the other banded teeth. Since there are so many of them, they do not move perceptibly when the appliance force is applied to the one tooth, hence they are called *anchor teeth,* or, as a unit, *anchorage* (Fig. 7-4).

All intraoral anchorage deals with reciprocal (equal and opposite) forces, therefore the term *reciprocal anchorage* is used widely. Anchorage is a function not only of

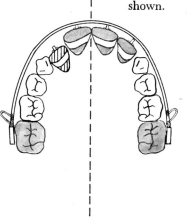

Fig. 7-4. Concept of anchorage units. A heavy round wire labial arch appliance is being used to move an upper lateral incisor out of cross-bite. The anchorage units are shaded; lateral incisor being moved out of cross-bite is cross-hatched; ligature wires tying labial arch wire to the four edgewise brackets on the banded incisors are not shown.

the number of teeth but also of the amount of surface of the roots of these teeth resisting movement. By this logic a permanent first molar would theoretically serve as a better anchorage than a bicuspid, and this holds true in practice.

Anchorage must be carefully planned because with minor tooth movement appliances it is difficult to correct undesired movement that may occur in the teeth used for anchorage. *The time spent in making constant measurements comparing the positions of the teeth in the original study casts to the child's own teeth during the course of treatment is a small price to pay for making sure that loss of anchorage or other undesirable movement is not occurring.*

TISSUE RESPONSES TO FORCES
Soft tissue response to forces applied to teeth

The health of the soft tissues surrounding the tooth, including the periodontal membrane, determines the success of the dentist in many cases of minor tooth movement. Teeth can be moved to new and more acceptable positions in the arches

only if careful attention is paid to the continued health of these tissues.

Gingival tissue response

The immediate clinical response to the application of a fairly large force to a tooth can well be a sudden blanching of the gingiva about the collar of the tooth. This may be seen when a spring is adjusted too harshly on a Hawley appliance, for instance, or when a ligature wire is tightened with too great a force while tying in an upper heavy labial arch. Almost invariably, if this whitening of tissue is seen, too much force is being applied against a tooth too quickly.

Longer-term gingival response to correctly adjusted appliance pressures should result in a tissue-appearance that markedly resembles normalcy. More than occasionally, the free gingival area around a tooth with a cemented band that has been in place for more than 3 months will show some reddening and slight edema. Usually this is *not* irritation caused by excessive movement of the tooth or even irritation by the gingival margin of the band as is commonly supposed, but rather it is a sign

Response in the root structure of the tooth

Not only is the bony socket resculpted under the influence of biomechanical forces, but also changes are noted in the structure of the root of the tooth being moved. Under the light, so-called physiologic, forces of well-constructed appliances, the changes in root structure may be limited to erosion of the cementum layer. Under heavier and more prolonged forces external root resorption may be observed.

SUMMARY

The responses of soft and hard tissues to various kinds of natural and biomechanical forces have been described. The natural forces reviewed are forces of eruption, lip and tongue muscular forces, forces originated by occlusion, and the alveolar growth factors. Abnormal forces have been singled out as causes of malocclusions. These include tongue thrust, thumb- and finger-sucking, and excessive mentalis muscle tension during swallowing.

Biomechanical forces are described as the forces generated against teeth in a continuous, interrupted, or intermittent fashion by minor tooth movement appliances. Periodontal membrane response and bone response to these forces are explained.

REFERENCES

1. Begg, P. R.: Begg orthodontic theory and technique, ed. 2, Philadelphia, 1971, W. B. Saunders Co., pp, 224-235.
2. Ewen, S. J., and Pasternak, R.: Periodontal surgery; an adjunct to orthodontic therapy, J. Am. Soc. Psychosom. Dent. Med. 2:4, 1964.
3. Fass, E. N.: A chronology of growth of the human dentition, J. Dent. Child. **36**: 391-401, Nov.-Dec., 1969.
4. Graber, T. M.: Symposium on Development of Malocclusion, University of Alabama Dental School, 1968.
5. Graber, T. M.: Orthodontics: principles and practice, ed. 2, Philadelphia, 1966, W. B. Saunders Co., pp. 508-514.
6. Hirschfeld, L., and Geiger, A.: Minor tooth movement in general practice, ed. 2, St. Louis, 1966, The C. V. Mosby Co., pp. 176-193.
7. Moyers, R. E.: Handbook of orthodontics, ed. 2, Chicago, 1963, Year Book Medical Publishers, pp. 256-260.
8. Ibid., pp. 114-118.
9. Norton, L. A., and Gellin, M. E.: Management of digital sucking and tongue thrusting in children, Dent. Clin. North Am., pp. 363-382, July, 1968.
10. Reitan, K.: Tissue rearrangement during retention of orthdontically rotated teeth, Angle Orthod. **29**:105-113, 1959.
11. Sim, J. M., and Vaughn, G. R.: A malocclusion survey of freshmen medical and dental students, unpublished data, Department of Speech Pathophysiology, University of Alabama, 1967.

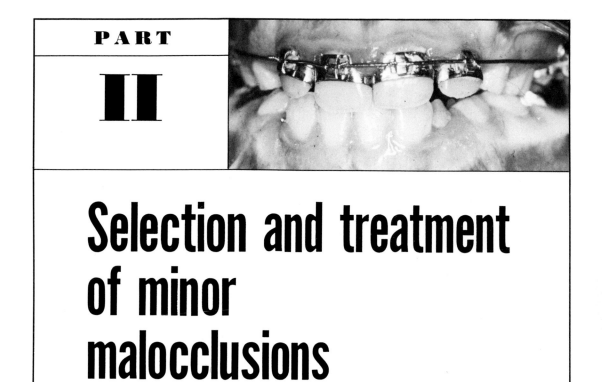

PART

II

Selection and treatment of minor malocclusions

8 | Preservation of arch form

One of the simplest and most direct kinds of treatment to preserve arch form in the permanent dentition is to conserve every single millimeter of space in the child's deciduous dentition and prevent any mesial drifting of the 6-year molars. Such a program of prevention of space loss or control of arch shape must not be undertaken hapazardly. The key concept of a control program such as this can be summed up in one word—*Measure.* Arch lengths must be measured, arch widths must be measured, and the widths of individual teeth must be measured.

However, before a dentist embarks on this kind of program, it is vitally important to establish just how much space is to be conserved and how it is to be measured. It is of little value to do a Moyers analysis or any other type of mixed dentition analysis (Chapter 4) to decide whether adequate space exists to allow normal eruption of the permanent teeth unless the dentist has a clear picture of what the shape and dimensions of the arch will be when the child reaches maturity. In other words, the dentist should be aware of his goals for each child he treats after he has measured a patient to determine the presence or absence of space loss in the child's quadrants.

The ultimate goal is to preserve each child's *best individual* arch form so that he may reach his full potential of good arch development and proper interdigitation of teeth as a young adult.

BILATERAL SYMMETRY AND ARCH FORM

Measures taken by the dentist to maintain arch form must also take into account the need to preserve not only arch space but also the bilateral symmetry of each arch. Preventive space control is nearly always helpful, but the broader views of the symmetry of upper and lower arches and the soft tissue facial profile of the child are also highly pertinent. The facial harmony that results from well-positioned teeth is commonly overlooked by dentists.

In general, the dentist seeks to *maintain* the arch space where it is normal, *regain* it where it has been lost by mesial drifting, and *control* it if the axial inclinations of the anterior teeth are being changed by environmental or muscular influences. Although the maintenance of proper arch space is important in both the upper and lower arches of the younger child entering mixed dentition, the lower arch presents the most critical challenge for the general dentist or pedodontist.

The preservation of the lower arch form is the key to a healthful, functioning dentition in most children. The lower arch is the foundation for a good occlusion, and any factor that causes loss of space or a distortion of the alignment in this arch should be immediately recognized. To improve the facility for such recognition, a quick recap of arch development is presented here.

Normal arch development

At age 4, if the child has all his primary teeth in good occlusion, and both upper and lower dental arches are in good alignment and have good interdigitation, it should be possible to make certain tentative predictions concerning the child's arch spacing and future adult occlusion. The only good method of preparing these tentative predictions is by the careful measurement of existing space in the arch, either in the child's mouth or, preferably, on study casts. The methods for accomplishing this are outlined in Chapter 4. The amount and direction of growth in the arches are also factors to consider.

There is considerable agreement that during the period of growth and development the child goes through between the ages of 6 and 13 years the following changes take place:

1. The maxillary arch length increases slightly, but mandibular arch length decreases.

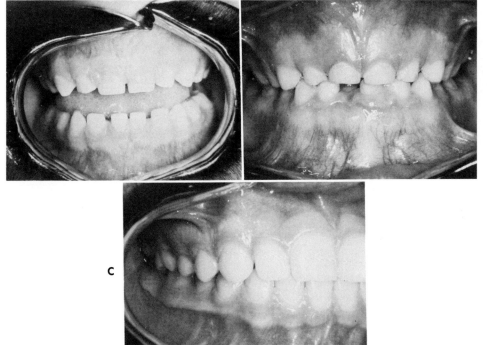

Fig. 8-1. A, Child, age 3 years, exhibiting space dentition. These interdental spaces can be expected to last into the mixed dentition period. It should be emphasized that interdental spaces do not grow wider as the child grows older. **B,** Child, age 6, in early mixed dentition stage. Note persistence of central diastema and primate spaces between the maxillary lateral incisors and cuspids and between the mandibular cuspids and first primary molars. **C,** Young adult exhibiting excellent Class I occlusion. Note that tooth size/arch space relationship has contributed to the proper interdigitation of the cusps of the teeth throughout the arches.

2. The height of the palatal vault increases.

3. The arch widths increase slightly.

4. The increase in the width of the dental arch is larger in the maxilla than in the mandible, and it is usually increased most rapidly during the eruptive phase of the permanent incisors and the canines (Fig. 8-1).

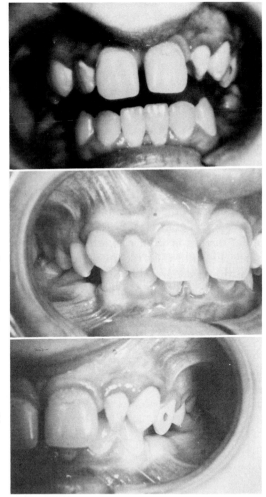

Fig. 8-2. Child, age 9½ years, demonstrating Class I, Type 1, genetic malocclusion. The tooth size/arch space discrepancy here is limited to the upper central incisors. Note rotation of upper left lateral incisor. This type of case is best handled by the orthodontist. **A,** Front view. **B,** Right view. **C,** Left view.

Factors causing abnormal arch development
Genetic factors in arch space potential

There are obvious cases where children have genetically acquired, too large teeth growing in a small jaw–facial complex. This will show up dramatically when arch circumferences are measured. Percentagewise, these genetic cases of Class I, Type 1, malocclusions are few, however, compared to the far greater number of children found in most dental practices who appear to have acquired a malocclusion from suffering either accidental loss of critically needed space or muscular distortion of the arch perimeters in such a fashion as to have a deleterious effect on the adult arches later. In those cases in which genetic factors appear clearly to be present, oversized teeth are causing problems of early exfoliation of primary cuspids, and lack of arch space is obvious, the child should be referred to the orthodontist as soon as the tooth size/arch space problem is diagnosed by the family dentist (Fig. 8-2).

When the child has one or more permanent teeth hereditarily or congenitally missing, a referral to an orthodontist is also in order. More children will have malocclusions caused by environmental disturbances, however. It is the children troubled by these factors who many times may be treated quite successfully by the generalist.

Environmental influences that can distort normal arch development

Several environmental influences that act to lessen or distort the arch space available for the permanent teeth can be seen as the child enters the stage of mixed dentition. If these influences are recognized and corrected early, the permanent teeth have as much opportunity to reach a normal alignment and occlusion as the genetic influences acting within the individual child will allow. The responsibility, then, for the general dentist is clear—to reduce to a minimum all environmental disturbances and to refer as soon as possible all genetically

to be kept in the child's mouth. The widespread use of the highly successful formocresol pulpotomy techniques (Fig. 8-5) has perhaps accomplished as much good as several thousands of dentists using preventive orthodontic appliances in their offices.

Distortion of arch space by oral habits. Almost all children who have oral habits of long standing exhibit damaged arches as the direct result of such habits. Thumb- and finger-sucking and tongue-thrusting can distort the symmetry of the anterior portions of upper and lower arches. A hyperactive mentalis muscle in a child who swallows improperly can serve to exert pressure against the newly erupted lower permanent inicisors, making them incline more lingually than is normal and taking away some of the space that should be available for the eruption of the lower permanent cuspids (Fig. 8-6). Such a child can wear an oral shield or other appliance to help train him away from sucking habits, tongue-thrusting, and hyperactive mentalis muscle swallowing patterns.

Ectopic eruption of lower permanent lateral incisors and 6-year molars. An obvious hereditary lack of lower anterior arch space may be combined with improper pressures of a hyperactive mentalis muscle action in a child age 6 to 8 years. The lack of arch space in such a child can be magnified by the presence of this environmental pressure acting against the labial surfaces of the newly erupted lower central and lateral incisors. The central incisors may be able to erupt normally but the lateral incisors, not being able to erupt normally, tend to be forced distally, so that they begin to resorb portions of the roots of the primary cuspids. A considerable amount of stability in this lower anterior region is lost when the deciduous cuspids are exfoliated prematurely.

Under ordinary circumstances the primary cuspids act as a restraining force to prevent the erupting permanent lateral incisors from moving distally. When the cus-

pids are lost by ectopically erupting lateral incisors the latter are free both to move distally and to incline lingually. The space loss that occurs is mostly the result of a flattening of the arc of the lower incisors. This can be prevented by placing a lingual arch early to help the lower anterior teeth withstand the battering force of the mentalis muscle contractions as well as to prevent the usual loss of dental midline that occurs when the lateral incisors lose the distal restraining force provided by the cuspids. (See Fig. 8-7.)

Ectopic eruption of the first permanent molars may also create a space loss problem. This, however, occurs in the posterior segment and is more clearly the result of a genetic pattern of molar eruption than of a

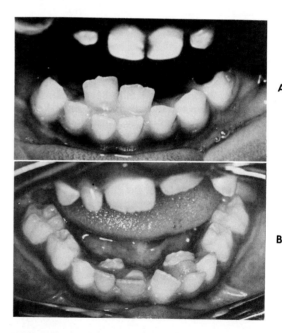

Fig. 8-7. A, Overretention of primary lower central and lateral incisors can cause the permanent incisors to erupt ectopically. Usually, if the primary teeth are not loose and a radiograph shows the roots are not being resorbed properly, they should be extracted so that tongue pressure can move them into their correct places in the arch. Appliance therapy is usually not necessary in these cases. **B,** Overretention of primary lateral incisors. Front view, open.

pattern influenced by environmental factors as in the case of the lower lateral incisors. (See section on axial inclinations later in this chapter.)

Functional anterior and posterior cross-bites. Upper anterior teeth erupting in cross-bite may cause a distortion of the premaxilla to the lingual in the maxillary arch. This results in a decrease in total upper arch length available for the later-erupting permanent teeth.

Posterior lingual cross-bites, especially those with functional shifts of the mandible on closure, can cause a distortion of the maxillary bone on the cross-bite side toward the palatal midline. This distortion in a palatal direction may act to decrease the total arch length and cause a space problem when the permanent bicuspids and cuspids erupt. Both anterior and posterior cross-bites should be treated as early as possible. (See Chapters 11 and 12.)

Overretention of deciduous teeth and ankylosis. A deciduous tooth will usually be exfoliated under natural circumstances at about the same time as its mate (called the *antimere*) in the opposite arch. Whenever a deciduous tooth is present in the arch long after its antimere has been lost, a radiograph is indicated to determine the underlying cause. Perhaps it will be seen that the root resorption pattern in the primary tooth is not progressing in the usual fashion. (See Fig. 8-8.)

If a primary tooth appears to be sinking, or submerging, into the alveolus, the little-understood process called ankylosis may be at work. Three things seem to occur when a primary tooth undergoes ankylosis and appears to submerge in relation to the adjacent teeth in the alveolus, as follows:

1. Root resorption by the permanent tooth slows down or ceases.

2. The natural growth along the crest of the alveolus does not act to carry the ankylosed tooth occlusally as it does the other unaffected adjacent teeth (Fig. 8-9, *A*).

3. There may be problems in the direc-

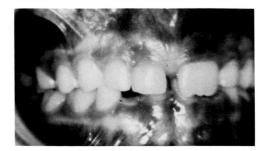

Fig. 8-8. Damaged upper primary central incisor has been overretained. This can cause a cross-bite due to forcing of permanent central incisor to the lingual. Primary central incisor should be extracted to allow normal eruption.

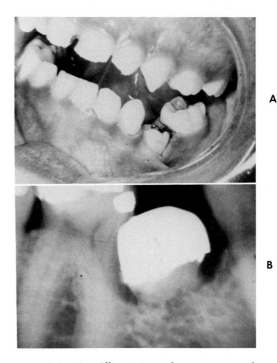

Fig. 8-9. A, Illustration demonstrates the amount of alveolar crest growth that can take place over a space of 3 years. The lower left first primary molar is ankylosed and is not being carried occlusally as the alveolar crest grows. **B,** This ankylosed second primary molar with no bicuspid erupting beneath it had a stainless steel crown placed on it in an attempt to restore occlusion. As the years passed, the other teeth have been carried occlusally while it has remained in its original position. Almost certainly extraction and a fixed prosthesis are indicated.

tion of eruption of the inhibited permanent tooth, ultimately producing an ectopic eruption pattern (Fig. 8-9, *B*).

A good solution to the problem of the ankylosed primary molar is to extract it when the problem is recognized and hold the space with a crown and loop space maintainer. Another solution that has been advanced is to anesthetize the ankylosed tooth and "rock" it with the extraction forceps, hopefully causing the ankylosis condition to disappear. At this time the extraction and space maintainer method appears to be the best way of treating this condition.

SPACE LOSS AND ITS CONTROL
Three types of space loss

Three rather distinct types of space loss are seen that may occur from environmental factors in a child who starts out with a normal occlusion in the primary dentition. These are as follows:

1. Premature loss by trauma or early exfoliation of one or more anterior teeth can cause a dental midline shift in one of the arches. This type of crowding of the developing permanent teeth originates in the *anterior* segment.

2. Severe caries attack or premature loss of a first or second primary molar may be followed by mesial drift of the 6-year molar. This type of crowding in the arch originates from the *posterior* segment.

3. A change in the axial inclination of the lower permanent central and lateral incisors due to abnormal pressures from the mentalis muscle during swallowing activities can cause the lower anterior teeth to be pressed lingually and can severely reduce the space available for the eruption of the permanent cuspids. This space distortion originates in the *anterior* segment.

Too often these important patterns of space loss go unrecognized and untreated until it is too late for preventive measures. The importance of knowing *how* the space was lost is seen when the dentist realizes that it takes a significantly more complicated appliance to provide treatment to reestablish a dental midline and to regain normal axial inclinations of lower incisors as compared to the therapy necessary to regain a small amount of space loss caused by a permanent molar's drifting mesially and encroaching on space needed for the erupting bicuspids.

Table 10. Summary of treatment to control arch space

Deciduous tooth lost prematurely	Consequences	Suggested appliance to control resulting arch space loss
Mandibular central or lateral incisor; mandibular cuspid	Midline shift in direction of lost tooth	Wait until *both* lower lateral incisors have erupted, then use F-R lingual arch with finger springs
Maxillary central incisor	Midline shift and possible delayed eruption of permanent successor	Simple acrylic partial denture supporting a replacement tooth
Maxillary or mandibular first molar	Mesial drift of E's and 6's	Crown and loop spacer; band and loop spacer; soldered lingual arch if bilateral loss occurs
Maxillary or mandibular second molar	Mesial drift of 6's; also may cause distal drift of D's and distal tipping of 4's	Crown and loop spacer cemented to D; band and loop spacer cemented to D; F-R lingual arch if loss is bilateral; removable appliance can be used if occlusion is a factor

Timing of space control measures in the deciduous dentition

Observations have been reported that show the greatest amount of space closure may occur during the first 6 months after the untimely loss of a primary tooth. In fact, a decrease in space will be evident in many patients within a matter of days.[7]

The matter, then, of when to use space maintainers is really answered by the previously mentioned report. The best time to insert a space maintainer is immediately after the primary molar is lost. When this is done, the dentist can truly say that he is controlling the space within the dental arches. He will avoid the unpleasant surprise at the child's next 6-month check-up of finding the loss of space may be as much as half the original dimension of the extracted tooth!

Space control during mixed dentition

For the children whose ages are 6 to 12 years, conservation of space in their arches becomes more a problem of *relative* space. The child may start out with an existing space of 23 mm. in one quadrant, occupied by the cuspid and the first and second primary molars, and lose 2 mm. somewhere along the line. If the permanent cuspid and first and second bicuspids can erupt nicely into the space remaining, certainly the dentist should recognize the fact and should not try to regain the lost 2 mm. by appliance therapy. This whole concept of close observation is not workable, however, unless the dentist is willing to measure arch spaces constantly in the child's mouth to keep a check on whether the available space is still adequate to receive the unerupted teeth. (See Fig. 8-10.)

Importance of measuring space in mixed dentition analysis

When a child who exhibits what appears to be normally spaced deciduous arches matures to age 7 or 8 years, the question may be asked of the dentist, "Does my child have enough room in his mouth for all his permanent teeth?" This question should never be answered carelessly without doing an arch space analysis, which, if done during the mixed dentition years is

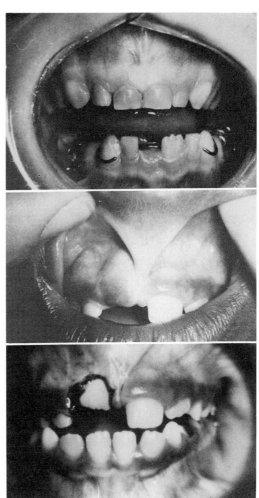

A

B

C

Fig. 8-10. **A,** Removable space maintainer can serve to preserve space in an arch where several teeth have been lost prematurely. The lower arch matures first and is the more important arch to consider when preserving space. **B,** Primary central incisor has been missing for so long that the keratinized epithelial tissue is preventing proper eruption of 1|. **C,** Surgical removal of the keratinized epithelium will allow normal eruption of 1|.

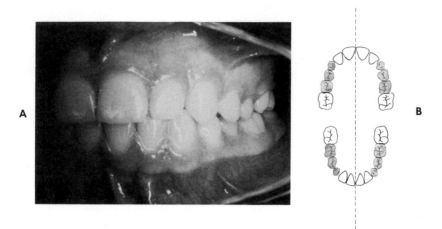

Fig. 8-11. A, Young adult exhibiting excellent Class I occlusion. Left view. **B,** The four quadrant areas where measurement of space is important for a good mixed dentition analysis. Shaded teeth indicate space areas that must be protected to ensure good occlusion.

called a mixed dentition analysis. (See Chapter 4 for review of the diagnostic quadrangle and methods of accomplishing mixed dentition space analysis.)

This analysis attempts in general to determine whether proper space is available for *three teeth*—the permanent cuspid and the first and second bicuspids—to erupt within each of the four quadrants (Fig. 8-11).

The clinical decision that faces the dentist is how best to determine how many millimeters of space the child will have in his dental arches to accommodate the remaining permanent teeth when they finally erupt. *It is a well-established principle that there is no physiologic provision for interstitial bone growth.* This means that there can be no increase in the amount of bone between the roots of adjacent teeth. Lateral growth anterior to the area of the first permanent molars is virtually complete before age 8. Thus it is considered that the total amount of dental arch space available for the eruption of the remaining permanent teeth will not be increased by growth after this time.[5]

If the dental arch circumference is measured from the mesial aspect of lower first permanent molar on one side around the arch to the mesial aspect of the first permanent molar on the opposite side, the dentist will have determined the maximum arch space a patient can anticipate in the absence of orthodontic intervention.

AXIAL INCLINATIONS OF TEETH AND THEIR TREATMENT TO PRESERVE ARCH FORM

The axial inclination of teeth is one of the more important factors to watch for as an arch develops. Many clues are available for the attentive dentist who wishes to detect early abnormal alignments of teeth.

Incisors. In the primary dentition, the maxillary and mandibular incisors erupt and appear to remain nearly vertical in their relationship both to the plane of occlusion and to the facial plane. There is only a slight overjet and overbite.

As the permanent incisors start to erupt, the crowns of both maxillary and mandibular incisors move into place considerably forward of their deciduous predecessors. During this transitional stage, a child may have what has been termed a "bucktoothed" appearance. Reasonable incisor protrusion at this stage does not always sig-

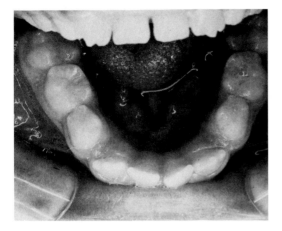

Fig. 8-12. When unsupported lower anterior teeth are being tipped lingually by muscle habits, the dentist should apply the 90-degree rule to clarify his diagnosis. (See Fig. 4-13.)

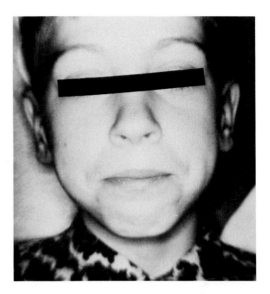

Fig. 8-13. Oral habits such as the excessive mentalis muscle contraction during the swallowing act can severely tip lower incisors lingually. By a wedging action the lower lip can also force the upper incisors labially, creating an abnormal overjet.

nify the development of a malocclusion. As the incisors continue to erupt during the transitional (mixed dentition) and the permanent dentition periods, a number of changes occur in the positions of the central and lateral incisors that somewhat reduce their early protrusive effect. The incisors become less protrusive relative to their bony bases, partly as a result of the development of the jaws and the alveolar process. The axial inclination of the maxillary incisor does not change significantly, as a rule. However, each lower incisor tends to upright itself during the process of maturation by tilting slightly lingually. An exaggerated lingual tipping of the lower incisors (to less than 90 degrees to the mandibular plane) is regarded as abnormal and is almost always brought on by unusual muscle pressures such as hyperactivity of the mentalis muscle (Fig. 8-12). This pattern was discussed previously in this chapter.

Significance of hyperactive mentalis muscle on axial inclination of lower incisors. The action of the mentalis muscle is directed almost entirely against the labial surfaces of the four lower incisors. This force is generated during the act of swallowing and can tip the incisors lingually, ef-

fectively decreasing the arch circumference and thereby lessening the available arch space for the eruption of the cuspids and the bicuspids. Proper treatment can help recover this lost arch length. Oldenburg[11] indicates that for each degree of axial inclination of lower incisors that occurs as they are tipped *orthodontically* in a labial direction, there will be a 1 mm. *gain* in lower arch length. (See Fig. 8-13.)

PREVENTIVE TREATMENT TO AVOID LINGUAL TIPPING OF LOWER INCISORS. The placement of an F-R lower lingual arch can act as the best preventive measure when the lower incisors appear to be in danger of being tipped lingually (Fig. 8-14). One or even two finger springs can supply the necessary pressure to slowly guide the incisors labially to their normal positions in the arch circumference. However, the treatment should not be started until both lateral incisors are well erupted. As explained before, it is embarrassing to have the laterals erupt *lingual* to the arch wire!

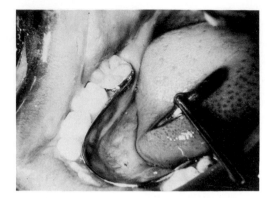

Fig. 8-14. Fixed soldered lower lingual arch can serve as a retainer to prevent distortion of an arch from excessive mentalis muscle contraction.

Cuspids. The maxillary cuspids during the primary and early mixed dentition stages will be found high in the body of the maxilla, with the crowns considerably forward of the roots. As they erupt, the cuspids come under the influence of the lateral incisor roots and are deflected downward in such a manner that during the last stages of eruption they assume a more vertical position. If cuspids do not axially align themselves properly, this is nearly always a reason for referral to the orthodontist.

Bicuspids. Intraoral x-ray films will show the positions of the unerupted bicuspids underlying the primary first and second

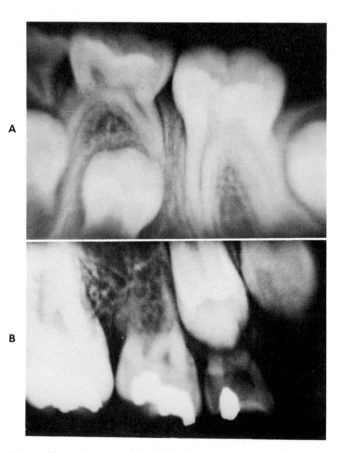

Fig. 8-15. A, X-ray film of 9-year-old child, showing normal resorption pattern of primary molars and no rotation of erupting bicuspids. **B,** X-ray film may well show that a bicuspid is missing. If such is the case, an orthodontist will help the dentist decide on the treatment.

molars. If these teeth appear rotated in the radiographs, usually little correction will occur during eruption, and they will appear in the mouth in a rotated position. Atypical axial inclinations of unerupted bicuspids are not uncommon, particularly in the mandibular arch where the bicuspids may have a distoangular position. Under the influence of pressures from adjacent teeth, most of these premolars will usually erupt into a normal position, provided, of course, that there is sufficient space for them within the arch. Caution must be used in examining bicuspids that are in the process of resorbing pulpotomized primary molars. More aberrant rotations and poor axial inclinations appear to occur among these premolar teeth than might be expected. (See Fig. 8-15.)

Molars. Characteristically, the primary molars are positioned vertically in their supporting bones, much like the deciduous incisors. The permanent mandibular first molar, before eruption into the lower jaw, tends to have a mesioangular axial inclination, with its crown lying mesial to the roots. If favorable growth occurs at the posterior portions of the body of the mandible, this tooth will upright itself so that at the time of maturity only a slight mesioangular axial inclination will be observed.

The upper permanent molars, unlike the lowers, before emergence have a marked distoangular axial inclination, with their crowns lying posterior to their roots. As the molars erupt, the distoangular axial inclination is reduced and may actually become a mesioangular axial inclination. This is particularly true of the first permanent molar. Because of this tendency toward distoangular axial inclinations, it would seem that fewer impactions of these teeth would be observed than in the case of the mandibular molars. The opposite is true, however. Occasionally, a mesioangular axial inclination can be observed on a first molar, which results in the resorption of the roots of the primary second molar and produces the typical picture described as "ectopic erup-

tion." *Ectopic* means "out of position." In this book, the meaning of *ectopic eruption* will be expanded to imply *both* abnormal tooth position *and* abnormal resorption of a primary tooth not normally resorbed during the eruption of the ectopic tooth. Usually, however, if insufficient room is available in the supporting bone, the maxillary molars tend to erupt to the buccal of the alveolar ridge.

6-year molars. Ectopic eruption of 6-year molars may occur in less than 3% of children, but when it occurs, it causes a problem in space control in the child's arch that nearly always has to be treated with the Humphrey appliance or any other appliance designed to guide this tooth for the remaining period of its eruptive thrust.

Although it is not rare, the ectopic eruption of a first permanent molar is uncommon. Young,[15] in reviewing 1619 children and looking for ectopic eruptions, found 52 children who exhibited a total of 78 ectopic eruptions. Of these, 75 were maxillary molars, but only 3 were mandibular molars. Most cases were Class I malocclusions, and the heredity factor appeared to be uncertain. The author defined ectopic eruption of the first permanent molar as occurring "when the permanent tooth is prevented from appearing in the oral cavity or is blocked from completely erupting by some portion of its mesial surface being blocked under the distal contour of the second primary molar."[*]

TREATMENT BY LIGATURE WIRE. One of the simplest methods of treating an ectopically erupting maxillary 6-year molar is to place a brass ligature wire between the second primary molar and the permanent molar (Fig. 8-16). This acts as an inclined plane to force the molar distally. Usually the deciduous molar becomes slightly mobile during this treatment because of the loss of part or all of the disto-

*From Young, D. H.: Ectopic eruption of the first permanent molar, J. Dent. Child. **24**:153-162, Oct.-Dec., 1957.

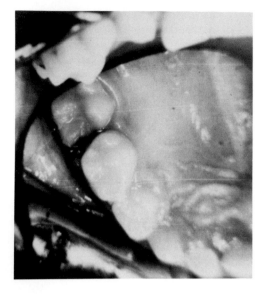

Fig. 8-16. Brass ligature wire (25 gauge) can be passed interproximally and twisted to create adequate space to seat a band comfortably.

buccal root and perhaps a portion of the lingual root. If the ligature wire does not succeed in moving the permanent molar distally but only loosens the deciduous molar further, this method should be abandoned.

TREATMENT BY HUMPHREY APPLIANCE. An ingenious fixed appliance has been described by Humphrey for moving distally an ectopically erupting first premanent maxillary molar. It consists of a molar band with a length of Elgiloy* wire soldered on the buccal aspect and contoured into an **S** shape to the distal area, then bent up into the central pit of the erupting permanent molar. A small cavity preparation may be made in the enamel to receive the wire and later filled with amalgam. By slightly opening the **S** spring, distally directed pressure may be placed against the ectopic molar. Two or three adjustments over a period of

*Available from Rocky Mountain Dental Products Co., Denver. See Chapter 14 for wire sizes and hardness options.

6 weeks should be sufficient to move the molar into its correct position distal to the second primary molar.

LABIAL FRENUM AND CENTRAL DIASTEMA

The existence of a large space between the upper central incisors is also one of the problems that will be seen by the general dentist. This is an unwanted space for some individuals. Parents will frequently ask the dentist to do something to close this space in their child's upper arch. Occasionally one of the parents will exhibit the same diastema. More usually they will not. It is one of the continuing mysteries of modern dentistry why so many competent dentists wish to do frenectomies for younger children when they may prove ultimately to be unnecessary. With the eruption of the upper cuspids, most of these spaces close by the mesial forces generated by the other teeth.

It has been noted that only in rare instances today is the frenum removed surgically. Blanching of the frenal tissue from the labial to the lingual side occurring when it is placed under tension is usually an indication of an abnormal frenum. In most instances the surgical removal of this tissue is not necessary. Surgery, indeed, may cause scar tissue to form in the interproximal space and serve as an additional obstruction to the closing of the diastema. As a test of normality, it is usually agreed that if a large diastema persists after the upper permanent cuspids begin to erupt, then the frenum may be considered to be at fault. Otherwise, it is considered a stage in the maxillary development of some children. (See Fig. 8-17, A and B.)

Other developmental factors can produce diastemas between the upper central incisors, such as the following:

1. A slight cleft of the interseptal alveolar bone, which can be detected in a radiograph.

2. A closed bite in which the lower incisors press deep into the palate and exert

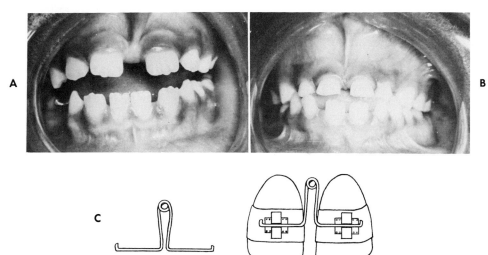

Fig. 8-17. **A,** Child, age 8 years, exhibiting a wide diastema with an associated heavy labial frenum. Before surgery is considered, upper cuspids should have erupted. **B,** This child, age 6 years, is the younger brother of child in **A.** Note that diastema is present even though frenum attachment is much higher. This demonstrates the genetic influences at work when spacing occurs. The wise dentist looks beyond the presence of a heavy frenum. See Table 11. **C,** "Safety-pin" appliance recommended for closing central diastema in a controlled fashion.

Table 11. Prediction table for natural closure of central diastema (accurate in 88% of cases)*†

If diastema measures (mm.)	1.0	1.3	1.4	1.5	1.6	1.85	2.1	2.2	2.3	2.4	2.7
Probability of closing without treatment (%)	99	95	90	85	80	50	20	15	15	5	1

*From Sanin, C., Sekigouchi, T., and Savara, B. S.: A clinical method for predicting of closure of the central diastema, J. Dent. Child. **36:**415-418, Nov.-Dec., 1969.
†Permanent maxillary central and lateral incisors must have fully erupted.

a labial pressure on the maxillary central incisors.

3. A discrepancy in the mesiodistal width of the maxillary and mandibular incisor teeth. All maxillary incisors may be too narrow, or the lateral incisors may be peg shaped. Quite frequently, however, the width of the maxillary incisors may be normal but the mandibular incisors may be proportionately wider by a fair amount. If this is true and the mandibular incisors do not jumble but retain a good alignment and proximal contact, they may wedge the maxillary incisors apart, producing spaces between them.[3]

Spacing due to any of the foregoing causes may occur between the maxillary central incisors and be wrongly diagnosed as an abnormal frenum. It probably is fair to state that there has been a decided swing away from the idea of surgical correction of diastemas in the younger child by orthodontists, pedodontists, and generalists.

Prediction of central diastema closure

Some dentists will want a method of accurately predicting whether the diastema seen in the younger child will be present in the adult a few years hence. Several methods have been brought forward, but they appear to be based mostly on office experiences. However, a recent study has given a clinically useful prediction table worked out from a research project involving 80 children who exhibited upper central diastemas.[12]

The authors indicated that the earliest age at which the presence of a diastema at completion of the permanent dentition could be predicted is the age of full eruption of the upper central and lateral incisors, or about age 7 to 9 years. If the diastema is measured at this time, Table 11 may be referred to, with an accuracy of 88% as claimed in the results of their study.

Treatment for closure of a central diastema

If a decision is reached that treatment is necessary to close a diastema between the upper central incisors, one of the simplest choices of appliances is to band each central incisor, weld or solder a tube to one band, and weld or solder a wire onto the other band that will fit into the tube. The appliance can be activated by either an elastic or ligation with a series of wires to close the space in a stepwise fashion over a period of time. Under normal circumstances, the time of treatment should take about 3 to 6 weeks, depending on the width of the space to be closed.

It has been noted[4] that two bands can be fitted to the central incisors, with attachments into which may be fitted and ligated a light resilient wire spring shaped on the order of a safety pin (Fig. 8-17, C). It is said that the movements of the teeth are better controlled in this way.

A light-wire labial arch may be also fabricated to close a diastema (Fig. 8-18). However, distortion of the unsupported wire in the posterior segments may result in uneven incisal alignment.

The ever-reliable removable Hawley appliance may be fabricated with two helical springs incorporated to produce pressures from the distal surfaces of each of the central incisors. One of the good features of the Hawley appliance is that it serves so well as a retainer after the movement is accomplished. The disadvantage is that it may not be worn as often as it must be to produce a good result in a short time.

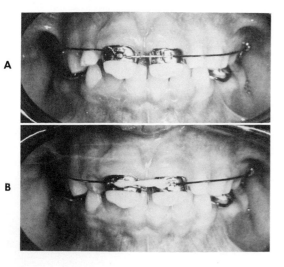

A

B

Fig. 8-18. Light-wire labial arch appliances for closing a diastema. These are only successful if the permanent lateral incisors are immediately available to exert a stabilizing pressure against the distal surface of the central incisors. **A,** Activated by ligature wire. **B,** Activated by elastic.

SUMMARY

The various treatment methods for preserving the arch form have been discussed. Some methods are preventive measures to enable the dentist to help the child conserve his natural arch space during the primary and mixed dentition ages. These include the restorative care necessary for primary teeth as well as the placing of fixed or removable space maintainers and fixed-removable lingual arches.

Another series of appliances are discussed for corrective treatment of the results of ectopic eruptions of lower lateral incisors and 6-year molars. The loss of arch length that results from ectopically erupting lower lateral incisors is described as being caused by environmental factors such as overactive mentalis muscle during swallowing, which may be corrected by re-retraining methods. The ectopic eruption of molars is described as a genetically caused potential space loss in the posterior part of the arch.

The treatment use of space-maintaining and space-regaining appliances is described. Chapter 12 should also be read regarding space control in dental arches and interceptive treatment methods to improve positions of 6-year molars.

REFERENCES

1. Baume, L. J.: Physiological tooth migration and its significance for the development of occlusion. 1. The biogenetic source of the deciduous dentition, J. Dent. Res. **29**:123-132, April, 1950.
2. Burstone, C. J.: Distinguishing developing malocclusion from normal occlusion, Dent. Clin. North Am., pp. 479-491, July, 1964.
3. Graber, T. M.: Orthodontics: principles and practice, ed. 2, Philadelphia, 1966, W. B. Saunders Co., p. 795.
4. Higley, L. B.: Maxillary labial frenum and midline diastema, J. Dent. Child. **36**: 413-414, Nov.-Dec., 1969.
5. Huckaba, G. W.: Arch size analysis and tooth size prediction, Dent. Clin. North Am., pp. 432-433, July, 1964.
6. McDonald, R. E.: Pedodontics, St. Louis, 1963, The C. V. Mosby Co., p. 315.
7. Moorrees, C. F. A.: The dentition of the growing child, Cambridge, Mass., 1959, Harvard University Press, pp. 36-39.
8. Ibid., pp. 85-86.
9. Moyers, R. E.: Handbook of orthodontics, ed. 2, Chicago, 1963, Year Book Medical Publishers, Inc., p. 71.
10. Nance, H. N.: The limitations of orthodontic diagnosis and treatment. I. The mixed dentition. II. Diagnosis and treatment in the permanent dentition, Am. J. Orthod. Oral Surg. **33**:177-223, 253-301, 1947.
11. Oldenburg, T. R.: American Society of Dentistry for Children Seminar on Preventive Orthodontics, Birmingham, Alabama, Aug., 1969.
12. Sanin, C., Sekigouchi, T., and Savara, B. S.: A clinical method for predicting of closure of the central diastema, J. Dent. Child. **36**:415-418, Nov.-Dec., 1969.
13. Sim, J. M., and Finn, S. B.: Operative dentistry for children. In Finn, S. B., editor: Clinical pedodontics, ed. 3, Philadelphia, 1967, W. B. Saunders Co., pp. 184-186.
14. Warrer, E.: Simultaneous occurrence of certain muscle habits and malocclusion, Amer. J. Orthod. **45**:365-370, 1959.
15. Young, D. H.: Ectopic eruption of the first permanent molar, J. Dent. Child. **24**: 153-162, Oct.-Dec., 1957.

quence of eruption of permanent teeth in the lower arch. If the child's sequence is favorable, his lower incisors are protected from being inclined lingually by the properly timed eruption of the lower permanent cuspids. However, if it is unfavorable, the inclination may occur. In addition, posterior space loss may occur if the second deciduous molar is exfoliated *after* the eruption of the 12-year molar has begun. The 6-year molar can be forced too far mesially by the untimely eruption of this *second* permanent molar, which may occur in some children earlier than the traditional age of 12 years.

The most favorable sequence of eruption in the lower arch begins at age 6 years and is as follows: 6-year molar, central incisor, lateral incisor, cuspid, first bicuspid, second bicuspid, and last, the 12-year molar. Most writers agree that the eruption of the central incisors before, or at the same time as, the eruption of the 6-year molars poses no violation of this favorable sequence.

The third permanent molars or wisdom teeth, erupt usually between the ages of 17 and 21 and are not considered to be a part of this childhood sequence. Discussion is continuing as to whether or not the third molars affect the positions of teeth already erupted. Probably only in unstable arches do they present a problem.

Therefore the most favorable mandibular eruption pattern may be outlined as follows: 6 1 2 3 4 5 7.

Mandibular cuspids should erupt after lateral incisors

It is important that the mandibular cuspid erupt before the first and second bicuspid. The cuspid's eruption "locks the arch," so to speak, and aids tremendously in maintaining the child's potential arch length by preventing the lingual tipping of the incisors. Lingual tipping of these teeth not only causes a loss of arch length but can allow the development of an increased overbite caused by the lingual tipping of the upper

incisors. Any pressures caused by abnormal lip musculature or swallowing habits that cannot be compensated for by the tongue may result in the lingual collapse of the lower incisor segment. The properly timed eruption of the permanent cuspids can prevent this.

As was indicated earlier, a lingual arch appliance may be placed if the deciduous cuspids are lost prematurely or the sequence of eruption progresses abnormally.[3]

Arch length endangered if 12-year-molar precedes second bicuspid

An added deficiency in lower arch length can develop if the 12-year molar erupts before the second bicuspid. This abnormal sequence of eruption causes a strong force to be exerted on the distal aspect of the first permanent molar, which can cause its mesial migration and encroachment on the space needed for the second bicuspid.

The fact cannot be stated too strongly that the natural and normal positions of the lower 6-year molars must be maintained. If a deciduous second molar is lost prematurely, a space maintainer should be placed immediately. If the condition is bilateral, then a passive lower lingual arch

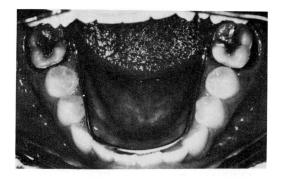

Fig. 9-3. This F-R lingual arch was worn for a period of 18 months and was removed and recemented twice during that period. It protected the 6-year molar from encroaching mesially on the area reserved for the second bicuspid. It also served as a maintainer of anterior arch form to prevent lingual inclination of the lower central incisors.

should be placed to protect the natural length of the prime arch. (See Fig. 9-3.) This will be discussed at length later in the chapter.

In the language of professional football, a strong "prevent defense" should be set up to protect the arch length being attacked by an offense coming from two directions: (1) collapse lingually of the incisor segment because of lack of protection on the distal flanks by the cuspids and (2) excessive mesial migration of the 6-year molar generated by the too early eruptive thrust of the 12-year molar.

In either of these cases, the best prevent defense is to place a lower lingual arch. It forms the best line of protection against loss of arch length "yardage."

SERIAL EXTRACTION OF PRIMARY CUSPIDS NOT RECOMMENDED

In one writer's opinion, "the *premature loss of one lower cuspid* [emphasis added], usually the product of the imminent eruption of the lower lateral incisor in the face of insufficient arch, making it encroach on

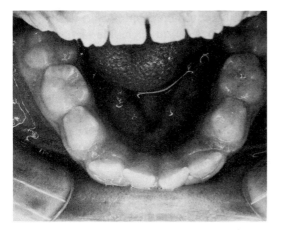

Fig. 9-4. Arch that has been "treated" to relieve crowding by serial extraction of lower primary cuspids. Note collapse of whole lower anterior segment lingually. Treatment indicated is immediate placement of a lower lingual arch with finger springs to reposition the lower anterior teeth in their proper ovoid arch.

the cuspid's territory, stands as a danger signal for an incipient malocclusion."[2] If one cuspid is lost from its too early root resorption by a lateral incisor, the dentist may feel committed to extraction of the remaining cuspid in an attempt to preserve the midline relationship. As discussed in Chapter 8, this procedure rarely achieves its goal. The seemingly simple measure of optional extraction of one or both deciduous lower cuspids cannot of itself solve the problem of insufficient arch length for the permanent dentition. It merely provides temporary space for the four lower permanent incisors at the expense of space that will be needed later for the permanent cuspids and starts the patient down the road of no return leading to the ultimate loss of four bicuspids.[3]

It must be realized, then, that the extraction of a single remaining primary cuspid to "make room" commits the unwary dentist to a route called "serial extraction." Not in all cases, certainly, but in many, the alternate choice to serial extraction is placement of a lower lingual arch. With judicious use of this appliance as discussed in Chapter 8, the dentist can recover a collapsed arch perimeter in the incisor area, realign the teeth labially, and also move the lower incisors so that the lower dental midline recovers its former relation in the midsagittal plane. A coupling together of the terms *lingual arches* and *serial extraction* should occur in the dentist's mind, so that he never serially extracts lower primary cuspids without thinking of placing a lingual arch for protection of the arch form (Fig. 9-4).

TWO MAIN CAUSES OF LOWER ANTERIOR CROWDING

To make a decision whether a child is showing definite warning signs of a future malocclusion, the dentist should ascertain whether the lower anterior crowding in Class I cases stems from a genetically caused lack of arch space (an imbalance of too much tooth material for the available

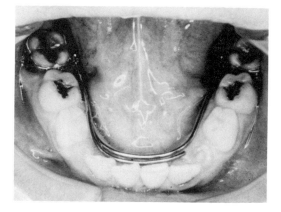

Fig. 9-7. This arch illustrates what happens when a hyperactive mentalis muscle is at work each time the child swallows. Note axes inclining to right side in lower incisors. This is being treated by F-R horizontal lower lingual arch with finger spring.

complished separately, but in some cases the diagnosis may indicate both are needed.

In most cases, treatment by expansion in these directions is directed toward gaining no more than 2 to 3 mm. of space in the prime arch length (the arch length that contained the primary teeth) without resorting to extractions. If more than 5 mm. is needed, then a consultation with an orthodontist would be a timely measure.

Objectives of treatment

There are four specific objectives that the dentist should accomplish if he finds a mild genetic lack of space in the lower arch. He may expand the arch buccally to gain an increase in arch length of 2 to 3 mm. as has been previously discussed. He also should seek to upright the lower incisors labially until a line drawn through their axes meets the mandibular plane at approximately 90 degrees. For each degree of uprighting, approximately 1 mm. is gained in the total arch length. He should reestablish the lower dental midline if it has been lost. Finally, he should maintain the positions of the lower 6-year molars so that no mesial drift occurs to lessen the prime arch length.

Expansion of lower arch buccally

Treatment of a lower arch by expansion when incisor crowding is severe and the cause is a genetic lack of space is probably outside the expertise of most dentists in general practice. In those cases where there is a *mild* crowding situation—2 to 3 mm. lacking in total arch length—careful buccal expansion of the arch has been recommended. Although certain appliances used in arch-expansion therapy have achieved a popular reception in Continuing Dental Education clinics given across the country in recent years, this kind of therapy has its pitfalls. Some writers properly indicate caution when buccal expansion is undertaken.

The picture of what he can and cannot do during expansion therapy must be clearly seen by each dentist who contemplates the treatment for his child patient. Expansion buccally of the lower arch by means of orthodontic appliances in either the deciduous or the mixed dentition is limited by the danger that the teeth may be moved off their supporting alveolar bone during such procedures. Contrary to popular teachings, the underlying bone is not stimulated to grow a larger supporting structure.[3] Orthodontic expansion of the lower dental arch through the cuspid area undertaken to accommodate the permanent incisors is limited to approximately 2 to 3 mm. gain in total arch length. Expansion greater than this may result in increased width (and length) of the arch, but when the retention appliance is removed, the excess

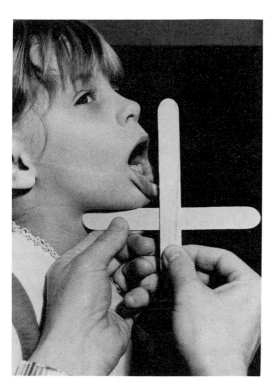

Fig. 9-8. Dentist is checking the approximate angulation of the lower central incisors in a child's mouth, using two tongue blades. The normal angulation to the mandibular plane is 90 degrees ± 5 degrees, according to Tweed. If lower central incisors are tipped too far lingually, lingual arch therapy is usually indicated in these Class I children.

expansion is generally lost and crowding of the incisors recurs.

There are exceptions to these general rules, since some patients may retain more of the expanded dimension than others, but this usually occurs in individuals with relatively flaccid oral musculature who have no tendencies toward closed-bite relationships and in whom the balance between the opposing forces produced by lips and tongue is not critical. To sum up, expansion can be a successful form of treatment if the dentist's expectation of arch space gain is not beyond 2 to 3 mm. and he maintains an attitude of reserved caution.[3]

Establishment of 90-degree axis for lower central incisors consistent with Williams diagnostic line

If the lower incisors have been crowded lingually, they will unscramble themselves when they are moved labially. Such movement tends to increase the arch length. However, there is substantial danger in this

approach to treatment if the following two important considerations are not met:

1. The central incisors should not be tipped labially beyond a position where a line drawn through their axes meets the mandibular plane at 90 degrees.

2. The incisal edges of the lower central incisors should not be moved forward of the Williams "diagnostic line." This extends from point A to pogonion.[8]

Tweed's 90-degree rule. It was stated by Tweed[7] and others that in most facially harmonious Class I individuals the axes of lower central incisors should stand at 90 degrees to the mandibular plane. A test may be accomplished at the chair to ascertain the approximate angle of the incisors (Fig. 9-8).

Williams diagnostic line.[8] The Williams diagnostic line can only be seen in a cephalograph of the child's skull. It is a line drawn from point A to the chin point, or pogonion. Williams stated that if the A-pogonion line passes through the incisal edges

type, in which the ends of the arch wire are fitted into tubes attached to the lingual surfaces of the molar bands. These appliances can be inserted or removed by the dentist but not by the patient.[5]

The emphasis in this chapter will be on the fixed-removable arch, which may be fitted against the lower teeth by a skilled dentist to function as an extremely versatile minor tooth movement appliance.

The fixed soldered lingual arch, commonly called a lingual "holding arch" (Fig. 9-11), may be used occasionally in cases where no movement of teeth is contemplated. Placement of such an arch acts as a lingual support and prevents the lower permanent incisors from being displaced lingually by the mentalis muscle action. Usually such a holding appliance will be kept in place until the lower permanent cuspids erupt enough to furnish the necessary stabilizing pressure against the distal surfaces of the lateral incisors.

If a fixed lingual holding arch is placed, it should be checked by the dentist 1 week after cementation and every 2 months

thereafter until it is obvious that the holding is no longer needed. It is strongly suggested that a fixed appliance be removed and the bands recemented at the end of each 6 months of wear. Such a procedure is helpful as a preventive dentistry measure. It allows the dentist to accomplish a thorough prophylaxis and do a topical fluoride application as well as make certain the cement bond between the tooth and band is not breaking down.

The use of the fixed-removable lower lingual arch is more common because of its versatility in treatment procedures. It is especially valuable when used to move or tip lower incisors to a more labial position. The F-R lingual arch may have either horizontal or vertical attachments on the lingual surfaces of the molar bands. In the

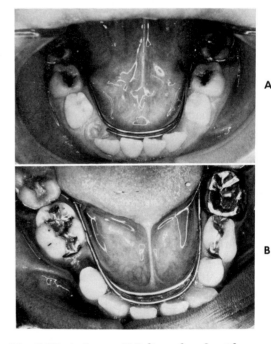

A

B

Fig. 9-12. A, Lower F-R lingual arch with *one* finger spring soldered to main arch wire. **B,** Different F-R lower lingual arch with *two* anterior finger springs used to position lower anterior teeth in a more labial alignment. The springs are adjusted every two weeks, usually with finger pressure alone. Occasionally the No. 139 (bird-beak) pliers are used.

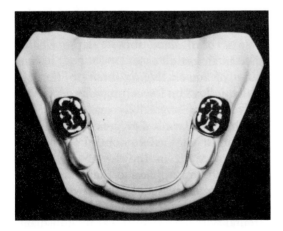

Fig. 9-11. Fixed soldered "holding arch" to maintain the arch form of the mandibular segments. Although these have been recommended much in the past, they are harder to make than an F-R lingual arch, which has another advantage in that the dentist may remove it to add an auxiliary spring if he wishes.

younger child the horizontal attachment is best because the 6-year molar has a shorter clinical crown height at this age.

Whether the choice is an F-R lingual arch with horizontal attachments or one with vertical attachments, the auxiliary springs used to move the lower incisors labially have approximately the same configuration (Fig. 9-12, *A*). A finger spring of smaller diameter than the main arch wire is spot-welded, then soldered, to the arch opposite the interproximal area between the first and second primary molars. The finger spring extends around to the distal surface of the lower lateral incisor on the opposite side of the arch. Usually the spring is contoured slightly labial to the arch wire position but follows the curve of the main arch wire closely. The spring may be made of 0.025 or 0.028 wire. In most instances a single finger spring is all that will be used, but bilateral springs can be made easily (Fig. 9-12, *B*).

When the desired labial movement of the lower incisors has been effected over a period of several months, a slight spacing will be noted between the incisors. Usually at this time the child's lower incisors will be seen in close relation to his upper incisors in the bite-closed position, and any existing overjet will have been decreased to near normal.

Retention factors

If the lower arch has been expanded buccally, the retention of the new arch configuration cannot be hoped for in every case. The dentist has already been warned that the cheek and lip musculature play a great role in those cases that appear to be unstable when expanded and end up by collapsing to the original arch shape.

Fewer retention problems are noted after the labial movement of lower incisors provided that the 90-degree rule and the Williams diagnostic line have not been disregarded. Best retention results are obtained by leaving the passive, adjusted lingual arch in place for 6 months after the active

treatment. At this time the lower permanent cuspids are usually erupting, and they will serve as the best retainers of arch shape at this stage.

TREATMENT OF CROWDING DUE TO OVERACTIVE MENTALIS MUSCLE

The treatment of crowding in the lower incisor region caused by the hyperactive movements of the lower lip during swallowing is not greatly different from that discussed in the foregoing section. The chief difference in treatment is that there is usually no need to expand the upper and lower arches as in the case of mild genetic crowding. Space is adequate, and it is the arch perimeter that is distorted.

Objectives of treatment

Essentially, the three objectives of treatment are (1) establish or reestablish normal arch perimeter in the lower incisor segment, (2) maintain or reestablish the lower dental midline in relation to the midsagittal plane, and (3) in some cases, retrain the child to swallow in a more normal fashion that does not cause a muscular pressure against the lower teeth.

Establish proper arch perimeter

The normal anterior perimeter of the lower arch may be checked by the brass or stainless steel wire method. When an appliance is fabricated to move the incisors labially to correct the arch perimeter, it is vital that the teeth not be moved labially off their denture base. The important concept here, however, is that the lower incisors are commonly seen to erupt in a fairly good position and then later be influenced by excessive lower lip pressure to tip lingually. Almost always, this tipping is greatest between the time the primary cuspids are lost and the time of the eruption of the permanent lower cuspids.

This tipping action of the lower incisors is most rapid in the child with a pronounced mentalis muscle spasm during the swallowing act. The incisors at this age are

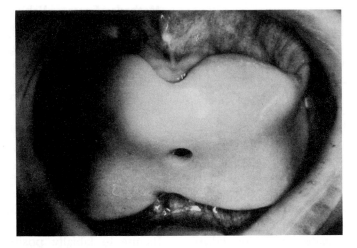

Fig. 9-14. Oral screen is one of the best appliances for the child to wear during swallowing or lip and tongue therapy. It forces the child to compress his lips and almost automatically acts to circumvent the "old" swallow and accompanying lip and tongue acrobatic movements and aids him in acquiring the "new" and more normal swallowing pattern.

Children like to play with a removable appliance, so it is a sound precautionary measure to add some positive psychological reinforcement along these lines at each appointment. Removable appliances may become lost or broken much more often than fixed ones. It is well that the parents are given to understand ahead of time the financial consequences of the loss of an appliance. (See discussion of this problem in Chapter 6.)

Use of oral screen to retrain a child's swallow. The use of a latex rubber oral screen appliance (the Rabinowitch habit appliance) is highly effective in changing a child's swallowing pattern. A custom-made acrylic or soft plastic oral screen will accomplish the same task, although more laboratory time is involved in making these latter two. The lip muscles must close around an oral screen in a totally new fashion, which aids the child in developing a more normal swallowing pattern. With practice, the new pattern can be learned in a period of 2 or 3 months. The oral screen is worn only at night, which is an advantage for the child who has trouble wearing an appliance during school hours. (See Fig. 9-14.)

In effect, the oral screen (also called the oral shield) acts to protect the lower incisors from excessive pressures produced by the mentalis muscle. At the same time, it seems to promote a greater tongue pressure against the lower anterior teeth during the swallowing act, which causes the lower incisors to move labially because of the unbalanced nature of the forces. The hope is that the teeth will stabilize in their new positions due to better balance of forces when the swallowing pattern becomes more normal.

The usual period of treatment is 3 to 6 months. If the swallowing pattern is indeed changed, the retention may be very good after such therapy.

An example of instructions to the child by the dentist to effect changes of the patterns of swallowing while the child wears his oral screen is as follows[1]:
1. Place your tongue tip flat on the "spot" (incisive papilla).
2. Close your back teeth together.
3. Close your lips together.
4. Now swallow.

Children learn this new swallowing pattern rapidly and well, and the resulting balance of muscular pressures acting against the teeth makes the effort worthwhile. The retention of the lower anterior teeth in their new positions is tremendously enhanced if this swallowing therapy is effective. It has been found that the dentist can teach a normal swallowing pattern much more rapidly using both therapy and an oral screen. With swallowing therapy alone, the change of tooth positions and establishment of muscular balance is less certain in most children.

SUMMARY

The two chief types of Class I malocclusions that demonstrate lower anterior crowding have been described, together with the etiologies of each. Treatment methods utilizing lower Hawley appliances (with and without jackscrews), lower fixed-removable lingual arches, and oral screens have been examined.

Also discussed is an office therapy approach to help the child whose lower incisors are being crowded lingually due to hyperactivity of the mentalis muscle in the lower lip. The treatment includes retraining the child to swallow in a more normal fashion in order to balance the muscular forces against the lower anterior teeth.

REFERENCES

1. Ehrlich, A. B.: Training therapists for tongue thrust correction, Springfield, Ill., 1970, Charles C Thomas, Publisher.
2. Gellin, M. E.: Indications and contraindications for the removal of primary teeth, Dent. Clin. North Am., pp. 899-911, Oct., 1969.
3. Mathews, R. J.: Malocclusion in the primary dentition, Dent. Clin. North Am., pp. 463-478, July, 1966.
4. McDonald, R. E.: Pedodontics, St. Louis, 1963, The C. V. Mosby Co., p. 127.
5. Moyers, R. E.: Handbook of orthodontics, ed. 2, Chicago, 1963, Year Book Medical Publishers, Inc., pp. 488-489.
6. Oldenburg, T. R.: Personal communication, 1970.
7. Tweed, C. H.: Clinical orthodontics, St. Louis, 1966, The C. V. Mosby Co., p. 42.
8. Williams, R.: The diagnostic line, Am. J. Orthod. **55**:458-476, 1969.

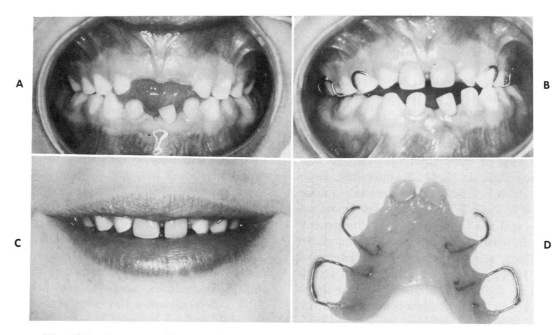

Fig. 10-1. Boy, age 4½ years. **A,** Injury a year previous had caused the loss of two upper primary central incisors and one lower primary central incisor. Child's speech showed difficulties with sibilants and his tongue was beginning to thrust through this opening to effect the seal for the swallow. **B,** Upper appliance supporting two upper central incisors has been fitted. Note the degree of open-bite that already exists from the beginning tongue-thrusting. This is slightly exaggerated by the clasps holding the bite open. **C,** Appliance in place in boy's mouth. Note that the presence of a diastema contributes to a natural appearance in primary incisor replacements. Labiodental speech sounds (*f* and *v*) improved immediately and became indistinguishable from normal. **D,** Appliance shown out of the mouth. It restores normality to the oral architecture at a time when child is actively learning speech and swallowing habits. Modified Crozat clasps were used. This type of clasp improves retention by the addition of a wire of 0.025 diameter soldered to the 0.028 molar clasp wire. The additional wire engages the mesial and distal undercuts of the primary molar in a better fashion than does any other clasp if the tooth is partially erupted or has a short clinical crown.

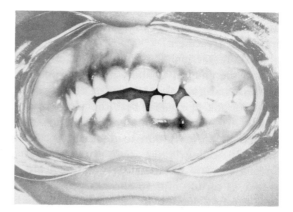

Fig. 10-2. Anterior open-bite in a 5-year-old child as the result of prolonged thumb-sucking. Tongue-thrusting has not been strongly developed. Treatment should be directed toward retraining the child away from the habit. Note that primary cuspids remain in contact in this *dental* open-bite. In a skeletal open-bite the opening of the bite extends to the bicuspid or molar area, as a rule. Note also geminated mandibular primary lateral incisor.

Examination for oral habits

In the examination for oral habits, the dentist is interested in observing whether a persisting thumb- or finger-sucking habit is present (Fig. 10-2); whether during swallowing there is a facial grimace or an excessive mentalis muscle contraction, a normal contraction of the temporalis and masseter muscles, and normal placement of the tongue against the teeth and palate; and whether the pattern of speech of the child is essentially normal. (See Fig. 10-3.) To observe these,* several steps can be taken:

1. Observe child at a time when he is not aware of your scrutiny to check the following.
   a. Facial profile. Is it essentially straight, concave, or convex?
   b. Lip positions at rest. Are they together or held apart?
   c. Positions of the lips during the swallowing act. Do they close together in a seal? Does the lower lip close the seal by pressing up behind the upper anterior teeth?
   d. Relative tensions of the upper and lower lips during swallowing. Is the upper lip passive or incompetent during the swallowing act?
2. Examine oral cavity for size and position of tongue at rest.
   a. Closely observe what the tongue does during the swallowing act, if possible. This cannot be done while holding the lips apart as has been suggested. *All* children thrust their tongues to make a seal for the swallow under these conditions.
   b. Observe symmetry of incisal positions of the upper central and lateral incisors. Asymmetry in this area may give a clue that the child sucks his right or left thumb or finger by preference. Tongue thrusts may also be in a lateral direction, creating an asymmetrical anterior open-bite.
   c. Measure dimensions of open-bite if it is present. Measure from the incisal edge of right upper lateral to

*See Table 1 for chart on which to enter these observations.

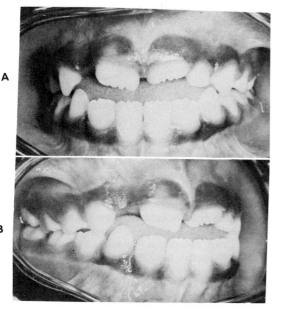

Fig. 10-3. Child, age 7½, with a developing anterior open-bite due to tongue thrust. Because of a tendency toward a hereditary Class III malocclusion, this oral habit may help the child achieve a better occlusion than would a more normal tongue position. **A,** Front view. **B,** Right view. Note the reverse curve of Spee developing in the lower arch, which is typical of anterior open-bite cases.

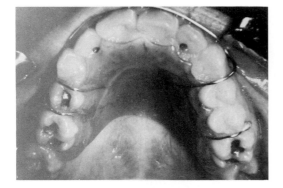

Fig. 10-6. Hawley appliance being used as a retention device after correction of protruding incisors. The acrylic has been removed from the appliance lingual to the incisors to allow lingual displacement caused by pressure exerted by the labial bow. Labial bow does not have the indent over the lateral incisors that is suggested for a well-fitted appliance.

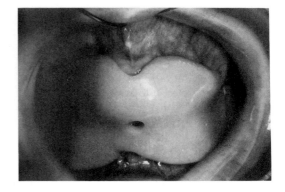

Fig. 10-7. Acrylic oral screen being worn by a 9-year-old child exhibiting upper anterior protrusion. This appliance has a "physiologic" action of using the labial muscles to move protruding teeth into a more normal relationship. It also improves the competency of the lips during the swallowing act as well as reducing the tendency of tongue-thrusting. The appliance should be worn on the same kind of schedule as any night appliance, at least 12 to 14 hours a day.

of the child's front teeth. Treatment time varies from 3 to 6 months in most cases, with retention time another 3 to 6 months.

Some additional considerations

If the upper Hawley appliance has a bite plane built into it lingual to the upper central incisors to correct an exaggerated curve of Spee, the bite plane should be flat and should not conform to the uneven incisal edges of the lower incisors. When it is made flat, it more effectively controls the incisal heights of the lower incisors during the treatment period. There is only minimal depression of the lower incisors during such treatment. Most changes in the curve of Spee are caused by opening the posterior bite in this case. The continued eruption of the posterior teeth act to change the curve of the occlusal plane.

An obvious precaution to observe in adjusting the labial spring of the Hawley appliance is to relieve the acrylic on the lingual aspect of the incisors so that the teeth are able to move lingually when labial pressure is applied (Fig. 10-6). For reten-

tion, the labial bow wire may be cut mesial to each cuspid U-loop, and hooks formed to support an elastic stretched across the labial surfaces of the upper incisors. The use of the newer light elastics can make the retainer nearly invisible during daytime wear.

Correction of protrusion by oral screen

The oral screen has established itself as one of the easiest to use yet most effective appliances for the correction of protruded upper anterior teeth. It has been termed a "physiologic" appliance, since it does not cause teeth to move by wires but generates its force against the upper anterior teeth by the pressure of the perioral musculature. These devices are fitted so that the child wears them held in place between his teeth and his lips (Fig. 10-7). Several types of oral screens are available, made of both hard and soft materials. (See Chapter 14 for types of materials available and Chapter 16 for details of fabrication.)

These appliances function best when worn each night from 12 to 14 hours. They exert an interrupted pressure on the anterior teeth, and treatment time will vary from 6 to 12 months. The child should be given a "home-wear chart" to help keep daily records while wearing this appliance (Fig. 6-1).

Using the ruler end of the especially prepared Boley gauge, the stepwise reduction of protrusion of the teeth (overjet) over a period of months can be measured directly in the child's mouth each time the dentist sees him (Fig. 10-4). It is important to keep chart notes on these measurements. Measured changes of the overjet can be entered once a month, so the progress in the case can be documented. If no changes are occurring in the incisor relationships, the dentist can infer that the appliance is not being worn as he has directed, since the oral screen has a continuing effect to reduce protrusion if worn properly by the child.

TREATMENT OF ANTERIOR OPEN-BITE

As has been mentioned already, anterior open-bites may be present in at least two quite different Class I malocclusions. The first exhibits protrusion with an exaggerated overjet, whereas the second exhibits protrusion with *little or no* overjet. It is important to separate the two types. A crowding situation may well be caused if an attempt is made to move the unspaced upper anterior teeth into normal alignment to correct a nonprotrusive open-bite. Many times these cases will be found to need extraction therapy to provide space to permit good alignment of teeth. It has been noted previously that preventive orthodontic therapy necessitating the extraction of bicuspids should be left in the hands of the orthodontist. (See Fig. 10-8.)

Oral screens
For open-bite with spaced, protruding upper incisors (Class I, Type 2, cases)

When an oral screen is placed over the labial surfaces of anterior teeth in which there is significant protrusion of the upper central and lateral incisors with interproximal spacing, a great deal of muscle-generated pressure can be exerted against the upper teeth by the closure of the lips over the oral screen. To lessen this pressure, particular attention should be paid to the *tissue* fitting of the upper and lower peripheries of the oral screen when the appliance is first fitted. All margins should be well polished (or smoothed if the screen is made of soft material) and have an indentation for both the upper and the lower frenum. In addition, if the oral screen is to be made of acrylic or heat-labile material, a thin film of plaster can be added to the labial surfaces of the upper central incisors on the models when the oral screen is being fabricated. This serves to lessen the initial pressure against the upper central incisors during the first week of wear and makes the wearing of this device considerably more comfortable for the child.

Later this plaster can be scraped away, and the pressures against the labial surfaces of these teeth increased by filling in new acrylic or reheating the plastic screen slightly. The addition of plaster seems a small thing, but the increase in comfort for the child wearing the appliance makes it worthwhile to consider doing.

For open-bite with unspaced upper incisors (Class I, Type 1, cases)

In the construction of oral screens for anterior open-bite cases where neither interproximal spacing nor upper protrusion exists to any great degree, the important factor to remember is that the appliance should be essentially a *tissue-borne* one, exerting little or no pressure against the teeth. If too much labial pressure against the unspaced teeth is incorporated into the appliance, the end result may be that the teeth will be moved into a crowded relationship or that the upper and lower incisors will be forced into an end-to-end relationship. Both of these results are undesirable.

The oral screen in open-bite cases should

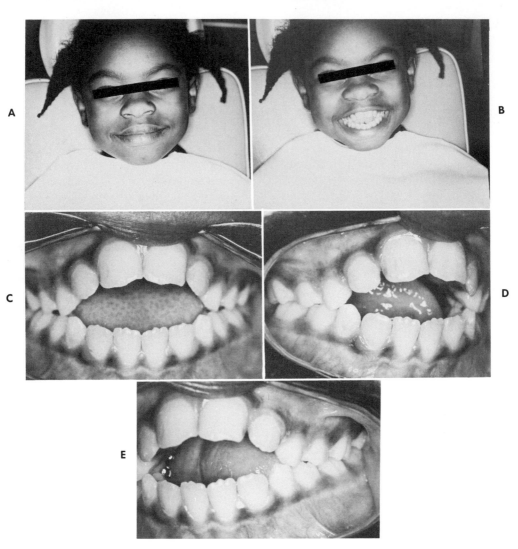

Fig. 10-8. Eight-year-old girl who was a long-term thumb-sucker and now exhibits a pronounced tongue-thrusting. **A,** She can close her lips but does not normally do so during swallowing. **B,** Her open-bite condition is apparent when she smiles. A definite anterior lisp is present. Because there is only slight spacing evident between the upper central and lateral incisors, a closure of the anterior open-bite could mean a crowding relationship would exist in the upper arch. A case such as this should be referred out because of the possible necessity of bicuspid extraction. **C,** Front view, closed. Note the reverse curve of Spee in the lower arch and lack of spacing in the upper arch. **D,** Right view, closed. Note overjet is not very marked. **E,** Left view, closed.

serve more as a tongue-thrust retraining device and less as a tooth-positioning device. The tongue thrust, constant sucking of the lower lip, and mouth-breathing are the chief entities that act to perpetuate the anterior open-bite in a child older than 6 years. If any or all of these habits are interrupted or altered toward the normal, the incisor teeth have a chance to grow together into a more normal incisal relationship. In part, this more normal relationship occurs as a result of better *lateral*

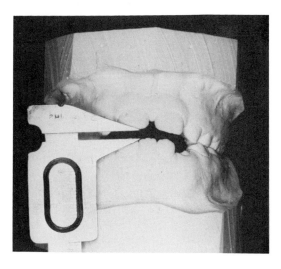

Fig. 10-9. On models, as shown here, or in the child's mouth the dentist may use the modified Boley gauge to accurately measure the exact amount of anterior open-bite. He can measure directly in the child's mouth at each check-up appointment the progress of closing the bite.

tongue pressures' being developed by the wearing of the oral screen. The lips can then close more naturally to act as a functioning portion of the muscular envelope and balance the pressures needed to produce normal positions of the anterior teeth.

If the open-bite in a child without excessive overjet and with unspaced upper anterior teeth exceeds 5 mm. (measured between the incisal edges of the upper and lower central incisors, Fig. 10-9) and the child is older than 10, he should be referred to an orthodontist. If the open-bite is less than this, treatment may be initiated, using the oral screen. The open-bite should close during treatment at a rate of 0.5 to 1 mm. a month if the child wears his oral screen 12 hours a day during sleeping hours.

Overall functions of an oral screen

Wearing a properly constructed oral screen during the evening hours and while sleeping can help the child accomplish the following:

1. Establish better lip competency and lessen the "slack-lipped" tendency so often seen in anterior open-bite cases.

2. Help restrain the tendency of the tongue to thrust forward through the open-bite area, and therefore help in the overall swallowing pattern. Also the oral screen forces the tongue to thrust more in a lateral fashion, more effectively balancing the action of the muscles of the cheek.

3. Restrict to a minimum the action of the mentalis muscle in the lower lip. This also helps to normalize the swallowing pattern.

4. Act as a deterrent to mouth-breathing. A more normal pattern of nasal airflow will be established, and the dryness of mouth and edema of the gingiva seen in these children after nocturnal mouth-breathing will be lessened.

5. Serve the child as a constant reminder of his habit-retraining exercises that have been assigned by the dentist.

Treatment of thumb- or finger-sucking

The pendulum of dental opinion has swung back and forth regarding the proper treatment course for children beyond age 6 who are habituated finger- or thumb-suckers. As a first step, it is perhaps better to relieve the child of as much parental pressure as possible at home regarding this habit. (See section in Chapter 3 dealing with this problem.)

It is necessary to avoid a too obvious, psychologically oriented probing of the needs of the child during the initial exam-

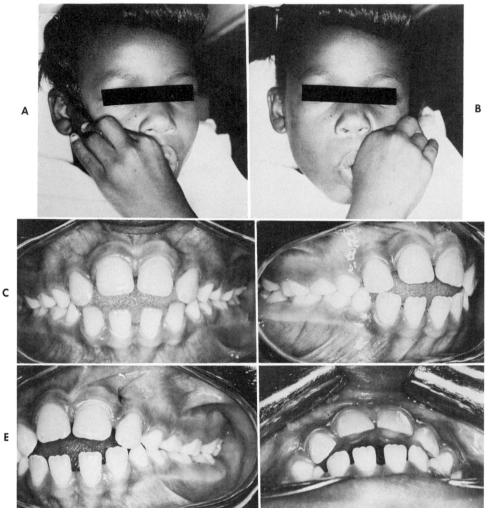

Fig. 10-10. A and **B**, Nine-year-old girl demonstrating she sucks her *right* thumb part of the time . . . and that she is also ambidextrous! Note that the hair-pulling is closely associated with this habit. Sometimes just talking with the child and getting her mother to change her hair-do will cause her to drop the habit. Cutting off braids has been suggested as a means of breaking the sucking habit, but this drastic measure should be a last, and not a first, resort. **C**, Even if the thumb-sucking habit is conquered, however, the tongue thrusting goes on, perpetuating the anterior open-bite (front view). In this case, an oral screen would be an ideal appliance. **D**, Right view. Note the interproximal spaces that exist between both upper and lower anterior teeth, which would permit the upper and lower incisors to be retruded to achieve a good incisal relationship. **E**, Left view. Mamelons still present on lower anterior teeth show a history of lack of incisal relationship since eruption. These are commonly present in anterior open-bite cases. **F**, Child's head tipped back to show moderate overjet.

ination procedure.[2,6] If the child appears immature in his relationships to those around him, he is often not a good candidate for correction measures, whether by appliances or by psychologic approach therapy. It must be stressed here that any preventive orthodontic appliance places a certain amount of psychic burden on each child. This extra stress may in some children produce the opposite result from what the dentist wishes by *increasing* the times and frequency of the thumb- or finger-sucking episodes.

It must be remembered that a thumb- or finger-sucking habit is *not* a dental emergency. Sometimes it is best to see the child in the dental office once or twice over a period of months before any correction is begun, so the child becomes adjusted to the suggestions of the dentist. This allows the dentist to reevaluate his thinking as to the level of cooperation on the part of the parents and child. He should be concerned with whether the structures in the child's mouth are being minimally, moderately, or severely affected by the habit. The less the severity of change, the less the need to initiate treatment. (See Fig. 10-10.)

Fixed appliances such as upper lingual "tongue screens" (described in section on use of fixed appliances in therapy of anterior open-bite due to tongue-thrusting) appear to be more effective in retraining the older child away from these habits. Usually a time period of 3 months is assigned as a goal toward which to work. If the child has made appreciable changes in his habits by that time, the appliance can be safely removed for a "testing period." If, however, gross signs of anxiety are aroused in the child, such as a return to bed-wetting, bad dreams, and frequent crying episodes, the dentist should consider removing the appliance. The wearing of any appliance demands a certain amount of maturity in the child. For the nervous, immature, or uncooperative child, the dentist would do well to defer treatment until the child is older.

Praise is the best therapy in working with all children. The praise should be sincere, and every opportunity should be given for the child to share in the procedures. If the appliance is one that is removable by the child, the parents should be mindful that the child wears his appliance exactly according to the dentist's instructions. However, continual, aggressive parental remonstrances directed toward the child at home can cause him to lose his usual ready willingness to please the dentist. Under these circumstances, some children will "lose" their removable appliances, usually just before the dental appointment. The dentist should remember that he is trying to correct a child's oral habit and is not trying to change the life-style of a whole family.

Graber[4] points out that it is usually the father who is most distressed at the child's abnormal sucking habits. This type of parent is also the one who usually fails to follow the advice of the dentist if an appliance is fabricated to be worn by the child.

Treatment failures

The following are two short case reports of failures to correct oral habits in my private practice. Fixed appliance therapy, only, was used for the first child, and hypnosis therapy, only, for the second. Perhaps a combination of the two approaches would have been better in each. Hindsight is usually considerably clearer than foresight in cases where psychological management is important.

Case 1. R. C., a 4½-year-old boy, treated for excessive thumb-sucking, using an upper fixed appliance.
The child entered the dental clinic apprehensively. After the dentist interviewed the mother, who was divorced, the child was also questioned at some length. He seemed eager to help the dentist even after it was explained that "some children were asked to wear a silver brace in their mouths to help them stop thumb-sucking." An appointment was made for taking impressions.
Impressions were taken, diagnostic proce-

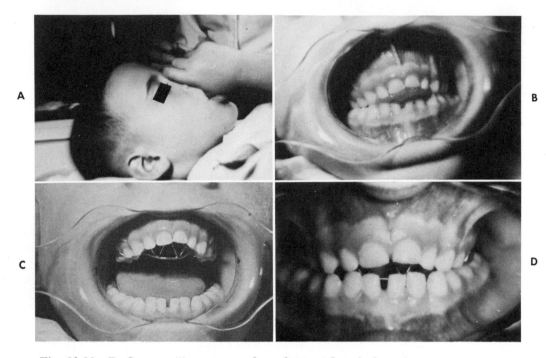

Fig. 10-11. R. C., age 4½ years, was brought into dental clinic for excessive thumb-sucking. **A,** He demonstrates the favorite position of his thumb against the palate as he grasps his nose during the sucking action. **B,** Note the development of an anterior open-bite and a bilateral posterior cross-bite, which are both almost certainly the result of the forceful sucking habit. **C,** Habit retraining device placed to help remind child not to suck his thumb. **D,** Fixed appliance in mouth and teeth closed in occlusion. Appliance has been worn for 8 weeks at this stage. Note anterior open-bite appears to have closed substantially from **B. E,** Continued forceful thumb-sucking by the child has driven the fixed appliance into the palatal tissue. Note swollen incisal papilla. **F,** Portion of the appliance has been embedded in his palatal tissue at end of 8 weeks. Outline of embedded wire is seen in this picture taken immediately on removal of the fixed appliance. **G,** Anterior open-bite has been reduced by approximately one half during 8 weeks' treatment. Because of continued thumb-sucking and other problems of behavior that seemed to be aggravated by the appliance, it was removed by mutual agreement of the parent and dentist.

dures were completed, and a case presentation made to the mother. At the third visit an upper fixed tongue-screen appliance was cemented in the child's mouth. The fit seemed to be comfortable. The child expressed eagerness to show it to his friends.

The child was seen at 2-week intervals for 8 weeks. The mother reported that the child had begun again to wet the bed almost nightly. He cried easily, did not eat well, and appeared to suck his thumb more often than ever.

The appliance was removed at the end of 10 weeks of treatment by mutual agreement of dentist and mother. The changes in the tongue pressure were being demonstrated, since the bite had begun to close, as evidenced by Fig. 10-11. Tolerance by the child of the appliance was poor in this case, even though he reported no discomfort.

Summary: Fixed appliance therapy for thumb-sucking in this immature, probably over-protected child was unsuccessful. More careful questioning of the mother would have elicited much of this information at the beginning and might have saved considerable effort and embarrassment on the part of the dentist.

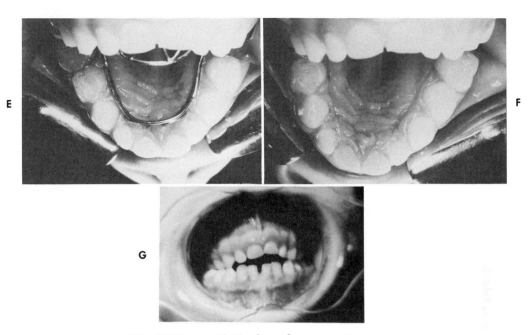

Fig. 10-11, cont'd. For legend see opposite page.

Case 2. G. H., a 10½-year-old girl, treated for prolonged thumb-sucking by use of hypnotherapy which I administered.

The girl was a smiling, apparently nonapprehensive patient. The father, a professional man, suggested the use of hypnotherapy to alleviate the prolonged sucking habit. The child was socially conscious of the immaturity of her response to induced anxiety but not concerned enough to stop the habit, which was producing an unsightly anterior open-bite of more than 6 mm. between the incisal edges of the upper and lower central incisors. It was agreed that each hypnosis session would be separated by a month's time.

Two hypnosis sessions later, the girl had not altered her habit noticeably. This was elicited both by questioning her and by measuring again the open-bite area between her upper and lower incisors. By mutual agreement the therapy was entered on her chart as unsuccessful.

About a year later the child was seen spontaneously to drop the habit.

Fixed-appliance therapy for anterior open-bite due to tongue-thrusting

Fixed appliances may also be considered in the treatment of anterior open-bite cases in which there is no present history of thumb- or finger-sucking but, instead, the child exhibits a constant pattern of tongue-thrusting. As a rule the child will be from 7 to 10 years of age. Older children almost certainly will have to undergo full-treatment orthodontics if a moderate-to-severe open-bite is present due to this problem at age 11.

In these older children, a muscular accommodation to their tongue-thrusting or tongue-positioning habit has been reached. The spaces that originally separated the upper anterior teeth may have been closed by the exaggerated mesial inclination of the teeth. Occasionally this may have moved the whole upper denture base forward, so that the occlusion comes to resemble a Class II, Division 1, malocclusion. Only in open-bite cases where the upper central and lateral incisors are *spaced* and the upper and lower cuspids are in good occlusion should treatment be attempted by the general dentist. If a fixed labial arch appliance is used in these *spaced* open-bite cases, a cervical extraoral force appliance will usually be found necessary to main-

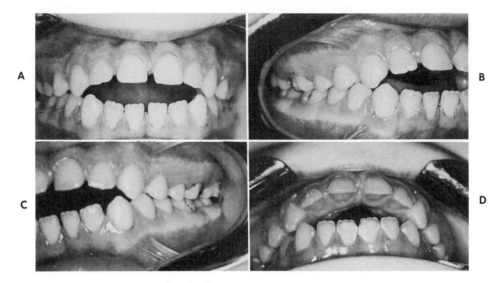

Fig. 10-12. Boy, age 14 years, exhibiting an anterior open-bite. In addition to a lisping problem, he presented an unattractive, open-mouthed profile. An oddity in such cases is the usual absence of severe decay pattern when anterior open-bite is present. Treatment with minor tooth movement appliances would probably be unsuccessful in such a well-established malocclusion. This child should be placed in the hands of an orthodontist. A, Front view. B, Right view demonstrating normal occlusion distal to the cuspids. C, Left view. Note that long-term tongue pressures have severely inhibited upper and lower anterior alveolar growth. D, Head tilted back to show marked overjet. Note presence of calculus due to mouth-breathing. (Other illustrations were made after teeth had been cleaned.)

tain the anchorage of the upper 6-year molars. Most of these types of cases should be referred to the orthodontist, even if the molar relationship appears to be Class I. (See Fig. 10-12.) The difficult *unspaced* open-bite cases in older children should be viewed as treatment failures waiting to happen. Don't let them happen to you!

Treatment for younger children

In spite of the failure in Case 1, it is believed that early treatment with a fixed appliance is valuable in some younger children who exhibit an open-bite caused by early thumb- or finger-sucking but later maintained by abnormal tongue-thrusting. In discussions concerning treatment for tongue thrust in younger children, it has been noted that a tongue-thrust appliance usually must be worn somewhat longer than a finger-habit appliance. Depending on the severity of the open-bite problems, 4 to 9 months may be required for the autonomous correction of the malocclusion. The observation has been made that not all preventive appliances are successful by themselves, and full orthodontic procedures are essential in some cases. If the dentist has been careful in his selection of a mature child, has studied the problem thoroughly to ascertain that he is dealing primarily with a tongue-thrust habit and not a basal and total malocclusion, and places the appliance early enough so that he can expect the permanent teeth to erupt and the alveolar bone to be laid down, his efforts should meet with routine success. The optimum age for placement of this

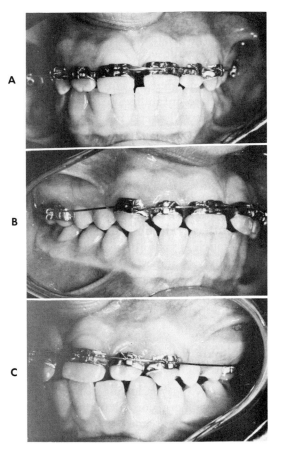

Fig. 10-13. Moderately protrusive dentition in a 9-year-old child under treatment. A mild anterior open-bite was present before treatment was started. **A,** Upper arch has been brought into a better alignment through the use of a fixed light labial arch. Upper molar anchorage has been maintained by use of a cervical extraoral force appliance, which fits into the larger of the two tubes in each double buccal tube. **B,** Right view demonstrates how this appliance combination can be used safely to maintain anchorage of the molars, keep good bicuspid alignment, and establish good incisal relationship. **C,** Left view exhibits the less balanced intercuspation of teeth in the opposing margins. However, after a period of time following treatment, teeth seem to "settle in," so the expectation is that intercuspation will improve in a case such as this.

type of appliance is between 5 and 10 years. If appliances are to be used after this age, corrective orthodontic appliances and the services of an orthodontic specialist will be more likely required.[3] (See Fig. 10-13.)

The fixed appliances most used for correction of tongue thrust are called tongue screens or, occasionally, "tongue traps." The latter term is not recommended, since it implies the use of a punitive device. The opposite is usually true, however, since most children are able to wear these two appliances with comfort.

When this type of fixed appliance is used, the tongue is forcibly retrained into new muscular positions and pressures. Its pressure is directed more laterally and less anteriorly. Within a few days to a week, as a rule, the tongue finds a comfortable

(and more correct) position to anchor its tip against the palate to begin the act of swallowing. It should be noted, however, that without the tongue pressures available to the *lower* anterior teeth, in certain instances a dangerous imbalance can be caused, allowing the mentalis muscle to force the lower incisors lingually.

Testing for the expected more normal swallowing pattern, the dentist will use his fingertips against the temples of the child to check for the desired contraction of the temporalis muscle, and against the angle of the jaw to check for the contraction of the masseter muscle. The activity of the mentalis muscle during the swallowing act should *subside* as the temporalis and masseter muscle contractions *increase* over a period of weeks.

but *before* the start of speech therapy. In the procedures the orthodontist rated the severity of the malocclusion, and the children were examined by the speech therapist to determine what dental sounds he would predict as defective and the degree of deviation. Each subject was asked to read the test sentences, and all defects were noted and graded by each examiner. Note that the consonant sounds are in *initial, medial,* and *final* positions in each sentence where possible.

Speech sounds used in the Rathbone-Snidecor articulation test*

1. *Postdental* consonants (tongue back of anterior teeth): *n, t, d, r, l, s, sh, z, zh, y*
   - *n* Her name was Ann and she lived near Dan.
   - *t* Terry counted the kittens and took three for his sister.
   - *d* Donald did not have the doll or the dog, but he did have an old radio.
   - *r* Roy watched the rabbit run around the chair.
   - *l* The lad lit the lamp and did his school work.
   - *s* The six sisters in red dresses sang school songs.
   - *sh* She washed the dishes and put them on the shelf at the shop.
   - *z* The boys were surprised at the zebra in the zoo.
   - *zh* Their father hid the television set in the garage.
   - *y* The young girl was amused by the three yards of yellow yarn which she found in the yard.

2. *Linguadental* consonants (tongue to incisal edges of upper anterior teeth): *th* (unvoiced) and *th* (voiced)
   - *th* (unvoiced) The thin thief stole the three thimbles, but could find nothing else.
   - *th* (voiced) That lathe belongs to my father and brother.

3. *Labiodental* consonants (lip and teeth sounds): *f, v*
   - *f* His father found the loaf of bread and coffee on the sofa.

   - *v* He has seven vests, one for every suit.

4. *Postdental combination* consonants (tongue back of anterior teeth; each sound is a combination of two sounds): *ch, j*
   - *ch* The teacher told the children to chew the cherries carefully.
   - *j* Jack ate the jam and drank his orange juice.

When read aloud by the child, the sentences in this list proved to be a valuable diagnostic instrument for determination of speech defects by the orthodontist. This assumption is based on the percentage agreement, 91.4%, reached by the orthodontist and the speech therapist in regard to the more common dental fricative sounds *s, sh, z, zh, th* (voiced), and *th* (unvoiced). When *all* dental sounds were considered, the percentage agreement was only 51.3%, a figure that could be expected as a result of the lack of speech training on the part of the orthodontist. Since there was no 1:1 relationship established between the severity of the malocclusion and of the speech defect, the use of study models alone in judging defective sounds was found to be insufficient in accuracy for the prediction of faulty dental sounds.

After 4 years, eight of the ten original subjects in the study were reexamined with the same speech test. Orthodontic treatment without speech correction reduced the number of faulty dental sounds from a mean of 6.4 to 1.5. Despite orthodontic treatment, residual speech errors were observed in the highly noticeable fricatives *s, z, sh, zh,* and *th* but to a lesser degree both qualitatively and quantitatively. The study casts indicate few, if any, reasons for these errors and point to the need for speech therapy.

The authors believe there are definite applications for speech testing in dental patients with malocclusions and recommend that the testing steps just outlined be followed in the orthodontist's office.

There has been a less complicated list of sentences to test for poor speech patterns published in a recent book by Erhlich.[1] She also recommends swallowing retraining be

---

*From Rathbone, J. S., and Snidecor, J. C.: An appraisal of speech defects in dental anomalies with reference to speech improvement, Angle Orthod. **29**:54-59, 1959.

accomplished in the dental office. To this end she has devised a list of interesting and practical suggestions that help immensely in teaching child patients new ways to swallow.

SUMMARY

Several alternative methods of treating children with Class I malocclusions exhibiting protruding and spaced upper anterior teeth are presented. Some of these children demonstrate an anterior open-bite relationship also, and both appliance therapy and methods of tongue and lip retraining are described to aid the child to bring his anterior teeth into a normal incisal relationship.

Moss' idea of the functional matrix of the soft facial tissues and how they act on the developing bony dentofacial complex of the child is reviewed, and treatment procedures are outlined to help the dentist use this concept in his minor tooth movement procedures.

The special considerations posed by speech problems are discussed, and two different testing methods are proposed that the dentist may accomplish in his office.

REFERENCES

1. Erhlich, A B.: Training therapists for tongue thrust correction, Springfield, Ill., 1971, Charles C Thomas, Publisher.
2. Finn, S. B., and Sim, J. M.: Oral habits in children. In Finn, S. B., editor: Clinical pedodontics, ed. 3, Philadelphia, 1967, W. B. Saunders Co., pp. 308-312.
3. Graber, T. M.: Orthodontics: practice and principles, Philadelpha, 1962, W. B. Saunders Co., pp. 571-572.
4. Graber, T. M.: Orthodontics: practice and principles, ed. 2, Philadelphia, 1966, W. B. Saunders Co., p. 308.
5. Moss, M. L.: The functional matrix. In Kraus, B. S., and Riedel, R. A., editors: Vistas in orthodontics, Philadelphia, 1962, Lea & Febiger, pp. 85-98.
6. Moyers, R. E.: Handbook of orthodontics, ed. 2, Chicago, 1963, Year Book Medical Publishers, Inc., pp. 560-574.
7. Ibid., pp. 109-112.
8. Rathbone, J. S., and Snidecor, J. C.: An appraisal of speech defects in dental anomalies with reference to speech improvement, Angle Orthod. **29:**54-59, 1959.
9. Spengemann, W. B.: Advantages of early (mixed dentition) treatment in Class I and Class II protrusion cases, Dent. Clin. North Am., pp. 529-540, July, 1968.
10. Winders, R. B.: Forces exerted on dentition by perioral and lingual musculature during swallowing, Angle Orthod. **28:**226-235, 1958. Reviewed by Noyes, H. J., in Yearbook of dentistry, Chicago, 1959, Year Book Medical Publishers, Inc.

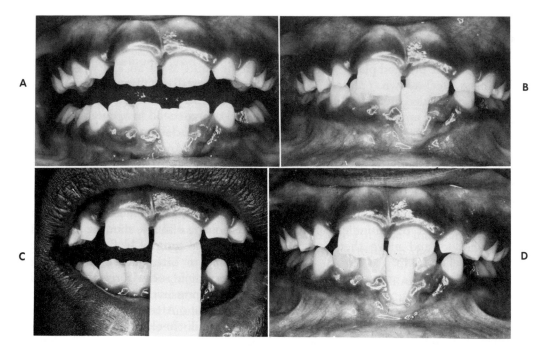

Fig. 11-3. One-tooth anterior cross-bite in an 8-year-old child. The inlocked upper left central incisor has caused excessive mobility in the lower left central incisor, resulting in noticeable periodontal damage on the labial aspect of the periodontium. It was decided that an "immediate" reduction of the cross-bite should be attempted, since there was mobility in *both* central incisors and the child could be placed in an incisal relationship by having his mandible guided into retruded position. **A,** Open view. **B,** Front view, closed. Blanching of tissue was evident on the labial aspect of the lower central incisor as the upper central incisor closed into its inlocked position. **C,** Narrow tongue blade being held in position by the child. He was asked to hold pressure against his teeth and to keep his jaw firmly closed for 20 to 30 minutes while he sat in the waiting room, supervised by the dental assistant. **D,** At the end of one half hour, the cross-bite in the incisors was corrected by the tongue blade and biting pressures. The child was told to go home and keep his teeth shut tightly together as much as possible over the weekend. On Monday the cross-bite tooth was still in the corrected position. The problem of crowding in the lower arch is evident, however, and should be treated later.

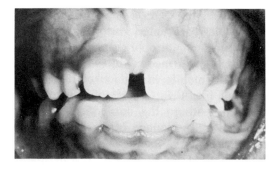

Fig. 11-4. Lower acrylic inclined plane placed in a child's mouth for treatment of two upper central incisors that erupted in cross-bite.

Lower acrylic inclined plane. The lower acrylic inclined plane (Fig. 11-4) is at once the most versatile and the most easily made appliance to use in reducing a one- or two-tooth anterior cross-bite. It may be fabricated on the lower model or it may be made directly in the child's mouth as a one-appointment procedure. When it is well contoured, polished, and cemented into place, *it should enclose the lower six anterior teeth* (if primary cuspids are present). This serves to prevent lingual movement of the lower incisors during treat-

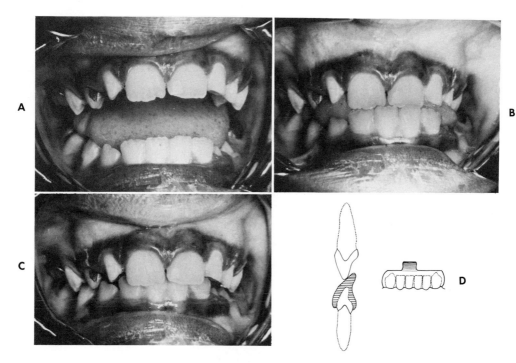

Fig. 11-5. Boy, age 7½, with an anterior cross-bite involving both upper central incisors, demonstrating Class I, Type 3, malocclusion. **A,** Front view, open. **B,** Front view, closed. Note mandibular shift on closure as compared with **A. C,** Anterior cross-bite has been corrected by use of a cemented acrylic inclined plane over a period of 3 weeks. Note that the mandibular shift is no longer evident. Front and side view of appliance. **D,** Drawing demonstrating how all 6 lower anterior teeth are included in the lower acrylic inclined plane. Note that portion of the plane contacting tooth or teeth in anterior cross-bite is approximately at a 45-degree angle to the axis of the lower central incisors.

ment. This appliance acts as an anterior guide plane applying slight labially directed pressure only to the upper tooth or teeth in cross-bite. The pressure on the tooth in cross-bite is controlled by the force with which the child closes his teeth to chew or swallow. The harder he bites, the more temporary discomfort he may have, but the faster the tooth in cross-bite will move labially into the normal bite position.

One of the best guides to determine whether the cross-bite has been reduced after the child has worn the lower acrylic inclined plane for a time is to check the opening between the posterior teeth in full bite closure. When the inclined plane is first cemented, the bite appears to be substantially open in the posterior segments when the child closes into full bite. Within a space of 2 to 3 weeks, however, the bite closes into contact posteriorly. When this is seen, the treatment of the anterior cross-bite may be regarded as completed in most cases and the appliance removed. (See Fig. 11-5.) The formerly inlocked incisors tend to remain in their new arch positions without further treatment because of the now normal pressures they exert against one another. When this is accomplished, the dentist may feel confident that he has performed an important and necessary service for the child.

Reversed stainless steel crown. By the careful fitting, then cementing, of an anterior stainless steel crown *backwards* onto an upper central incisor in cross-bite, a

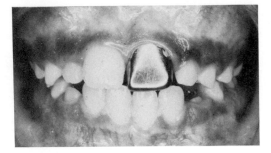

Fig. 11-6. Anterior stainless steel crown fitted and cemented to an upper left permanent central incisor that is inlocked. Worn for a period of 2 to 3 weeks, appliance will reduce the child's one-tooth anterior cross-bite.

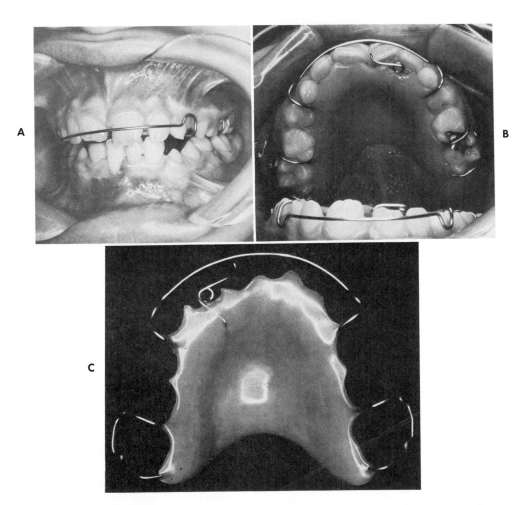

Fig. 11-7. A, Upper Hawley appliance with a helical spring moving 1| out of cross-bite. No bite plane is needed to open the bite in most of these cases. Note the periodontal involvement on the labial surface of 1|. A Stillman's cleft is forming as the result of the torquing forces generated as the incisors lock together. **B,** Appliance with helical spring in child's mouth. **C,** Appliance removed from child's mouth. Note lack of indentation in labial bow for lateral incisors. This can create a "denture smile."

metal guide plane can be established (Fig. 11-6). When the child bites down, a gentle force results that acts to move the lower incisor lingually and the inlocked upper incisor labially. One advantage of this procedure is the easy, one-appointment visit. A disadvantage is that the cement holding the stainless steel crown may become loosened during the usual treatment interval of about 2 weeks. In addition, the fitting of the crown onto a partially erupted central incisor may be somewhat difficult.

Banded metal incline. An alternate choice to fitting a stainless crown backward is the fabrication of a banded metal incline to fit over one or two upper central incisors. This procedure requires some skill with contouring pliers and a spot welder. A band is first contoured and fitted onto the middle third of the exposed crown of the incisor. Then a metal strap made of the same band material is bent at an acute angle and fitted over the incisal area and spot-welded to the band both labially and lingually. The device can be fitted and cemented to provide increased stability, and the angle of the metal guide plane can be adjusted to make it somewhat more versatile than the reversed steel crown previously described.

Active appliances

Upper Hawley appliance. The versatile Hawley appliance, useful in so many minor

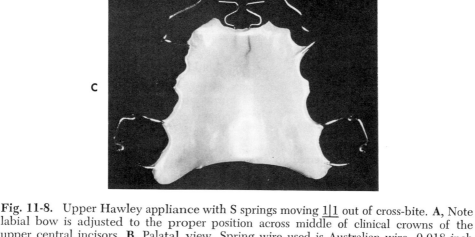

Fig. 11-8. Upper Hawley appliance with S springs moving 1|1 out of cross-bite. **A,** Note labial bow is adjusted to the proper position across middle of clinical crowns of the upper central incisors. **B,** Palatal view. Spring wire used is Australian wire, 0.018 inch in diameter. **C,** Appliance removed from child's mouth. Note proper configuration of labial bow to "indent" across lateral incisors and avoid a "denture" look. Adams clasps are made with 0.025 wire.

Table 12. Summary of treatment methods for anterior cross-bites

Method used	Length of treatment	Age of child (years)
Tongue blade	2 hours to 2 weeks	7 to 8½ (Fig. 11-3)
Lower acrylic inclined plane	2 to 4 weeks	7 to 9 (Figs. 11-4 and 11-5)
Stainless steel crown (placed backwards) or banded metal incline (on upper central incisor)	2 to 3 weeks	7 to 9 (Fig. 11-6)
Upper Hawley appliance with springs	2 to 10 weeks	7 to 10 (Figs. 11-7 and 11-8)
Heavy labial arch	3 to 16 weeks	7 to 10 (Fig. 11-10)
Light labial arch	3 to 16 weeks	8 to 10 (Fig. 11-11, B)

amalgam plugger with a serrated face. A broken explorer with a small notch cut in its end may also be utilized.

As the weeks of treatment pass, it may be found that the light arch wire must be recontoured slightly in the area labial to the incisors in cross-bite in order to maintain the active wire pressure needed to move the inlocked teeth labially. The bite does not have to be opened to accomplish this labial movement of incisors to take them out of cross-bite.

As a rule, the light-wire arch will move teeth more quickly with lighter forces involved than the heavy wire arch. The ideal forces for moving anterior teeth are of the order of 2½ to 3 ounces.

Retention after treatment. The retention of the incisors in their new positions is enhanced by leaving the appliance in place for 6 weeks to 2 months after minor tooth movement is completed. When upper lateral incisors are being moved out of cross-bite, some rotation of the teeth may need to be accomplished. To do this, a wider bracket may be substituted, or another ligature wire may be tied to an auxiliary loop that is spot-welded to the labial surface of the band at the greatest distance from the arch wire. The ligature wires are removed and replaced every 2 weeks. To successfully treat rotated teeth, they must be overrotated about 20 degrees dur-

ing the treatment phase because there is a strong tendency for these teeth to relapse to their former positions if this rule is not followed. (See discussion of tissue response to biomechanical forces, Chapter 7.)

SUMMARY

The use of six appliances in the treatment of anterior cross-bites seen in children 7 to 10 years of age has been described (Table 12). The tongue blade, lower acrylic inclined plane, and the reversed stainless steel crown are used as inclined planes and do not need adjustments during treatment. The upper Hawley appliance, the heavy labial arch, and the light labial arch are more sophisticated adjustable appliances, useful when more than one tooth is in cross-bite. The clinician is warned, however, that when more than two upper incisors are in cross-bite, there is danger that the child may be exhibiting the first clues of Class III malocclusion and referral to an orthodontist should be considered.

REFERENCES

1. Hitchcock, H. P.: Recognition of Class III malocclusions and treatment of Class I, Type 3, malocclusions, Dent. Clin. North Am., pp. 399-408, July, 1968.
2. McDonald, R. E.: Dentistry for the child and adolescent, St. Louis, 1969, The C. V. Mosby Co., pp. 355-361.

12 | Treatment of posterior cross-bites

It may sound odd, but many dentists have made the claim that they graduated from dental school without ever having diagnosed a posterior cross-bite (Class I, Type 4, malocclusion) exhibited by a child. Yet posterior cross-bites share the spotlight with anterior cross-bites in that they are among the most commonly occurring malocclusions that may be identified in any large population of children.

REVIEW OF ETIOLOGY OF POSTERIOR CROSS-BITES

The cause of a posterior cross-bite in a specific child patient may not be able to be determined with any great degree of accuracy. A large body of opinion holds that most of these cross-bites stem from a genetic pattern, with an overlay of complications resulting from environmental factors. Despite the disagreement that prevails concerning their etiology, there is substantial agreement as to the treatment course of these malocclusions.

McDonald[3] infers that some cross-bites may be of muscular origin and suggests that unequal tongue forces or abnormally low tongue positions such as seen in mouth-breathing children may be causative factors. However, Mathews,[2] in his excellent review of malocclusions occurring in the primary dentition, places the burden of the etiology of a deciduous molar cross-bite on the maxillary deciduous cuspids. He explains that a functional cross-bite (described in this book as a unilateral lingual cross-bite) may have its beginnings when the maxillary cuspids erupt without sufficient intercuspid width to clear the lower cuspids on closure. Consequently the child learns to bite in an eccentric (functional) closure to avoid discomfort. This more comfortable but improper biting relation is then perpetuated as the posterior teeth erupt. Emphasized by Mathews is the concept that the treatment of such a unilateral functional cross-bite is directed toward *bilateral* expansion of the upper arch. Mathews's concept is followed in this chapter in the treatment of cross-bites in younger children, 4 to 10 years of age.

The initial diagnosis of these malocclusions at an early age is best accomplished by following the steps in the diagnostic quadrangle and using the length of dental floss and modified Boley gauge as described in Chapter 4, then referring to Table 14. The dental floss is held in the midsagittal plane of the child's face, and the upper and lower dental midlines and the mandibular shift on closure are identified. The Boley gauge is used to measure across the palate from the buccal surface of one 6-year molar to the buccal surface of the other. This may be done in the child's mouth or on the diagnostic cast. If the 6-year molars have not erupted and cross-bite is present in the primary molars, the distance is measured across the arch between the buccal surfaces of the upper second primary molars.

Steps 1 and 3 in the diagnostic quadrangle are the most important when diagnosing the posterior cross-bites—step 1 to determine the molar relationships on each side of the arch and step 3 to determine deviations of dental midlines from the midsagittal plane and the presence of a mandibular shift on closure. (See p. 55 for a review of the complete steps of the diagnostic quadrangle.)

DESCRIPTION OF MOLAR RELATIONSHIPS IN POSTERIOR CROSS-BITE CASES

Usually judged in mesiodistal plane. In the other five types of Class I malocclusions discussed in this book one of the first concerns of the dentist is to establish relationships of 6-year molars if the patient is in the mixed dentition years. Usually left unstated is the fact that this examination is made to determine the molar relationships in a *mesiodistal* plane of reference.

The usual molar relationships for which the dentist is alerted are Class I, Class II, and Class III. There are, however, two additional mesiodistal molar relationships seen in children, which may be described as *end-to-end* (or *end-on*) and *super–Class I*. The end-to-end molar relationship may be a temporary one, with the molars poised halfway between Class I and Class II relation. The super–Class I molar relationship is halfway between Class I and Class III.

The spectrum of possible mesiodistal molar relationships is *Class III, super–Class I, Class I, end-to-end,* and *Class II.*

Must be judged both in mesiodistal and buccolingual planes. In posterior cross-bites the usual mesiodistal molar relationships that are determined as the child closes into his bite cannot be trusted. This is due to the rotation of the mandible that occurs in some cross-bites, particularly the lingual unilateral cross-bite. The rotation is caused by the cuspal slopes of the *lingually* malposed maxillary molar and the other *lingually* posed teeth in the posterior segment.

In the case of a cross-bite on the left side, the child's mandible shifts to the left, rotating the lower teeth distally on the left side and mesially on the right. This commonly produces what appears to be a molar relationship that could be described as super–Class I on the right and end-to-end on the left.*

To get a more correct picture of the true molar relationships, grip the child's chin and guide him slowly into his mandible-retruded position. In this way the child's inherent Class I molar position will be more clearly seen on both sides of the arch, although buccolingually the cusps of the molars may be in a cusp-to-cusp relationship that cannot be sustained by the child as he closes his teeth together by himself. Instead he will slide up the cuspal slopes into his convenience bite, which is termed the *lingual unilateral posterior cross-bite.*

PREDICTING POSITIONS OF BLOCKED-OUT TEETH

When space has been lost in a posterior segment, a permanent tooth may erupt labial or lingual to its normal position in the arch. Such a one-tooth *dental* cross-bite may be only a localized malocclusion. The positions expected to be assumed by such

---

*This may be tested in your own mouth. If you can close your teeth so they simulate a cross-bite on the left side. Hold your fingertips over your condyles and note the distal rotation of the left condyle that occurs.

Table 13. Direction in which blocked-out teeth will usually erupt

Blocked-out teeth	Direction
Maxillary	
Permanent cuspid	Labially
First bicuspid	Buccally
Second bicuspid	Lingually
Mandibular	
Permanent cuspid	Labially
First bicuspid	Buccally
Second bicuspid	Lingually

blocked-out teeth may be predicted with some accuracy (Table 13).

Working out the puzzles that cross-bites represent is a continuing problem for the general dentist. To separate out the uncomplicated cross-bites he may wish to treat is a challenge that should not be taken lightly, since some posterior cross-bites can indicate genetic patterns in the child's dentofacial complex that should be placed in the orthodontist's hands for specialized treatment. Others may appear to be genetic but will, from a treatment point of view, be regarded as functional cross-bites, which may be treated successfully by the generalist or pedodontist.

TIMING OF TREATMENT

Ideas concerning the proper timing for treatment of posterior cross-bite have changed over the years. Researchers have shown that when the positions of primary teeth are changed under the influence of orthodontic appliances, the developing permanent tooth buds beneath these primary teeth tend to follow them and erupt into the changed positions. This is, of course, directly applicable to the problem of treatment of posterior cross-bites in the deciduous dentition. However, the dentist will be wise to avoid promising the parents that reducing a cross-bite in the primary dentition will solve all the problems that will be present in the permanent dentition.

There is now a broad general agreement among orthodontists that cross-bites, whether anterior or posterior, functional or skeletal, should be treated as soon as it is practical to do so. This necessarily is dependent on the immaturity of the child patient and his level of acceptance of the process of impressions, radiographs, and the fabrication and wearing of an appliance in his mouth.[3] (See Table 15.)

POTENTIAL DAMAGE RESULTING FROM UNTREATED POSTERIOR CROSS-BITES

The potential damage that may result in the maturing child when a posterior cross-bite is left untreated is not limited to unusual wear facets on the posterior teeth. It involves additionally a warping of the bony alveolar ridges in the oral cavity and also promotes a pattern of asymmetry in the bones making up the structure of the face.* Moss' functional matrix theory of facial bone development indicates that the tensions and pressures of the envelope of soft tissues surrounding the developing, malleable, immature facial bones actually help shape these bones. Therefore if abnormal tensions and pressures of the masticatory and other facial muscles are applied to the dentofacial bony complex for a long period of time, the symmetry of the face of the child can be altered significantly beyond the range of what is accepted as normal.[4] The results of these abnormal tensions and pressures of muscles are clearly seen in children who have developed posterior cross-bites over a prolonged period of time. The alveolar ridges may respond to the unequal occlusal pressures present in posterior cross-bites. In lingual cross-bites the maxillary arch may be constricted palatally, whereas the mandibular arch, responding more slowly due to the denser bone, may be warped in a buccal direction on the side of the ex-

*During long-term cross-bites, changes in the function of the temporomandibular joint may be noted.

pressed cross-bite. These patterns differ with the number of teeth involved in the cross-bite. Therefore the family dentist should attempt early identification of cross-bites and make an effort to judge their treatment complexity. It must be stressed how important is that "second look" at young patients already undergoing operative procedures in a practice. After a seminar emphasizing diagnosis and treatment of cross-bites, a dentist of my acquaintance found 21 cross-bites in the space of 5 weeks among children in his regular practice.

DESCRIPTION OF CROSS-BITE COMBINATIONS AND THEIR MEASUREMENTS
Former designations of cross-bites

Two distinct types of posterior cross-bites have been emphasized by most writers.[6] The etiology of each is said to be identified by whether or not the mandible shifts perceptibly as the child closes into his occlusion. A posterior cross-bite is considered *functional* (also called a *convenience pattern* or *habitual pattern* of occlusion) if a mandibular shift during the final 2 to 3 mm. of closure is noted (Fig. 12-1). If the child's mandible does not shift as he closes into his final occlusion, the posterior cross-bite demonstrated is said to be *genetic* (also termed *skeletal* or *anatomic*) (Fig. 12-2). Traditionally, it has been suggested that the generalist and the pedodontist should treat only functional cross-bites and should refer to the orthodontist those cross-bites of genetic, or skeletal, origin.

The problem of identifying which posterior cross-bites with these inherently confusing designations are treatable by the generalist is twofold.

First, a so-called functional posterior cross-bite usually is considered to be treatable by the generalist. However, the malocclusion may persist for several years in a child, escaping the notice of the parents and perhaps even of the dentist. As the child's alveolar ridges warp under the oc-

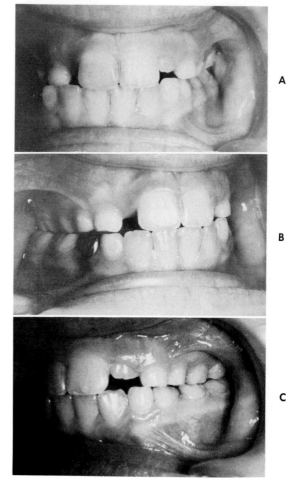

Fig. 12-1. *Functional* posterior cross-bite in mixed dentition. Compare upper and lower dental midlines and note the mandibular shift *toward* the side where the unilateral cross-bite is evidenced. Most posterior cross-bites expressed unilaterally are really bilateral, with a functional shift to one side. Diagnosis is Class I, Type 4. **A,** Front view. **B,** Right view. Note primary cuspids on right side are somewhat worn down and not pointed as cuspids appear in many unilateral cross-bites. **C,** Left view.

clusal forces, the original mandibular shift during closure (identifying it as a functional cross-bite) tends to disappear. With the mandibular shift gone, does it now become a *genetic* cross-bite? Patently this is not true. It remains a functional cross-bite, the pressures of which have stimulated an

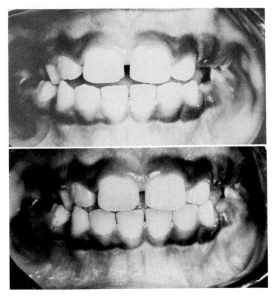

Fig. 12-2. Genetic posterior unilateral cross-bite. Compare this figure with Fig. 12-1 and note that there is no mandibular shift on closure. **A,** Front view, slightly open. **B,** Front view, closed. If a mandibular shift is present, it will occur in the last 2 mm. of closure.

abnormal direction of growth in the bony tissues to create a much more complex orthodontic problem. In older children when mandibular teeth are seen to have acquired dental malpositions from long-term functional cross-bites, the treatment of these malocclusions is best accomplished by the orthodontist. If the child is young enough to still have the malpositions of teeth limited to the upper arch, then he will be able to be treated by the generalist.

Second, there is a fairly broad agreement that most posterior cross-bites are genetic in origin. And yet cross-bites proved as genetic formerly were considered as necessary to be referred. To show how specious this reasoning is, take an example of an upper 6-year molar that may erupt in lingual cross-bite spontaneously, qualifying it as a genetic cross-bite. No mandibular shift may be noted on closure. And yet in almost all cases such a "genetic"

cross-bite may be treated by the general dentist quite successfully.

Obviously needed is a new system of diagnosing cross-bites and identifying those which may be treated without complications by the generalist and the pedodontist.

New system for describing cross-bites

A new approach to the problem of categorizing treatable posterior cross-bites was explored in Chapter 3. This new system appears to answer most of the problems that arise in separating out those cross-bites which may be treated in the generalist's practice.

With this new system, three kinds of posterior cross-bites may be identified as they are expressed in the child's functional occlusion (i.e., as he brings his teeth together in his comfortable closed bite): the *lingual cross-bite,* the *complete lingual cross-bite,* and the *buccal cross-bite* (Fig. 12-3).

Each of these three is named according to the relative buccolingual positions of the upper posterior teeth as they relate in functional occlusion with their opposing lower teeth. Each of these kinds of cross-bite may be expressed functionally only on one side of the arch, qualifying it to be termed *unilateral,* or on both sides of the arch, which makes it then *bilateral.* It is important to restate here that the child seen with a functionally *unilateral* posterior cross-bite in reality has a *bilateral* constriction of his palate, which produces the cross-bite. Treatment in this case consists of bilateral expansion of the upper arch to reduce the cross-bite.

Table 14 makes clear the approximate amounts of expansion that need to be considered in each kind of cross-bite. (See also Fig. 12-3.) This figure is based on the formula that a *lingual* unilateral cross-bite involving an entire posterior segment indicates a bilateral palatal constriction. The amount of measurable palatal constriction is approximately one half the buccolingual thickness of the molars that are in cross-bite, or about 3.5 to 5 mm.

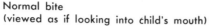

Normal bite
(viewed as if looking into child's mouth)

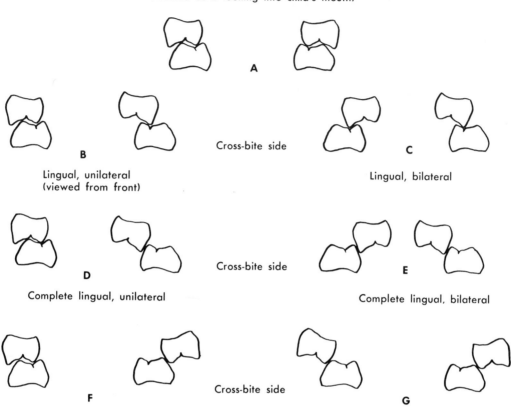

Fig. 12-3. The six possible posterior cross-bite molar relationships. Note that molars in cross-bite are toward the center of the page in the unilateral cases shown on the left.

Table 14. Approximate amounts of maxillary expansion or constriction needed in treating posterior cross-bites

Type of posterior cross-bite	Expansion (mm.)	Constriction (mm.)	Length of treatment (months)
Unilateral			
Lingual	3.5 to 5		3 to 4
Complete lingual	8 to 10		6 to 8
Buccal		3.5 to 5	2 to 3
Bilateral*			
Lingual	8 to 10		6 to 8
Complete lingual	15 to 20		6 to 12
Buccal		8 to 10	6 to 8

*All posterior cross-bites expressed *bilaterally* should be referred to an orthodontist, with the possible exception of bilateral lingual types.

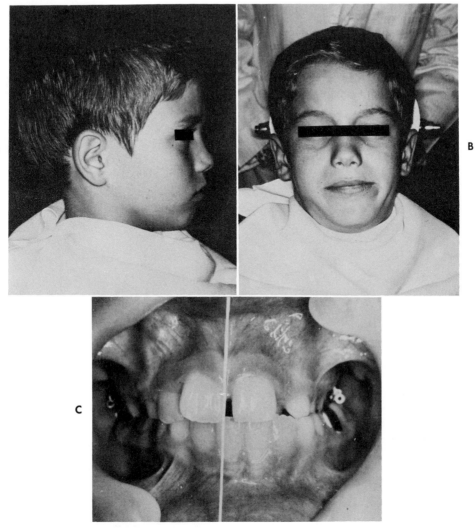

Fig. 12-4. Boy, age 8½, exhibiting a functional posterior cross-bite, Class I, Type 4. **A,** Profile view. **B,** Front, full-face view. Note his chin is shifted to the left, giving him an odd, "truculent" look. **C,** Front view. Note how the dental floss held in midsagittal plane discloses a mandibular shift to the side of the cross-bite, as expected, but also that the upper dental midline has migrated slightly to the left. Visible are double buccal tubes preparatory to fitting a heavy wire labial arch with lingual extension arms. (See Fig. 12-10.)

The *complete lingual* unilateral cross-bite represents a palatal constriction in the amount of the full buccolingual width of the molar that is in crossbite. This is approximately twice that of the lingual crossbite, or about 8 to 10 mm.

In a *buccal* cross-bite there exists the opposite situation to a palatal constriction.

There is, instead, *expansion* of one half the width of the molar, or an added dimension of 3.5 to 5 mm. across the palate, which will need to be reduced during treatment. Treatment in this case will consist of constricting the width of the upper arch to the proper dimension. The approximate amount of constriction may be estimated by referring to the entries in Table 14.

Accurate intermolar measurements as aid to diagnosis

Measurements taken across the palate will also separate the unilateral from the bilateral cross-bite, since the bilateral cross-bite demonstrates a palatal constriction approximately twice that of a unilateral one.

By measuring with a Boley gauge across the palate (buccal surface of one molar to buccal surface of the opposite molar) the existing dimension may be compared to the hoped-for dimension after bilateral palatal *expansion* (or *constriction* in the case of *buccal* posterior cross-bites) to produce cross-bite correction. The intermolar dimension of the lower arch is an important measurement to establish also. In measuring 100 cases with normal occlusion, I found that the normal intermolar dimension of the *upper* arch may be obtained by measuring the *lower* arch from the buccal surface of one 6-year molar to the buccal surface of the opposite 6-year molar and adding 2 mm. It must again be emphasized that this rule-of-thumb formula to estimate in millimeters the palatal expansion needed in the upper arch is applicable only in younger children whose cross-bite has been present for a short period of perhaps less than 3 years. Usually treatment of children beyond the age of 10 years will be referred to the orthodontic specialist, since by this age the alveolar bone of the mandible has responded to the unusual forces present in the cross-bite and has itself undergone change.

TREATING THE SIX COMBINATIONS OF POSTERIOR CROSS-BITES

In treating the six combinations of posterior cross-bite there are necessarily duplications in the uses of appliances. Important in each one of the six combinations, however, is the difference in the *distance* the teeth will have to be moved to reduce the cross-bite malocclusion and produce a normal occlusion (Table 14).

Lingual cross-bites expressed unilaterally

Lingual cross-bites are expressed by the child as a convenience, or functional, cross-

Fig. 12-5. Girl, age 7½ years, exhibiting a functional posterior unilateral cross-bite. There is a decided shift of the mandible to the side of the cross-bite on closure. The anterior openbite is the result of a tongue thrust during swallowing. Her speech was tested after a pronounced lisp was noted by the dentist. After consultation with the speech therapist it was agreed that the dentist should reduce the cross-bite first, then speech therapy would be instituted. The cross-bite correction was accomplished using a palatal expansion plate, but no follow-up pictures are available. **A,** Front view. **B,** Right view. **C,** Left view.

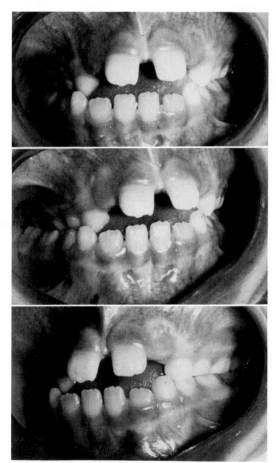

A

B

C

bite on only one side of the arch and are among the most common malocclusions seen in children (Figs. 12-5 and 12-6). During bite closure a mandibular shift will nearly always be present as the child seeks to avoid cuspal prematurities. As treatment progresses, there may be a period of time when the child is without a comfortable, stable bite, due to changing cuspal relationships. When it is borne in mind that the general treatment is bilateral expansion of the upper arch over a period of several months, this is more true when all the teeth in the posterior segment are seen to be in lingual cross-bite. Occasionally only the second primary molar or the 6-year molar will be found to have erupted in lingual cross-bite. In such cases there will be no discomfort during the bite change.

One-tooth lingual cross-bites

When only one maxillary molar is found to be in lingual cross-bite, it is assumed that only this one upper molar is out of

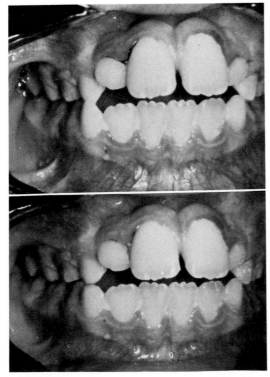

A

B

position. Therefore the treatment should include an application of forces that, ideally, will move only the tooth which is out of position. The forces brought to bear against the tooth should remain until the malposed tooth has moved to where it occludes in a normal fashion with the opposing molar. Retentive forces, only, are then held against the tooth until it has stabilized in its new position. Usually retention is considered to be necessary for a 3-month period.

Bands, hooks, and cross-elastics. For a one-tooth lingual cross-bite the most efficient method of reducing the malocclusion is the use of bands, hooks, and cross-elastics. The upper tooth in cross-bite and the lower opposing tooth are fitted carefully with bands. A hook (or button) is spot-welded or soldered on the palatal side of the upper band. On the lower band the hook is placed on the buccal side in the same fashion. (See Fig. 12-7.)

An orthodontic latex elastic, size $\frac{3}{16}$-inch medium, is placed so that it engages the hooks and is worn by the child day and night at all times except during meals. Under normal conditions most one-tooth lingual cross-bites may be reduced to normal occlusion in a space of 3 weeks to 3 months by such a course of treatment.

No adjustments are necessary during treatment, although a heavier elastic may be incorporated after the first 2 weeks if the child is having the problem of biting through the smaller one. Also, two elastics may be worn at one time if the dentist deems it advisable, once the movement of the upper molar is begun.

When placing the elastic on the hooks, the child is asked to slip it onto the index

Fig. 12-6. **A,** Boy, age 8 years, has a locked bite due to the right primary cuspids' being in cross-bite. Simple disking may improve his lateral excursions and, it is hoped, the health of his gingival tissues. **B,** Same boy, shown after disking procedure on the cuspids has freed the locked bite.

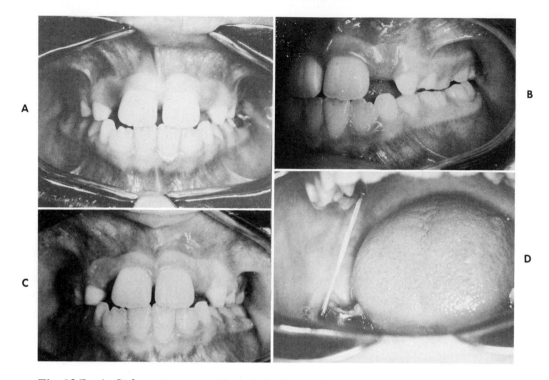

Fig. 12-7. A, Girl age 8 years, with a skeletal cross-bite involving the upper left 6-year molar. At this age the use of cross-elastics should reduce the cross-bite in 2 to 6 weeks. In this case it took 3 months, probably because it was my daughter. **B** and **C,** Same girl, age 8 years, 3 months. Cross-bite reduction has been accomplished. Left view and front view. **D,** Lingual buttons spot-welded to the molar bands may be used instead of hooks. Shown here is a boy, age 8, being treated for lingual cross-bite involving 6|.

finger of his writing hand so it is about ¼ inch from the fingertips. By "wiping" the ball of his finger over the upper hook, then twisting and crooking his finger slightly, he can stretch the elastic down to the lower hook and engage it. The child learns to do this rapidly and should be praised for his dexterity.

Cross-bite elastics should be renewed each day the child wears them. This is best done in the morning before school. A small supply should accompany him to school in case he loses his elastics while replacing them after eating lunch or chews them in two during classes.

Although it would seem as if this cross-elastic appliance would necessarily produce equal and opposite forces that would move the molar in cross-bite buccally and the normally positioned lower molar in a lingual direction, this is not the case. The softer and more cancellous upper alevolar bone allows the upper tooth to do almost all the movement under the forces generated by these elastics. The firmer mandibular bone and the inherent angulation of the mandibular molar combine to resist the forces that are acting to dislodge it. In a practical fashion, then, the upper tooth is seen to move out of cross-bite into a more normal bite, with negligible change in the position of the lower banded molar.

Posterior segment lingual cross-bites

A lingual cross-bite involving the whole posterior segment and expressed as a unilateral lingual cross-bite as the child closes fully into his occlusion is a common malocclusion in children. Usually the primary cuspid is seen to be in cross-bite also in these cases. It is in these children that a mandibular shift of 2 to 4 mm. to the cross-bite side is seen as they close into their convenience, or functional, bite. This shift on closure is most easily identified by holding a 15-inch length of dental floss in the midsagittal plane of the child's face while his teeth are apart and then having him close into his bite *slowly*.

The presence of the mandibular shift on closure is one of the clues that the cross-bite is in reality due to a bilateral constriction of the maxilla, even though functionally in the child's bite it is expressed as a unilateral cross-bite. Another clue will be the comparison of intermolar measurements between upper molars and between lower molars. The proper intermolar dimension of the *upper* arch is obtained by adding 2 mm. to the intermolar dimension of the *lower* arch. (See Table 14 and Fig. 12-3.) Once it has been determined that the amount of expansion of the upper arch needed is of the order of 3.5 to 5 mm., the appliance to produce the expansion may be selected. In general, the greater the amount of expansion needed in the upper arch, the more the choice would favor a removable appliance. The split-palate removable appliances produce forces that act against the soft tissue of the palate as well as the upper posterior teeth. These forces acting slowly will expand the palate by molding the alveolar ridges in a buccal direction. If adjusted to provide harsher forces, such appliances can cause "palate splitting" to occur, which results in a separating (visible by radiograph) of the bony suture in the midline of the palate.

It is not advocated here that the generalist or the pedodontist follow the rapid, palate-splitting method of upper arch expansion to reduce posterior cross-bite. Too few definitive studies have been published to show that this method should be used by any but an orthodontic specialist.[1] The slower, palatal expansion method accomplished over a period of 3 to 6 months appears at this time to be better suited to the capabilities of the generalist and pedodontist unless he has received special training in rapid expansion techniques.

Three appliances may be used to produce slow expansion of the upper arch. The fixed, banded, heavy labial arch and the Porter (or W) appliance may be utilized to provide expansion up to 5 mm. The acrylic split-palate appliance utilizing a jackscrew may be used for those cases where the desired amount of expansion exceeds 5 mm.

Split-palate removable appliance. The upper split palate removable appliance is much like an upper Hawley appliance with the labial bow removed and a spring-loaded jackscrew or a heavy wire (0.040) bent in the form of a long narrow U embedded in the midline of the palatal portion of the appliance. There are slight advantages to each kind of expansion device, but both are adjusted in approximately the same fashion and each produces the same result.

Adjustments of jackscrew type. The jackscrew type of split-palate appliance incorporates a small thin jackscrew that is spring-loaded to maintain its adjusted position and permit an overall expansion of exactly 4.5 mm. to the limits of the jackscrew drive (Fig. 12-8). The screw drive is activated by a small pin that acts as a wrench to force the shaft to rotate and expand the two halves of the appliance. This ensures bilaterally directed pressures against each side of the palate.

The wrench pin is inserted into the distal side of the drive shaft and pressed in a mesial direction to produce an expansion of the crack cut in the midline of the appliance. Each forward turn of the jackscrew opens the midline 0.25 mm. This allows the dentist to instruct the parents in the method of using the wrench and asking them to make a "one-turn appliance adjustment every Sunday morning." Over a month's time this will produce about a 1.2

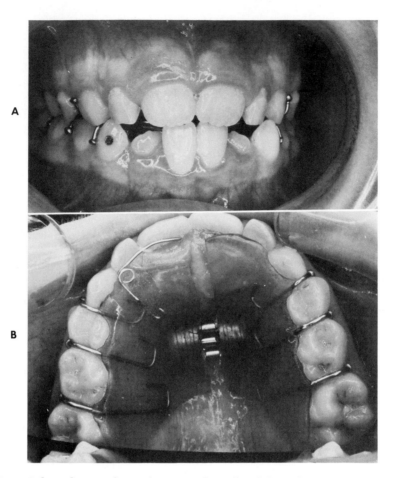

Fig. 12-8. Split-palate appliance being used to effect bilateral expansion. **A,** Front view. Note that "ball clasps" are fitted interproximally to increase retention. **B,** Palatal view. Adjustments may be made by turning the driving screw one half of a full turn every 2 weeks. *Rapid palatal expansion resulting in a separation of the maxillary midline suture is not recommended!* Note that a helical spring has been added to move the upper right central incisor labially.

mm. expansion of the palate. During a period of 3 months an expansion of about 4.5 mm. should be accomplished. In most lingual unilateral cross-bite cases this amount of slow palatal expansion should come very close to reducing the cross-bite.

If the expansion proceeds at the normal pace of 1.2 mm. a month and an expansion of 4.5 mm. is achieved, reaching the limit of the screw drive, a careful examination of the occlusion should be done. If a small amount of further expansion is found to be needed, the appliance must be remade.

A new alginate impression of each arch is taken (for diagnostic purposes), and the new split-palate appliance is adjusted to provide continued expansion as before.

Retention after treatment. When the proper dimension of expansion has been reached, the child may either continue to wear the appliance "as is" for a retainer, or the separated area in the middle of the appliance may be filled in with acrylic and the solid appliance worn as a retainer for a period of 3 months. Under normal circumstances the child will be seen each 2 or 3

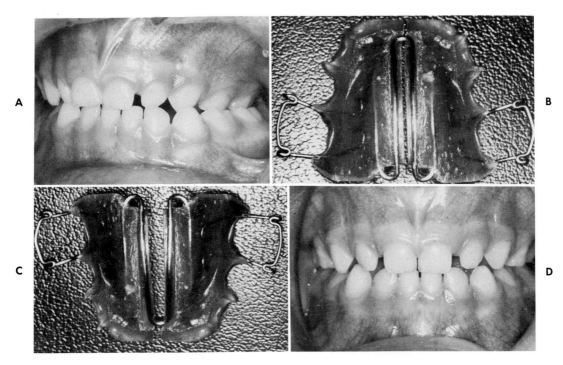

Fig. 12-9. A, A 5-year-old child, with an expressed unilateral posterior cross-bite involving |B C D E. There is a 3 mm. mandibular shift that cannot be seen when the midlines are compared at this angle. **B,** Upper U-loop palatal expansion appliance used to treat this posterior cross-bite in the deciduous dentition. Appliance is shown as it was fabricated and before activation of the U-loop expansion device. **C,** Same U-loop expansion appliance at the end of 4 months' treatment time. **D,** Front view after treatment, showing that posterior cross-bite has been corrected. Note the midline discrepancy has been almost totally corrected. (Courtesy Dr. Theodore R. Oldenburg, Chapel Hill, N. C.)

weeks in the dentist's office so that he may check the treatment progress. *At each visit he will take an intermolar measurement of the upper arch of the child, using the modified Boley gauge.* This will allow him to monitor the progress of the expansion of the arch by comparing each new measurement with the one taken as the previous office visit. Nearly all uncertainty regarding the progress of the case is removed if these measurements are conscientiously taken and entered in the dental chart at each appointment.

After a retention period of 3 months some recontouring of teeth may be done. Usually this is limited to disking the primary cuspids on the side of the cross-bite,

but occasionally the deciduous molars may need cuspal adjustment for better occlusion. Seldom will the 6-year molar need to be recontoured in such a fashion.

Adjustments of U wire spring type. Occasionally the dentist will feel that the split-palate appliance should be designed utilizing the narrow U wire spring in the midline of the palate instead of the jackscrew (Fig. 12-9). The U wire design has two advantages over the jackscrew: (1) it may be made with less palatal bulk so that the child's tongue pattern in swallowing and speech is not disrupted as much and (2) the U wire may be adjusted beyond 4.5 mm. without having to remake the appliance as in the jackscrew type.

One precaution must be observed with the U wire type, however. The U-shaped wire is quite easy to open carelessly, and a warp in the appliance is achieved that makes it difficult to fit. In other words, a wire that can be adjusted in two dimensions absolutely must be adjusted in only one—to make it wider. If this is not done, no amount of wire bending will seemingly return it to its original fit, and the appliance may have to be remade.

Since there are no measurable jackscrew turns to keep track of, the parents cannot adjust this type of appliance at home, and the dentist will see the child every 2 weeks for routine adjustments. Each time he sees the child he will measure the intermolar dimension of the upper arch as well as the expanding space in the middle of the appliance. Cross-checking these two measurements will enable him to keep a close watch on the progress of the child's upper arch expansion.

Retention after treatment. When sufficient expansion has been accomplished, an alginate impression is taken with the appliance in place, and on the plaster cast the expansion space in the middle of the appliance is filled in with acrylic and polished. Ideally the child will wear this as the retainer appliance for a period of 3 months.

Heavy labial arch appliance. The heavy labial arch appliance may be used to reduce a lingual unilateral cross-bite in either the primary or the mixed dentition. It is a versatile appliance to use and easily adjusted, but it has the disadvantage that the forces it generates tend to act more against the teeth themselves than against the alveolar ridges. This may produce a buccal "splaying" of upper molars during the bilateral expansion to correct a lingual cross-bite. Teeth tipped excessively in a buccal direction present a poor angulation for good occlusion.

In primary dentition. The use of the heavy labial arch to reduce a cross-bite in the primary dentition has the following advantages: (1) it is a fixed appliance and cannot be removed by the child (although don't challenge a child to disprove this!); (2) only the second primary molars need be banded; and (3) the forces creating the expansion in the upper arch may be measured with a Dontrix gauge. (See Fig. 12-10.)

The labial wire of the appliance may be made of 0.040 or 0.036 wire. This fits into a comparably sized buccal tube that has been spot-welded on the buccal surface of each band fitted on the deciduous second molars. A hook is soldered on the arch wire at the mesial opening of the round buccal tube to act both as a stop and as a hook to allow the arch wire to be ligated around the distal end of the buccal tube and so be stabilized in the child's mouth as a fixed appliance.

On the palatal side a lingual arm of 0.036 wire extends mesially to the mesial aspect of the cuspid. This wire is contoured so that it is closely adjacent to the primary first molar and cuspid. As the labial wire is adjusted to expand the arch, the lingual arms act to carry the teeth that they contact in a buccal direction.

ADJUSTMENTS. For the first week of wear the appliance is adjusted so that it is passive in the child's mouth. There is little or no discomfort, and for the 4- to 6-year-old child it is usually a simple matter to adapt to the presence of the appliance. Since the labial wire is visible in his smile, the child can be asked at the first appointment how many people he has shown his appliance to. This question usually opens up a Pandora's box of names of the child's friends and relatives and serves as a nice bridge toward continued rapport.

At the first and each subsequent 2-week appointment the labial wire is removed by cutting the ligating tie wire at each molar buccal tube and recontoured so that it has a 3 mm. expansion dimension built into it. This may be seen when one end is inserted into the buccal tube and the other end compared to the tube position. When the heavy labial arch is used in this fashion, about 4 ounces of force are generating the expansion movement in the upper arch. This may be checked by finger-con-

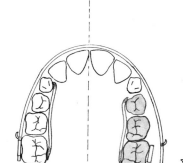

Fig. 12-10. A, Child's lingual cross-bite being treated using heavy wire labial arch. This appears to be the most versatile of all appliances to use in treatment of posterior cross-bites, due to its easy removal for adjustment. In the younger child only the two molars are banded, as a rule. In the older child, the central and lateral incisors are usually banded for added anchorage and stabilization of the labial wire. **B,** Drawing showing heavy labial arch appliance unsupported by anchorage to upper anterior teeth. Note arch wire is sprung about 3 mm. buccally to produce the force to move teeth on shaded side of arch out of cross-bite. Compare lengths of soldered lingual arms and note that there should be greater movement in a buccal direction *on the cross-bite side* than on the anchorage side. *a,* Hook of 0.020 wire is soldered to the arch wire to serve both as a stop and as an attachment to secure the ligature wire twisted around the end of the arch wire. *b,* Alternative to *a,* soldered U-loop spring that serves as an adjustable stop as well as an attachment for ligature tying.

touring the labial arch wire to fit passively into the buccal tubes and tracing the wire's inside outline on a piece of paper. The arch is then recontoured to expand it 3 mm., and the Dontrix gauge is used horizontally against the paper to test the amount of force needed to return the expanded spring to its original traced outline on the paper.

RETENTION AFTER TREATMENT. After the completion of arch expansion over a period of about 3 months the labial arch wire is left ligated in place as a passive appliance for 2 additional months to ensure retention. Such an appliance has proved to be one of the most trouble-free in use in my practice.

In mixed dentition. For use in mixed-dentition lingual cross-bites the heavy labial arch undergoes a slight modification. The four upper anterior teeth are usually banded for stabilization of the arch wire. The positions of the bands and the single edgewise anterior brackets centered on their labial surfaces are most important. The reason for this is that adjustment steps in a gingivoincisal direction are difficult to incorporate in a heavy wire arch to take care of discrepancies in the level of the brackets.

ADJUSTMENTS. Other than the factor involving bracket levels, this labial arch appliance is adjusted exactly the same as the one to reduce lingual cross-bites in the primary dentition. As the adjustment periods progress, however, it will be found that the U-loop adjustment springs on this mixed dentition appliance may need to be opened slightly as the expansion of the arch progresses. This relieves the pressure against the anterior teeth.

For each adjustment it is suggested that the appliance be removed by cutting the four ligative ties holding the labial wire to the anterior brackets. Then the expansion adjustment of the arch wire may be done before the wire is religated into place. The U-loops may each be expanded perhaps 1 mm.

As described in the chapter on anterior

cross-bites, lip balm or other emollient may be necessary for the child when he is first wearing the heavy labial arch appliance. Chapped or abraded lips can be very uncomfortable during the first week.

RETENTION AFTER TREATMENT. The retention period of 3 months poses no problems in the use of this appliance. The labial arch appliance may be left in place for this period, or a Hawley appliance may be fabricated to serve as a retainer. Since final impressions and casts are to be accomplished anyway, the Hawley appliance is usually the best choice for the retention period.

Porter, or W, *appliance.* The Porter, or

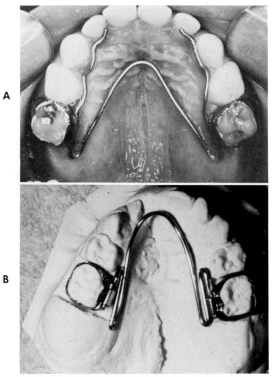

Fig. 12-11. A, Fixed Porter appliance. This appliance must be removed from the child's mouth to be adjusted properly and must then be recemented. **B,** Fixed-removable Porter appliance on a plaster cast of child with a surgically corrected cleft palate. Such an appliance can be removed for adjustment during the treatment of a posterior cross-bite.

W, appliance has the advantage of being a fixed appliance and is particularly effective in treating a lingual cross-bite requiring bilateral expansion in the primary dentition. Although it is usually made as a fixed soldered appliance, with the disadvantage that it cannot be removed from the child's mouth for adjustments, it is a far superior appliance when made with molar lingual tubes to serve as a fixed-removable appliance (Fig. 12-11).[5,7]

Two of the chief disadvantages of this appliance are the difficulty in bending the lingual wire to the configuration necessary and the difficulty in adjusting it, either in or out of the mouth, to achieve the proper minimal pressures needed to expand upper deciduous arches slowly. Most dentists find themselves having achieved the expansion at much too rapid a pace for the health of the teeth and their periodontium.

Adjustment of these appliances should take place once a month, with most of the adjusting pressure gained by *equal* adjustments of mesial bends in the arch wire. Admittedly this take some skill, but many dentists believe that this is the only appliance to use in deciduous cross-bite cases. For those in the mixed dentition it does not work as well and is not recommended.

Lingual cross-bites expressed bilaterally

Bilaterally expressed lingual cross-bites are not common malocclusions. As the child closes into his occlusion, there is seen to be either no mandibular shift or a minimal one. The correction of such a malocclusion may be carried out by the generalist or the pedodontist, using either type of split-palate expansion appliance just described in the section dealing with lingual unilateral cross-bites. This may be accomplished during either the primary dentition or the mixed dentition.

Split-palate appliance. The fabrication and adjustment of the split-palate appliance is carried out exactly as previously described except that the expansion necessary to produce a proper occlusion is of the order of 8 to 10 mm. and will take a correspondingly longer time to accomplish. A period of 6 months' treatment must usually be allowed for, with an additional 6 months for retention. (See Table 14.)

Since this implies a period of 1 year during which the dentist will be actively treating or checking closely for retention, the child must be younger than 10 years when the case is started, or the pubertal growth period can be encroached upon. To attempt this in an older child is to deny the orthodontist his opportunity for using the time of best growth potential for the corrective treatment of malocclusions.

Complete lingual cross-bites expressed unilaterally

Complete lingual cross-bites that are expressed unilaterally by the child are quite unusual and will be seen infrequently by the general dentist. The etiology is usually a genetic malpositioning of some of the upper posterior teeth. In this malocclusion one or more of the upper posterior teeth on one side occlude completely lingual to their opposing teeth in the lower arch. Referral is best in such cases.

In almost all cases the maxillary teeth in cross-bite are seen to be positioned closer to the midpalatal line than the paired teeth in the opposite side of the arch. Clearly the treatment indicated is not the simple bilateral expansion of the maxillary arch. Instead, treatment by the specialist will be aimed at expanding a selected segment of alveolar bone and its enclosed teeth in a buccal direction over a distance of 10 to 12 mm. (See Table 14.)

For the task of moving a portion of the posterior segment buccally a modification of the split-palate appliance is needed. Again, as in the case of the lingual unilateral cross-bites previously described, either the offset jackscrew or the U spring of 0.040 wire can be incorporated into the appliance.

Offset jackscrew split-palate appliance. The offset jackscrew appliance is a removable appliance that can be prepared so that the force generated by expanding the drive of the jackscrew can be applied to only a portion of the alveolar ridge and teeth of an upper posterior segment. By splitting the appliance in an unequal, or offset, fashion, the selected segment is moved outward while the entire remainder of the arch, both soft and hard tissues, acts as the anchorage.

Adjustments. In this instance the design of the appliance must be accomplished only after the diagnosis has been double-checked. Should teeth on the opposite side of the arch from the complete lingual cross-bite begin to move, then chaos could result, and certainly the case would be mistreated rather than treated.

The adjustments of the jackscrew are therefore better made in the dentist's office than by the parents at home. Two or three single adjustments of the jackscrew every 2 weeks will succeed in producing about 1 to 1.5 mm. of buccal movement of the segment in cross-bite each month. Because the distance the segment must be moved is always at least twice the distance of the screw-drive, the appliance must be remade at least once and perhaps twice. This probability should be planned for when a case is presented to the parents at the beginning. Certainly not every generalist or pedodontist will want to accept such a cross-bite for treatment. The depth of experience and skill needed to treat this is decidedly greater than that for the much simpler unilateral lingual cross-bites in which only a relatively small amount of bilateral expansion is required.

U wire spring split-palate appliance. The U wire spring split-palate appliance demonstrates its versatility in the case of complete lingual cross-bite expressed unilaterally. If the U wire spring is properly formed and the U shape of the wire is kept narrow (2 to 3 mm. across the U), then the potential for expansion of a selected posterior segment of teeth may be as much as 10 mm. before the appliance must be remade.

Differing from Fig. 12-9, *B* and *C*, the U-loop of wire is embedded in the split-palate appliance to the cross-bite side of the midpalatal line. The acrylic is split (cut with a metal wheel, see Chapter 15) palatally from a position mesial to the cuspid so that it meets a cut of perhaps 5 mm. made parallel to the midpalatal line but toward the cross-bite side.

By opening the U wire loop, a force is generated only against the teeth in complete lingual cross-bite, while the anterior teeth, the posterior teeth on the other side of the arch, and the palatal tissue serve as anchorage.

Adjustments. Just as with jackscrew appliances used to treat posterior cross-bite cases, this appliance should not be opened more than 1 to 1.5 mm. at any one adjustment. With careful use, it will not only move the selected teeth buccally so that the cross-bite is reduced but will also exert forces against the alveolar bone at the same time. This results in a better occlusion and less buccal "splaying" of the teeth that have been moved out of cross-bite.

Each adjustment is best done with the No. 139 pliers. It is tempting to use the thumb and fingers to spread the split-palate appliance apart. Unfortunately this results too often in a three-dimensional adjustment, and the appliance may not be able to be fitted back into the child's mouth properly. Of all of the appliances described in this book, perhaps the U wire spring type of split-palate appliance deserves the reputation of being most difficult to adjust. This is even more true of the one just described used to treat a complete lingual cross-bite unilaterally expressed by the child.

Complete lingual cross-bites expressed bilaterally

The treatment of complete lingual cross-bites expressed bilaterally by the child is best left to the specialist in orthodontics. The reasons for this become clear when the intermolar measurements are compared

in Table 14 and the sketch of such a cross-bite is seen in Fig. 12-3.

The expansion needed in the palatal arch of such a child is 15 to 20 mm. In some cases it is even more. The expertise of generalists usually does not extend to tooth movement of this magnitude.

A series of split-palate appliances may be used by the orthodontist to gain the necessary palatal dimension in such cases. As a rule the treatment may extend over more than a year's time.

Buccal cross-bites expressed unilaterally

Cases in which one tooth or a whole posterior segment of teeth erupt in buccal version to the opposing lower teeth are less often seen than the lingual unilateral and lingual bilateral cross-bite cases whose treatment has already been described. Most often seen will be one-tooth buccal cross-bite cases.

One-tooth buccal cross-bites

The most commonly seen cases of one-tooth buccal cross-bites in posterior segments involve the upper 6-year molar or the upper first bicuspid. Both types may be treated in much the same fashion.

In the case of a 6-year molar that has erupted in buccal version to its opposing lower molar, the term *ectopic eruption* might be pertinent. However, the use of this term usually indicates a *mesial* inclination and not a *buccal* inclination.

Being the most distal tooth in the upper arch at this age, the maxillary 6-year molar can erupt in a buccal position and be moved to a normal bite position fairly easily, since there is no problem involving inadequate space in the arch. Although other appliances may be used to treat this one-tooth buccal cross-bite, the cross-elastic is perhaps the best approach.

Bands, hooks and cross-elastics. The use of bands, hooks, and cross-elastics in a buccal cross-bite involving one tooth is quite parallel to the use of this appliance in correcting a one-tooth lingual posterior cross-bite. The sole difference is that the hooks to engage the elastics are placed exactly oppositely to those in treatment of lingual cross-bite. Thus in the buccal cross-bite the upper hook is placed on the *buccal* surface, and the lower is placed on the lingual surface of the molar band. (Compare with Fig. 12-7, *D.*)

After 3 to 4 weeks of having the child wear the cross-elastics at all times except when he is eating his meals, a change in the buccolingual relationships of the two molars should be discernible. For a child older than 7 or 8 years the buccal cross-bite correction process takes a longer time. If after 3 months of wear the maxillary molar has not moved sufficiently in a lingual direction to create a normal Class I situation, a change of appliance might be in order.

First bicuspid may erupt in a "dental" cross-bite

In an older child the maxillary first bicuspid may erupt in what has been termed a "dental" cross-bite.[3] Commonly this is seen to be the result of a lack of proper space in the upper arch to contain the erupting permanent cuspid and the first and second bicuspids. The most common cross-bite into which the upper first bicuspid erupts is a buccal one.

To successfully treat such a cross-bite the dentist must usually solve two problems: (1) regain enough arch space mesiodistally to permit the cuspid and two bicuspids to occupy their normal positions in the arch and (2) when space is available, move the first bicuspid lingually into its normal bite position.

The first problem may be solved by the use of an extraoral force cervical appliance or an upper Hawley appliance with a distalizing spring placed against the molar. Both these devices can be adjusted to provide selective force to distalize the mesially tipped or drifted 6-year molar that was the culprit which caused the lack of space for the buccally erupting bicuspid.

The second part of the problem cannot be solved until enough space is gained in the arch circumference to contain the added mesiodistal dimension of the buccally located biscuspid. This tooth may be moved lingually by either of the fixed labial arches, of course. However, if the Hawley appliance with a distal spring is used to exert force against the 6-year molar, then the same appliance may be used to move the bicuspid lingually. All it takes is the addition of an S spring of 0.025 wire to create the force needed for movement.

It must again be urged that no lingually directed force be applied to move the bicuspid that is out of alignment unless the space in the arch is adequate to contain the tooth. First, gain the space mesiodistally, and then the malposed tooth may be moved lingually.

If the buccal cross-bite involves more than one tooth, it should be clearly a case to be referred to the orthodontist. Almost certainly a facial dysplasia may be present when one whole upper quadrant is in buccal cross-bite.

Buccal cross-bites expressed bilaterally

In most cases of a buccal cross-bite expressed bilaterally, there is what appears to be micrognathia of the mandible. The entire upper arch appears to enclose the lower arch when the child attempts to occlude.

Although heavy labial arches may be used to treat certain upper *spaced* dentitions exhibiting this sort of occlusion, the problem here is usually seen to be one of genetic mismatching of the upper and lower arch sizes. More of these malocclusions are seen in retarded than in normal children, although such a malocclusion must certainly not be thought of as diagnostic for mental retardation. Such is not the case, as any orthodontist will tell you. These cases should be handled only in the orthodontist's office because of their genetic complexities.

Table 15. Summary of treatment methods for posterior cross-bites

Method used	Length of treatment	Age of child (years)
Disking of primary cuspids	2 to 4 weeks	2 to 6 years (Fig. 12-6)
Cross-bite elastics, hooks on banded molars	2 to 8 weeks	4 to 9 years (Fig. 12-7)
Heavy labial arch appliance	6 to 12 weeks	4 to 10 years (Fig. 12-10)
Porter (W) appliance	8 to 12 weeks	4 to 8 years (Fig. 12-11)
Split-palate appliance	8 to 12 weeks	4 to 10 years (Figs. 12-8 and 12-9)

SUMMARY

Posterior cross-bites have been described as having six possible combinations under usual circumstances. Of these the lingual unilateral, the lingual bilateral, the complete lingual unilateral, and the buccal one-tooth cross-bites are recommended for treatment by the generalist and the pedodontist. The lingual unilateral cross-bite, as it is expressed by the child in his convenience bite, has been described as a true *bilateral* constriction of the maxillary arch in most cases of younger children, causing a mandibular shift toward the cross-bite side during closure.

In older children the shift of the mandible may disappear as the maxillary and mandibular alveolar bony ridges distort under the pressures of the teeth occluding in an aberrant bucco-lingual fashion. If at all possible, the uncomplicated posterior cross-bites should be treated as soon as they are recognized in the child. They may be treated in the primary dentition as well as early and middle mixed dentition ages, but treatment by the generalist later than 10 years of age may cause an encroachment on the "prime time" of the pubertal period of growth. Treatment after this time should be deferred to the orthodontist. (See Table 15.)

REFERENCES

1. Graber, T. M.: Orthodontics: principles and practice, ed. 2, Philadelphia, 1966, W. B. Saunders Co., p. 561.
2. Mathews, J. R.: Malocclusion in the primary dentition, Dent. Clin. North Am., pp. 463-478, July, 1966.
3. McDonald, R. E.: Dentistry for the child and adolescent, St. Louis, 1969, The C. V. Mosby Co., pp. 361-364.
4. Moss, M. L.: The functional matrix. In Kraus, B. S., and Riedel, R. A., editors: Vistas in orthodontics, Philadelphia, 1962, Lea & Febiger, pp. 85-98.
5. Moyers, R. E.: Handbook of orthodontics, ed. 2, Chicago, 1963, Year Book Medical Publishers, Inc., p. 335.
6. Ibid., pp. 159-160.
7. Ibid., pp. 495-496.

13 | Treatment of mesially drifted 6-year molars

The loss of critical millimeters of space in the posterior segments of a child's arches can all too easily go unnoticed by the family dentist. The term *critical* is used accurately, because the loss of too much space may prevent the child from having sufficient arch space to allow the unimpeded eruption of the three teeth with which the dentist interested in space analysis is constantly concerned—the permanent cuspid and the first and second bicuspid. This professional inattention may leave no reasonable alternative at a later time other than four-bicuspid extraction and full-treatment orthodontics.

The conscientious dentist must be aware of the need for a series of measurements to determine the difference between the *existing space* he sees in the child's mouth and the *needed space* that will be required to allow a normal eruption sequence. Merely to "observe" a child who has lost critical space in the posterior segment is a waste of time. Moyers states pointedly that he has never seen a space-loss case under "careful observation" that progressed any better than a space-loss case at which no one was looking.[8] The point he makes is that space-regaining treatment should begin immediately after the realization on the part of the dentist that space loss is occurring in any posterior segment.

The tooth that can most often cause the loss of space is the 6-year molar. It accomplishes this by drifting mesially and encroaching onto the territory needed for the second bicuspid to erupt. The mesial drift of the 6-year molar is only the final act in a series of events that may initiate space loss, however.

THREE BASIC FACTORS PERMITTING MESIAL MOLAR DRIFT

In general, three basic factors may allow the 6-year molar to drift mesially and cause crowding in the bicuspid-bicuspid-cuspid (BBC) segment of the arch:

1. *Carious attack* in the mesial and distal areas of the primary molars. This may destroy enough of the substance of the crowns of these teeth to cause space loss.

2. *Ectopic eruption* of a 6-year molar. This seems to be the result of a genetic factor causing the erupting molar to be directed so far mesially that its eruption acts to resorb the distal root portions of the second primary molar and perhaps bring about the early loss of this tooth.

3. *Too early extraction* of primary molars by the dentist with no provision for

195

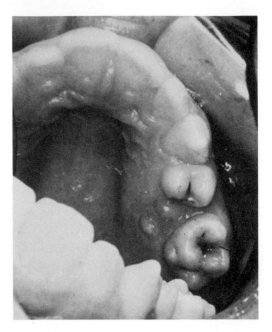

Fig. 13-1. Upper arch of 10-year-old boy whose upper left 6-year molar has drifted mesially. This was the result of the too early extraction of ⌊E, with no spacer being subsequently placed. ⌊5 has been blocked out palatally because it was the last succedaneous tooth to erupt in the quadrant. Treatment with either an upper Hawley appliance with a helical spring or an extraoral force appliance *might* enable the dentist to regain the space necessary to move ⌊5 into the arch.

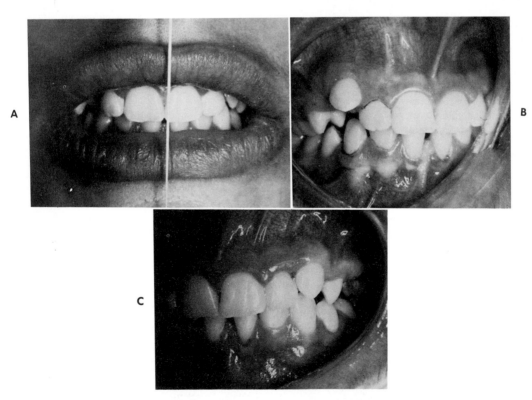

Fig. 13-2. Boy, age 11. **A,** Dental floss is held to simulate the midsagittal plane. This test shows that upper and lower dental midlines have not appreciably deviated. **B,** Right view shows crowding out of 3⌋ due to lack of space in quadrant. Questioning the parent revealed that D⌋ had been extracted several years previously, with no space maintainer having been placed. Amount of space lacking in this case was 3.5 mm., which could probably be regained using unilateral pressure against 6⌋ with an extraoral force appliance over a period of 6 to 9 months. **C,** Left view shows normalcy of occlusion on opposite side of arch.

placing a space maintainer (Figs. 13-1 and 13-2). Space loss of this sort may be termed iatrogenic (caused by the dentist).

When the basic arch relationships of the child is classified as Angle Class I and the only arch deformity is the drifting of a 6-year molar more than 1 mm. mesially, then the Dewey-Anderson classification is Type 5. (See Chapter 3.)

ESTIMATING AMOUNT OF SPACE TO REGAIN AFTER SPACE LOSS

As described in Chapters 4 and 8, there are several approaches to measuring the *amount* of space that has been lost. The key word is *measure*. Only by careful measurements can arch space analysis be accurate. It should be emphasized that if an upper molar has drifted mesially and caused *more* than 3 mm. loss of arch space, then some thought must be given to the possibility of an orthodontic consultation. The same limitation might be placed on the generalist if a lower molar has drifted mesially and caused more than a 2 mm. space loss.

There is an uncomplicated method of measuring with the Boley gauge the exact amount of space loss if it has occurred in only *one* upper or lower quadrant and no other deciduous teeth have been lost in posterior segments. The dentist may measure on the intact side of the arch the sum of the widths of deciduous teeth C D E and compare this measurement to the quadrant that has suffered loss of space. The difference in the two measurements will be the amount of space he must recover in his treatment procedure on the side that has suffered the loss of arch space. (See Chapter 4.)

Also, a grid may be made from a protractor. When aligned with the midpalatal line, the grid can indicate the amount of mesial drift that has occurred in one molar as compared to its antimere (Fig. 13-3).

APPLIANCES USED TO MOVE 6-YEAR MOLARS DISTALLY

To obtain distal movement of the 6-year molar, the following appliances can be used:

1. The upper or lower Hawley appliance with a helical or dumbbell spring in position against the mesial surface of a molar that has drifted forward
2. A lower F-R lingual arch with U-loops as compensating springs to gain pressure distally against the molars
3. An extraoral appliance (cervical ap-

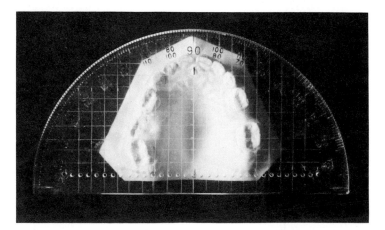

Fig. 13-3. Grid with 5 mm. squares scratched on a protractor has been placed over an upper cast. Distance the mesially drifted molar has moved can be demonstrated by comparing its position to that of its antimere in the opposite arch.

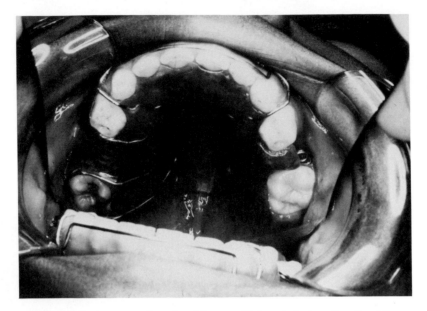

Fig. 13-4. Upper left 6-year molar of a 10-year-old boy is being distalized by an upper Hawley appliance with a posterior helical spring.

pliance or headgear) for the upper arch

4. Brass separating wires placed interproximally as an aid for gaining space in the whole quadrant or to distalize an ectopically erupting 6-year molar

It is substantially more difficult to move *lower* 6-year molars distally with appliance therapy than to accomplish the same movement with *upper* molars. The four appliances just described may be used, but extraoral force should not be used on the *lower* molars without an orthodontist's supervision. Therefore the lower Hawley appliance and the lower F-R lingual arch are the two obvious choices for controlled distal movement of lower molars.

Upper Hawley appliance. To move an upper 6-year molar distally with a Hawley appliance, a compressed helical spring is formed at a right angle to the alveolar ridge immediately adjacent to the mesial surface of the 6-year molar to be moved (Fig. 13-4). The spring is arranged so that it can be adjusted to maintain distally directed pressure over a distance of 3 to 4

mm. A spring made of 0.028 yellow Elgiloy or 0.020 Australian wire (see Table 17 for source of these materials) will produce the desired movement if it is positioned properly in the appliance and adjusted at intervals of 2 weeks.

For the molar across the arch from the mesially drifted molar, any one of a series of clasps can be used with the upper Hawley appliance. The Adams clasp, the modified Crozat clasp, or the C (circumferential) clasp are all recommended. (See Chapter 15.)

Lower Hawley appliance

With a helical spring. The lower Hawley appliance should have a labial bow with adjustment loops built into it labial to the cuspids. The wire passes *distal* to the cuspids over the ridge and is embedded in the body of the appliance on the lingual side of the alveolar ridge. This helps "unitize" the lower anterior teeth and so assists the whole lower arch in acting as a total anchorage unit. The wire for the labial bow may be made of 0.025 or 0.028 yellow Elgiloy. The helical spring posi-

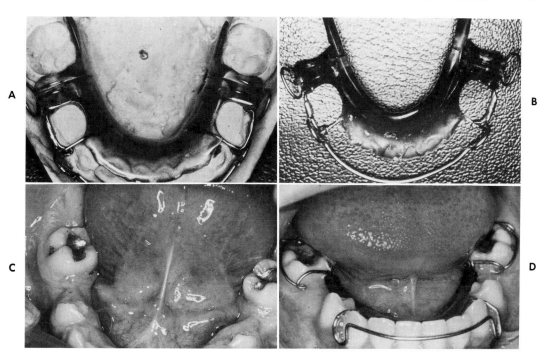

Fig. 13-5. Child, age 9, whose lower 6-year molars have both drifted mesially, encroaching on the arch space needed by the lower second bicuspids. A, Lower Hawley appliance with two dumbbell springs has been fabricated (shown on model). Note that acrylic is split through center of spring so adjustment of the spring will generate pressure distally against each 6-year molar. B, Lower Hawley appliance removed from child's mouth. C, Child's lower arch after 6 months of treatment with lower Hawley appliance. D, Another lower Hawley appliance in place, serving as a retention device. Retention must be maintained in these cases until the second bicuspids erupt through the crest of the alveolar ridge. (Courtesy Dr. Theodore R. Oldenburg, Chapel Hill, N. C.)

tioned against the mesial surface of the molar to be moved distally is made of either 0.028 Elgiloy or 0.020 Australian wire, the same as with the upper Hawley appliance.

The molar clasp on the opposite molar may be made of 0.036 blue or yellow Elgiloy if the C clasp is used. A combination of 0.028 and 0.025 yellow Elgiloy may be used for the modified Crozat clasp. The choice is 0.025 yellow Elgiloy if an Adams clasp is to be utilized. (See Table 17 for sources of these materials.)

The helical spring for the lower Hawley appliance may be made in two configurations, depending on the experience of the dentist. The *double* helical spring requires slightly more time to bend, but it is kinder to the periodontium of the tooth being repositioned. These helical springs should be adjusted with little or no pressure exerted distally against the molar during the first week of treatment. At the second visit and thereafter at intervals of 2 weeks, the springs should be adjusted to produce slight distal pressure against the 6-year molar. Constant measurements of the child's arch during treatment, with the modified Boley gauge, will give the dentist an exact indication of his progress in moving the molar distally. Usually it takes 2 to 4 months to move a lower molar a dis-

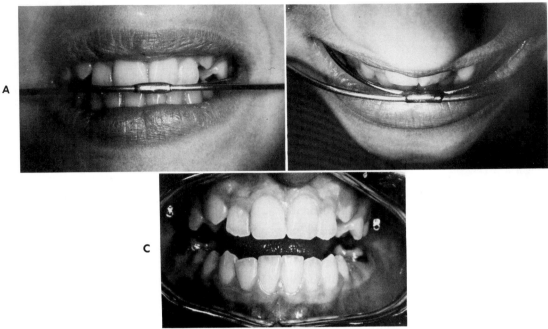

Fig. 13-7. Girl, age 10½ years, who exhibited *bilateral* lack of space to erupt upper cuspids. On the right side 2.5 mm. space was lacking; on the left, 3 mm. A, Extraoral force appliance, front view. This is a straight-pull cervical appliance (also called Kloehn cervical gear) that works best with younger children. The dentist using such an appliance should have training in its use. B, Cervical appliance shown is usually fitted so that at least 3 mm. clearance to the labial of the upper anterior teeth is available. This clearance will diminish as the molar(s) move distally. C, Double buccal tubes are attached to upper molar bands preparatory to fitting cervical extraoral force appliance. Treatment approach was to distalize both upper 6-year molars to a super–Class I position. D, Front view, closed. Note there has been a slight midline shift to the left in the upper arch. E and F, Age 11 years. E, Right view, demonstrating the upper right in labial position and overlapping of distal margin of 2|. F, Left view, showing |3 erupting into a labial position because of a lack of space. G, Age 11 years 4 months. Light labial arch is being used during treatment of the maxillary arch to establish a better position for the upper central and lateral incisors. Cuspids now have sufficient space into which to erupt.

accomplished by an auxiliary appliance such as a fixed light-wire labial arch. (See Fig. 10-9, *B*.)

2. *Tip* the crowns of one or both 6-year molars distally to their former position when they have undergone mesial tipping due to loss of one or both upper second primary molars.

3. *Bodily move* one or both maxillary 6-year molars distally.

4. *Retard maxillary growth* if a minimal but constant force is held for a long pe-

riod of time (months, or even years) against the upper 6-year molars in a distal direction. This can usually be done from about the eighth year to the tenth year, during which the maxillary growth potential acts in a forward direction. In a child whose maxilla seems to be too far anterior on the skeletal base and does not match the mandible (as in Class II malocclusion), a dramatic improvement in occlusion may result after wearing properly fitted and adjusted cervical gear for a

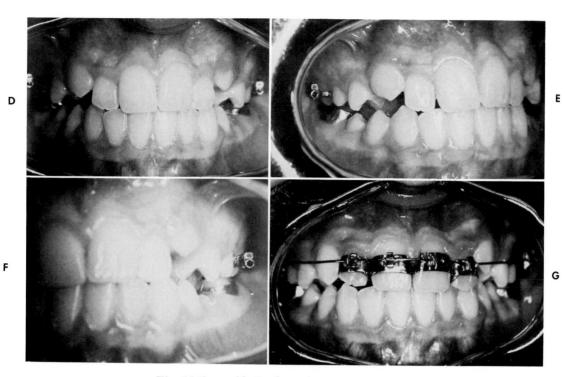

Fig. 13-7, cont'd. For legend see opposite page.

period of even 6 months to a year. Only a trained orthodontist or pedodontist should attempt the treatment of a Class II malocclusion by the use of cervical gear.

Also, such a cervical appliance must be worn *every night* for 12 to 14 hours by the child for it to be effective, which limits its application. Lack of parental discipline and the children's obedience patterns in some households will defeat the purpose of such an appliance before it is placed in the child's mouth. As has been emphasized before, no dentist can afford to charge a fee for an unsuccessful appliance.

One of the reasons for writing this section is to remove the aura of mystery that seems to surround the use of cervical gear and similar extraoral force appliances, which can so effectively control the positions of the upper molars as well as inhibit growth in the maxilla. It is not expected that anyone could become proficient in

the use of such appliances solely by diagrams and drawings. In a sense, this type of appliance should be more understood than used by the general dentist.

Because a large amount of *distally* directed force against permanent molars can be generated by this appliance with no reciprocal pressures against the other teeth, it is quite different in its treatment application from the other appliances outlined in this book. This section, however, should give the attentive reader a broad outline of how the forces generated by such appliances act to move or maintain the positions of upper molar teeth. If this goal seems limited, please remember that the limitations of this book have been clearly outlined in the preface.

At the end of this chapter will be found a section discussing the controversy over whether or not stimulation or inhibition of growth of the maxilla and mandible can occur and the future role the general dentist may play in such treatment for children.

Early distal positioning of deciduous molars can affect bicuspid positions. Many men have questioned the wisdom of correcting certain Class II malocclusions by the *early* use of extraoral force directed against the upper second deciduous molars. It has been asked, "What happens to the unerupted bicuspids?"

Mathews[6] notes that over thirty years

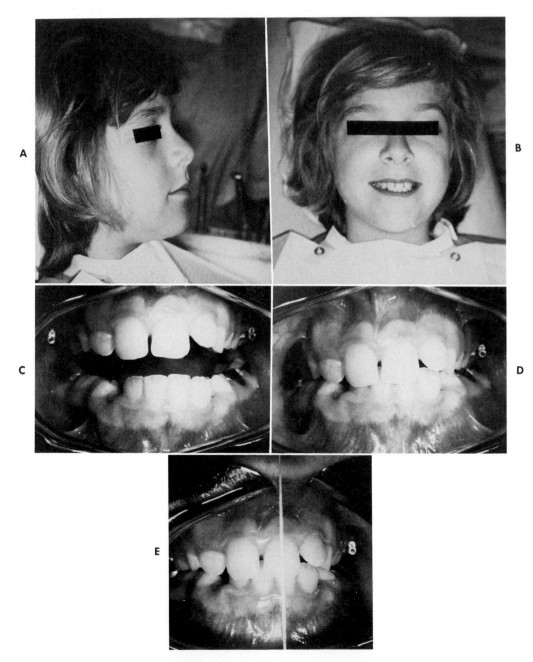

Fig. 13-8. For legend see p. 206.

ago Breitner demonstrated *movement of the unerupted permanent tooth buds* (italics added) when the overlying tooth was moved orthodontically. Mathews goes on to explain that the significance of this experiment apparently was not immediately realized by orthodontists. Serial cephalometric films have demonstrated beyond doubt that the positions of unerupted permanent teeth are influenced by orthodontic movement of the overlying deciduous teeth. (This also has obvious implications

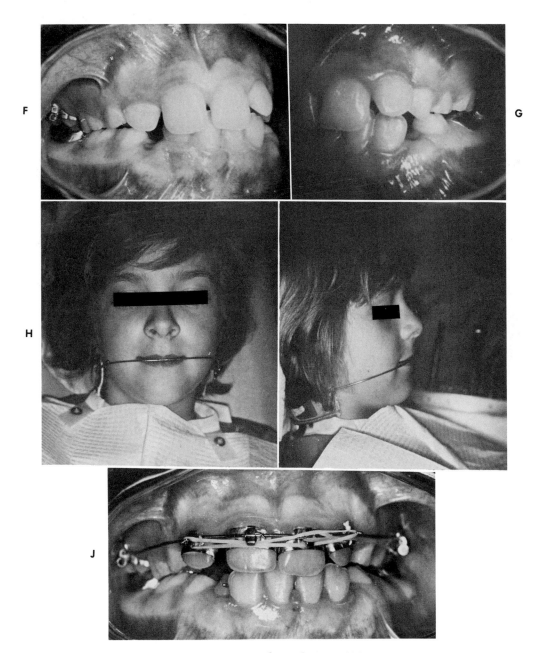

Fig. 13-8. For legend see p. 206.

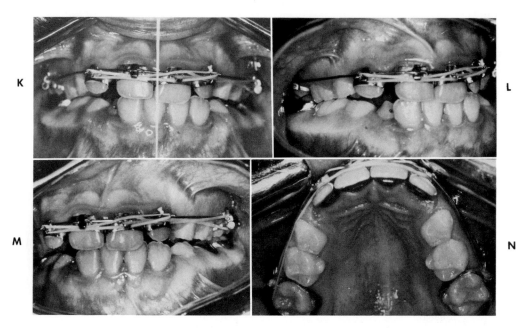

Fig. 13-8. Girl, age 10½ years, exhibited a congenitally missing C|. The upper dental midline had shifted rather dramatically to the right (see arrow rule, Fig. 4-10). The upper right 6-year molar had not drifted mesially. The lower anterior teeth had inclined lingually under the force of a hyperactive mentalis muscle as a result of her swallowing pattern, crowding the lower permanent cuspids. A mixed dentition analysis showed arch space was available for all permanent teeth to erupt if both collapsed arches were restored to normal arch perimeters. To accomplish this, anchorage positions of the upper 6-year molars has to be maintained. A, Side profile. B, Front view, smiling. C, Front view, open. D, Front view, closed. E, Front view, with midsagittal plane established by dental floss. Note severe midline shift in upper arch. Lower midline shift is slight. F, Right view. Note upper molar bands have been fitted with attached double buccal tubes and also fitted for a vertically attached F-R lingual arch. Note that 2| abuts against D| with no space left for the cuspid to erupt. G, Left view. Note lingual inclination of lower anteriors. H, Girl shown wearing cervical extraoral force appliance to provide anchorage while wearing an upper light-wire labial arch appliance. I, Side view showing "low pull" position of cervical gear. This appliance was worn 12 to 14 hours a day during treatment. J, Four months later the positions of the upper and lower anterior teeth have responded to the pressures exerted by the appliances. Upper midline has been corrected almost entirely by combined use of upper light labial arch and light elastics. In the use of the elastics, a major portion of the upper arch served as anchorage to move one or two teeth at a time. K, Midlines are checked each visit by use of dental floss. L, Right view. Note shift of 1 | 1 2 to the left under pressure of light elastics "trolleying" teeth along the light labial arch wire. A large diastema has been opened up between 2| and 1| as the result of selective pressures. M, Left view. Maxillary arch in process of becoming normal in its perimeter. N, Full palatal view demonstrating how arch has been restored to near-equal symmetry in both quadrants. Mixed dentition analysis accomplished at this stage, using combination analysis method (Chapter 4), showed that all permanent teeth could erupt into this arch. Treatment time was 11 months to this point. The author was called into the Armed Services at this time to serve as a pedodontist in the Army Dental Corps. The case was taken over by an orthodontist. Further pictorial records are not available.

when the early treatment of posterior cross-bite is contemplated.) This finding has practical significance for both the general dentist and the orthodontist. For example, if a Class II malocclusion in a 5-year-old child is corrected by multiple banding of the maxillary arch and the biting relation reduced to Class I by using occipital extraoral traction with care to avoid tipping the teeth distally, one may expect the unerupted bicuspids and 6-year molar to be "carried along for the ride" in a distal direction. Extraoral force utilizing occipital traction is beyond the scope of this discussion. However, the generalist should realize that this possible treatment pathway exists and is open to the orthodontist.

If the orthodontist were to institute early treatment at age 5 for a severe Class II malocclusion, it would almost certainly be necessary to institute a second period of treatment in the late mixed or early permanent dentition to adjust the alignment of the maxillary incisors and cuspids. The significant gain for the patient would lie in the early establishment of correct anteroposterior alignment of the posterior teeth, thus eliminating or markedly reducing the need for extraoral traction in the adolescent years.

Precautions in the use of extra-oral force. Having explained what the simple cervical gear will accomplish, now let me sound a clear warning. Only an orthodontist or a specially trained pedodontist should attempt to alter maxillary growth potential to resolve the problems in Class II malocclusions. This is true also in those cases where mesial drift of 6 | 6 has caused a loss of more than 2 to 3 mm. of space needed for the proper eruption of 5 | 5. The general practitioner should have had advanced training before using *any* cervical gear because of the problems inherent in fitting the appliance properly and adjusting it during the patient's visits. There is also the possible danger that excessive distal pressure against the upper molars can cause necrosis of the periodontal membrane. A pressure of 2 to 4 ounces is suggested for the first 2 weeks' wear, after which the pull may be increased to 8 ounces (as measured by a Dontrix tension gauge, described in Chapter 14).

In some instances, an extraoral force appliance is used to enhance the anchorage of upper 6-year molars during the utilization of an upper fixed light labial arch appliance. Particularly when elastics are being used to "trolley" teeth along the arch wire, the anchorage requirements are increased (Fig. 13-8).

Treatment of ectopically erupting 6-year molars

Ectopic eruption is treated as a loss of posterior space in this chapter *if* the second primary molar has been lost during the eruption of the 6-year molar. Ectopic eruption is seen to be usually a unilateral problem, although occasionally it can occur bilaterally.[1] It almost always involves the maxillary first permanent molars. In a recent study only 3 out of 78 instances of ectopically erupted first permanent molars occurred in the lower arch.[9]

The first appliance therapy that must be accomplished is to tilt the mesially erupting molar back to its more normal axial alignment. This is best done by using an upper Hawley appliance with a helical spring made of highly resilient Australian wire, size 0.020. After this has been accomplished, a cervical neckband may be fitted so that extraoral force may complete the distal movement of the molar that is too far to the mesial. As can be seen, this very much parallels the treatment already outlined for children who have lost a second primary molar and whose permanent molar has drifted mesially, encroaching on the future space needed by the upper second bicuspid.

Let a warning be sounded that treatment of an ectopically erupted 6-year molar is not an easy task. It takes good timing, good appliance therapy, and close supervision of the child. Three of the appliances sug-

Fig. 13-9. Child, age 7, with Humphrey appliance in place. Humphrey appliance may be used for the treatment of an ectopically erupting upper 6-year molar. It consists of a molar band to which has been soldered an **S** spring of yellow Elgiloy wire. The distal end of the **S** spring is bent at a 90-degree angle, and the sharpened tip inserts into the central pit of the upper 6-year molar.

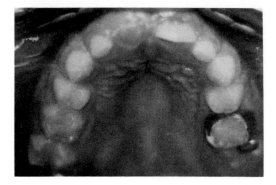

gested here for use are *removable by the child and are worn at his option.* Motivation must be of the highest order for the child and his parents to carry out the wishes of the dentist. Fortunately, younger children are more amenable to suggestions and routines of this sort than are teenagers, as a rule.

Humphrey appliance. If the second primary molar has *not* been lost, an interesting fixed appliance has been proposed by Humphrey.[3] An S-shaped wire can be formed from 0.028 yellow Elgiloy wire and soldered to the buccal surface of a band fitted to the second primary molar being loosened by the ectopically erupting 6-year molar (Fig. 13-9). The sharpened end of the S-wire fits into the central pit of the ectopically erupting permanent molar. Adjustments to open the spring are made in the child's mouth without removing the appliance.

Ectopic lower molars

A lower F-R lingual arch appliance with *vertical* attachments is the choice for use in *lower arch* ectopic eruption cases involving mandibular 6-year molars. Treatment is essentially the same as described previously for *mesially drifted* lower molars. If accomplished early (at age 7 or 8), the treatment consists mostly of *tilting* the ectopically erupted 6-year molar distally over a period of 2 to 4 months.

Occasionally a lower Hawley appliance is used with a helical spring engaging the mesial surface of the ectopic molar to exert distal pressure. The obvious precaution here is that *the child must wear the appliance constantly.* If the removable appliance is not worn as directed by the dentist, the molar quickly lapses back to its former ectopic position and will ultimately block out the erupting second bicuspid. Once the proper axial relation of the molar has been reached, it should be realized that the retention period is a longer one (waiting for the second bicuspid to erupt) than for many other minor tooth movement cases. A lower F-R lingual arch is an ideal retention device for these cases after treatment.

Use of separating wires to gain small amounts of lost space

When a partially erupted second bicuspid does not have quite enough room in the dental arch to erupt into proper alignment, a series of interproximal separating wires can be used to regain the necessary space. This method can gain as much as 1.5 mm. of space within the quadrant over a period of a week or so, which in many cases will allow the normal eruption of the second bicuspid.

This method of using separating wires appears to work far better in the upper arch than the lower. Since only a few minutes of chair time are involved, the regaining of the necessary space may be attempted in this fashion if the bicuspid has erupted part way but is being blocked out of normal eruption due to a measurable lack of space.[2] The space occupied by the antimere bicuspid in the opposite side of the arch may be measured for comparison.

Soft brass wire of 0.020 dimension (28 gauge) is used for these separating wires. First, a 2-foot length is rolled off the spool and cut. In the laboratory, wetted pumice (laboratory grade) is held in one hand, and the 24-inch brass wire is drawn repeatedly through the fingers coated with the wet pumice. This polishes the wire brilliantly by cleansing away all surface discolorations.

In the preparation of the brass wire in lengths and configurations convenient for use, a ⅜-inch wooden dowel or a fountain pen has the proper diameter for wrapping the brass wire around evenly, so that it becomes a coil. By cutting the wire coil with a scissors, the dentist can quickly make a whole series of correctly sized brass ligature rings. These should be soaked in alcohol, dried, and stored in a small, clear plastic box. When they are readied for use, each ring should be reshaped slightly to resemble a fish hook. Also, in some instances the end that is to be inserted interproximally between the teeth should be flattened and sharpened. This makes it pass more easily between tightly adjacent teeth. With the *side jaws* of the How pliers, the end of the wire may be flattened; then with a pin and ligature pliers the flattened area may be cut at an angle, so that a pointed end is formed. There is no question that this aids in the rapid placement of these separating wires. Painting topical anesthetic on the interproximal gingiva may also help the dentist in placing separating wires for the slightly apprehensive child.

CONTROVERSY OVER THE STIMULATION OF GROWTH IN THE MAXILLA OR MANDIBLE

A better method for reducing some Class II malocclusions to Class I would be to somehow stimulate the growth of the mandible in the condyle areas. In spite of the claims of European orthodontists, many American dentists remain unconvinced that any great degree of growth stimulation can be promoted on a selective basis in either the maxilla or the mandible of a child.

Regarding this argument concerning stimulation, Mathews[6] explains that "bite jumping," using either removable appliances or Class II elastics with fixed appliances, is often resorted to in an effort to stimulate the mandible to grow and thereby eliminate a Class II malocclusion. In spite of claims of the contrary, Mathews believes that no evidence exists for such differential stimulation of growth of facial parts. To explain the bite correction that European orthodontists appear to accomplish with their functional jaw (orthopedic) appliances to correct Class II malocclusions by stimulating the mandible to grow forward, it is said that the correction is similar to the case of headgear therapy. With the use of headgear therapy for Class II malocclusions, it is not always possible to demonstrate distal growth of the maxillary buccal teeth, yet the biting relation of the teeth has been corrected. In actuality, many prominent orthodontists, Moyers and Graber among them, are in the process of rethinking this whole growth-stimulation problem. Although this controversy seems far removed from general dental practice, even now many continuing dental education courses are teaching the use of Bimler, monobloc, and Andreson appliances to generalists. It seems almost inevitable that the use of such appliances by generalists will increase, paralleling a similar increase among European generalists. In a pragmatic fashion, such appliances are used because they work.

COMPARISON OF GROWTH INHIBITION IN MAXILLA AND MANDIBLE

In contrast to the argument concerning growth stimulation is the case for growth inhibition. Moore[7] appears to bolster the growth inhibition argument strongly as the result of a study of records of orthodontic treatment which indicate that *distal* or *posterior* force applied to the maxillary molar teeth may cause actual distal movement of the maxillary teeth. He indicates that under such force the profile length of the maxilla of the child clearly does not increase or increases only negligibly. On the other hand, he believes that a similar force applied to the mandible does not produce like results. Apparently because the mandible is a free-floating bone, distally directed force is not capable of inhibiting mandibular growth, nor is a force applied in the reverse direction capable of accelerating mandibular growth.

• • •

The general practicing dentist usually has too little experience to judge the claims and counterclaims in either growth stimulation or growth inhibition areas of orthodontics. Probably a good rule to follow in growth stimulation considerations is that a child cannot grow beyond his potential, regardless of any stimulation measures the dentist may initiate.

SUMMARY

The treatment of mesially drifted 6-year molars is discussed. It is suggested that three basic factors permit the mesial drifting of erupting or newly erupted 6-year molars: carious attack on the deciduous molars, ectopic eruption of the 6-year molars, and too early extraction of deciduous molars with no space maintainer being subsequently placed by the dentist.

The uses of the removable upper and lower Hawley appliances are described in distalizing 6-year molars, as well as the use of the F-R lower lingual arch. The cervical extraoral force appliance is also discussed in the treatment of mesially drifted upper 6-year molars, with precautions expressed against its inappropriate use in untrained hands. The possible future role of appliances to stimulate jaw growth and of growth-inhibiting appliances is advanced.

REFERENCES

1. Barber, T. K.: Minor orthodontic guidance in the mixed dentition. Paper presented at Pedodontic Seminar, University of Alabama Dental School, Dec., 1967.
2. Hitchcock, H. P.: Preventive orthodontics. In Finn, S. B., editor: Clinical pedodontics, ed. 3, Philadelphia, 1967, W. B. Saunders Co., p. 296.
3. Humphrey, W. P.: A simple technique correcting an ectopically erupting first molar, J. Dent. Child. **29:**176-178, 1962.
4. King, E. W.: Extra-oral appliance treatment; the neckband, Dent. Clin. North Am., pp. 479-488, July, 1966.
5. Kloehn, S. J.: An appraisal of the results of treatment of Class II malocclusion with extraoral forces. In Kraus, B. S., and Riedel, R. A., editors: Vistas in orthodontics, Philadelphia, 1962, Lea & Febiger, p. 234.
6. Mathews, R. J.: Malocclusion in the primary dentition, Dent. Clin. North Am., pp. 463-478, July, 1966.
7. Moore, A. W.: Observations on facial growth and its clinical significance, Am. J. Orthod. **45:**399-423, 1959.
8. Moyers, R. E.: Seminar: Advanced orthodontics for the general practitioner, Southern Illinois University School of Dental Medicine, Edwardsville, Ill., Jan., 1972.
9. Young, D. H.: Ectopic eruption of the first permanent molar, J. Dent. Child. **24:**153-162, 1957.

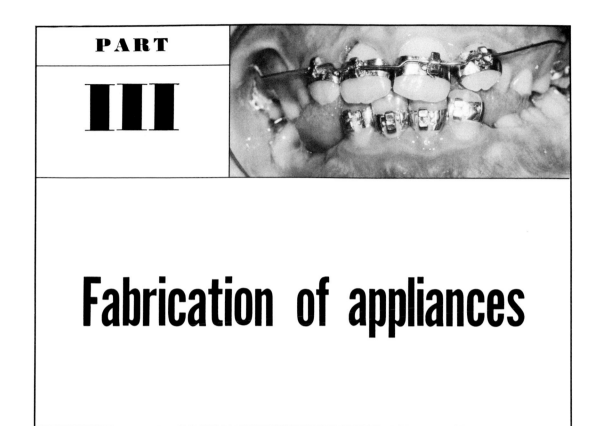

Fabrication of appliances

14 | Selection of instruments and appliance components

When one thinks of instruments used for minor tooth movement, there comes to mind the picture of the drawer full of gleaming pliers issued and paid for in dental school. In most dental students' experience, most of these were seldom used in dental school, and perhaps several have not been used since. For the dentist interested in minor tooth movement these pliers can be a treasure chest of valuable instruments. They are valuable, however, only to the extent he is willing to reshape their jaws or otherwise modify them to suit his specific needs.

For most dentists, though, the thought of modifying instruments to a shape or use different from that which the maker intended is a form of heresy. Instruments are viewed somewhat like stone tablets from the mountain. They must not be changed. In reality, *each* of these instruments can be reshaped to meet specific appliance fabrication needs, and in many instances the cost of new pliers can be avoided.

HOW TO SELECT PLIERS

As in operative dentistry or oral surgery, it is better to have one versatile instrument that, when familiarity is acquired, will do many tasks well. It is better to train one's hand to perform a few tasks well with one pair of pliers than to do many things poorly using several sets of pliers.

Let us examine the components of good wire-bending pliers. No wire-bending pliers should ever be autoclaved or steam sterilized. Some of them are made of carbon steel, which may rust. Others are made of stainless steel but have carbon steel pins through the jaws, which may deteriorate. In selecting instruments for wire bending, the following considerations should be kept in mind:

1. Are the pliers commercially available, or can they be modified from an existing instrument?

2. Are the pliers made of stainless steel, which can be cold sterilized or dry-heat sterilized, or are they made of plated metal, which will rust?

3. Is the instrument for limited use, or is it a truly versatile one that can perform many tasks?

4. Should the working tips of the pliers be made of hard carbon steel or of the softer and more easily deformed stainless steel?

213

I-2 Orthodontic blowpipe, National, available from Unitek Corp., order No. 603-014; cost $15.00. May also be ordered through a dental supply dealer. Uses any kind of natural or bottled gas.

The metal flame-back (black) is an added nicety. Use thick-walled ⅛-inch black hose for best results.

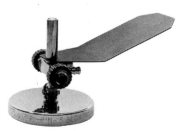

CAUTION: This fine instrument is capable of minute adjustments of flame intensity *if* it is not clogged with melted wax from inlay or denture wax-ups. Use it only for soldering stainless steel or gold appliances.

Fig. 14-3. If the flame of the orthodontic blowpipe is adjusted exactly to a height of ¾ inch so that a slight hissing sound may be heard, the adjustment is proper for flame soldering. (Courtesy Unitek Corp.)

I-3 No. 139 bird-beak (Angle) pliers, Rocky Mountain Dental Products Co., order No. I-139; cost $14.50.

Most versatile of all orthodontic pliers. The bird-beak pliers can be used for the most intricate clasp- and wire-bending. If carbon steel pliers are used, little deformation of their jaw tips will be seen even after years of hard use. This is not true in the case of stainless steel pliers whose jaw tips may become separated if wires of too large diameter are bent.

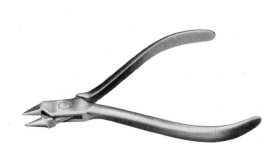

Fig. 14-4. Bird-beak pliers, the most versatile instrument the dentist can use for wire bending. (Courtesy Rocky Mountain Dental Products Co.)

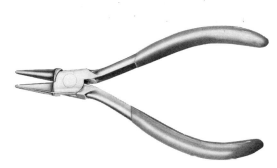

Alternate: Light bird-beak pliers, Unitek Corp., order No. 800-416; cost $14.50.

Suitable companion pliers for the No. 139, but they should be limited to use on lighter wires.

Fig. 14-5. Light-wire bird-beak pliers are used for bending wires 0.020 and smaller. (Courtesy Unitek Corp.)

I-4 No. 110 straight lip-safe How pliers, hard carbide-sprayed beaks, Rocky Mountain Dental Products Co., order No. I-110; cost $14.50.

Used mostly for inserting the fixed-removable lingual arch and the heavy and light wire labial arches and for small adjustments of certain light wires. Also, they may be used to twist and tighten wire ligatures that tie arch wires to edgewise brackets or round buccal tubes. Tying ligature wires is much better accomplished by using I-13, the ligature-tying plier.

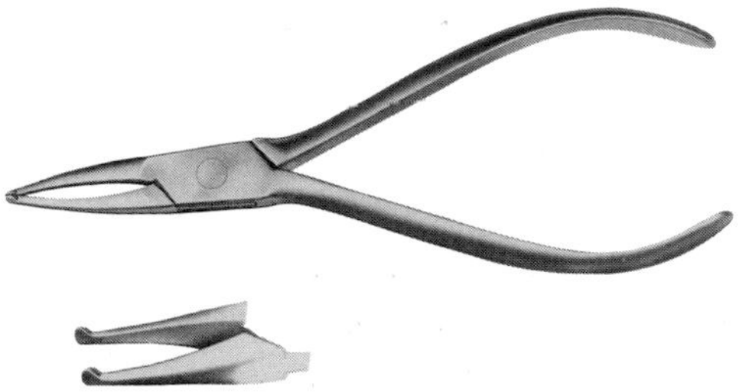

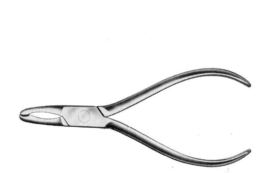

Fig. 14-6. *No. 110 How pliers insert and remove lingual arches and labial arches. They can also be used to twist ligature wires to place if ligature-tying pliers (I-13) are not available. (Courtesy Rocky Mountain Dental Products Co.)*

I-5 No. 114 contouring pliers, stainless, Rocky Mountain Dental Products Co., order No. I-114; cost $12.00.

Used to contour slightly inward the gingival margins of bands and stainless steel crowns to achieve a better fit. The jaws may be altered by selective grinding so that they are thinner across the jaws and permit the contouring of smaller bands.

Alternate: Crown- and band-contouring pliers, Unitek Corp., Order No. 800-417; cost $14.50.

Excellent pliers, better for molar bands and stainless steel crowns. They place a more tightly controlled contour at the margin than any other pliers.

Fig. 14-7. *No. 114 contouring pliers shape the gingival margins of bands and crowns for better fit. (Courtesy Rocky Mountain Dental Products Co.)*

I-6 No. 53 clasp-contouring pliers, stainless, Rocky Mountain Dental Products Co., order No. I-53; cost $11.50.

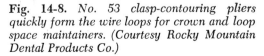

Used to form fixed space-maintainer wire loops easily and quickly. They can also be used to form shallow adjustment loops to shorten lingual arches or other arch wires.

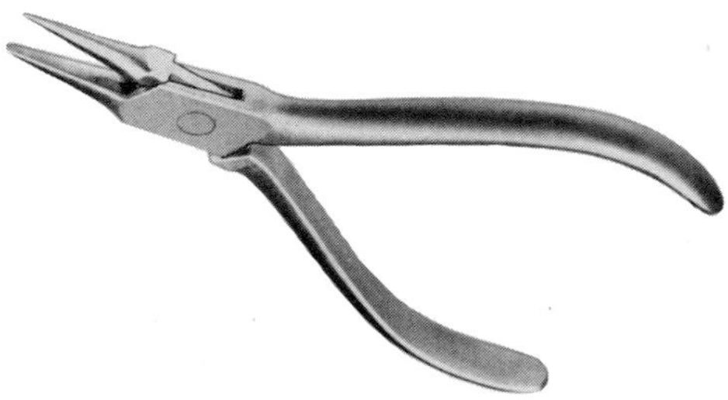

Fig. 14-8. *No. 53 clasp-contouring pliers quickly form the wire loops for crown and loop space maintainers. (Courtesy Rocky Mountain Dental Products Co.)*

C-3 450-band introductory kit, narrow, seamless bands without lugs for right and left maxillary *lateral incisors,* assorted sizes, Unitek Corp., order No. 123-131; cost $140.50. Walnut kit box is included at no extra cost.

Both of these introductory kits will provide an extremely wide variety of sizes of anterior bands shaped for right and left teeth. By belling the bands slightly, one may use the central bands in those few instances where upper and lower permanent cuspids need to be banded for minor tooth movement. Also, the smaller sizes among the lateral bands may be used in operative dentistry for children's anterior *primary* teeth during restorative banding procedures when mesial and distal decay areas are present.

Alternate: Same as C-2 alternate.

C-4 Roll band material, 0.003 × 0.150, Rocky Mountain Dental Products Co., order No. B-83; cost $2.15 per roll.

Alternate: Ribbon band material, 0.003 × 0.150, Unitek Corp., order No. 100-330; cost $2.15 per roll.

This all-purpose band material can be used to fabricate most bands for upper anterior teeth if there are certain tooth sizes not available in the custom seamless band kit.

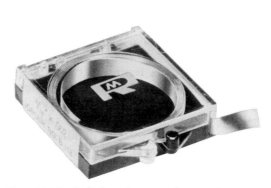

Fig. 14-22. *Roll band material may be used to fabricate an anterior band. No. 110 How pliers may be used to pinch the band preparatory to spot-welding the seam. (Courtesy Rocky Mountain Dental Products Co.)*

C-5 Round arch wire, Elgiloy wire, Rocky Mountain Dental Products Co., order from following wire size table:

Size	Order No.	Cost
0.040 blue Elgiloy	E-237	$3.40/10 lengths
0.036 blue Elgiloy	E-236	3.40/10 lengths
0.036 yellow Elgiloy	E-208	3.40/10 lengths
0.032 yellow Elgiloy	E-276	3.40/10 lengths
0.028 yellow Elgiloy	E-206	3.40/10 lengths
0.025 yellow Elgiloy	E-205	3.40/10 lengths
0.020 yellow Elgiloy	E-284	3.40/20 lengths

NOTE: The Elgiloy series of wires tends to be softer and more easily formed into arches, clasps, and springs than standard round wires. They may be easily tempered, passivated, or annealed using the No. 660 or comparable electric welder. Each wire size comes in 14-inch lengths, with 10 or 20 in a package.

Alternate

Unitek standard wire

0.036	211-360	$1.90/pkg.
0.032	211-320	1.90/pkg.
0.028	211-280	1.90/pkg.
0.025	211-250	1.90/pkg.
0.020	211-200	1.90/pkg.

Alternate to 0.028 and 0.025 Elgiloy wire

0.020 Australian wire	TP Laboratories	$3.00/roll
0.018 Australian wire	TP Laboratories	3.00/roll

C-6 Stainless ligature wire, dead-soft, 0.009, 4-ounce spool, Unitek Corp., order No. 200-092; cost $3.20 per spool.

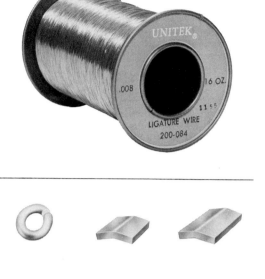

Fig. 14-23. *This light soft wire is used to tie (ligate) labial arch wires to brackets. The size shown is 0.008, but 0.009 or 0.010 wires are equally suitable. (Courtesy Unitek Corp.)*

C-7 Wire solder, 25 gauge, Rocky Mountain Dental Products Co., order No. H-24; cost $3.75 per spool.

C-8 Bar solder, standard, Rocky Mountain Dental Products Co., order No. H-21; cost $2.05 per foot.

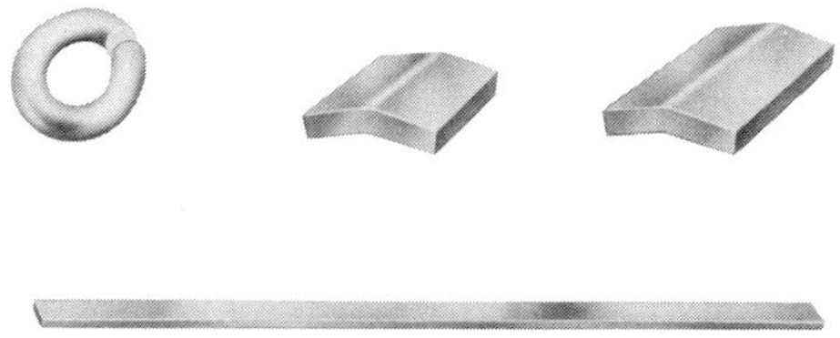

Fig. 14-24. *Silver solder may be used in wire or bar form. The small circlets pictured may be formed by wrapping the solder wire around 0.036 wire to form a tight coil spring and then cutting across the coil spring with pin- and ligature-cutting pliers. Bar solder is cut into ⅟₁₆- and ⅛-inch pieces and is used mostly for crown and loop space maintainers. The pieces of bar solder may be bent by squeezing them in the jaws of the No. 53 pliers. (Courtesy Rocky Mountain Dental Products Co.)*

C-9 Solder flux, Rocky Mountain Dental Products Co., order No. J-41; cost $1.45 per bottle.

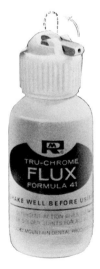

Fig. 14-25. *Solder flux should be shaken to make the mixture flow with the consistency of loose honey. It should be used **liberally.** (Courtesy Rocky Mountain Dental Products Co.)*

C-16 Solid aluminum Iden orthodontic impression trays, TP Laboratories; cost $21.00 for set of 12 upper and lower, assorted sizes.

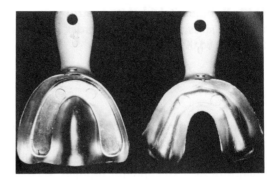

These trays must be rimmed with wax for alginate impressions. However, the added hydrostatic force available during impression taking makes for better impressions. Dental assistants will enjoy the ease with which these trays may be cleaned.

Fig. 14-31. *Solid aluminum Iden orthodontic impression trays. The chief advantage of using these trays is that they may be easily and quickly cleaned and sterilized by the dental assistant.*

C-17 Sectional lingual arches, 0.036, Rocky Mountain Dental Products Co., order No. A-205; cost $3.20 for set of 10.

Arches are bent one-half arch at a time and then soldered in the middle to make a complete lower lingual arch. A connector tube (A-11) is usually slipped over the arch ends as they join in the middle (lingual to the lower central incisors) to facilitate soldering. The lingual vertical tubes to fit these arches are described (A-3).

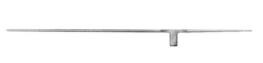

Fig. 14-32. *Sectional arches are easily paired to form a vertical lingual arch. A connector tube is necessary to join the ends at the middle (Fig. 14-48). (Courtesy Rocky Mountain Dental Products Co.)*

C-18 Prefabricated Ellis lingual arches, 0.036, short post with adjustment loop, Rocky Mountain Dental Products Co., order No. K-254; cost $12.20 for 20 assorted sizes.

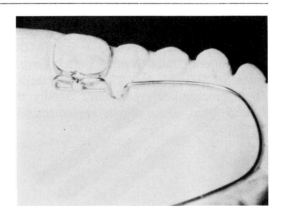

This arch is easily fitted on a study model if the dentist is able to passivate it after forcing it to place in the lingual tubes. The vertical lingual tubes to fit these arches are described later (A-3).

Fig. 14-33. *Ellis type prefabricated lingual arches with adjustment loops are highly versatile appliances. Caution must be used to match the proper size vertical tube (Fig. 14-41) to the arch wire size. (Courtesy Rocky Mountain Dental Products Co.)*

C-19 **Hotz preformed** vertical lingual **arches,** 0.036, Unitek Corp., order No. 305-150; cost $33.80 for a set of 20 assorted sizes and 40 lingual sheaths.

One of the easiest of all lingual arches to fit on a study model. It is also easy to insert into, and remove from, a child's mouth. One disadvantage is the large size of the lingual sheath, which occasionally causes gingival and tongue irritation. (See Fig. 17-6.)

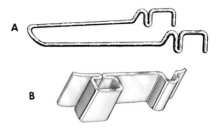

Fig. 14-34. *Hotz vertical lingual arches,* **A,** *may be used only with the Hotz preformed lingual sheaths,* **B.** *Sheath shown here would be spot-welded to lower right molar band. (Courtesy Unitek Corp.)*

C-20 **Tru Chrome polishing compound,** Rocky Mountain Dental Products Co., order No. J-42; cost $1.00 per tube.

Helpful in polishing all stainless steel and solder joints to a high luster.

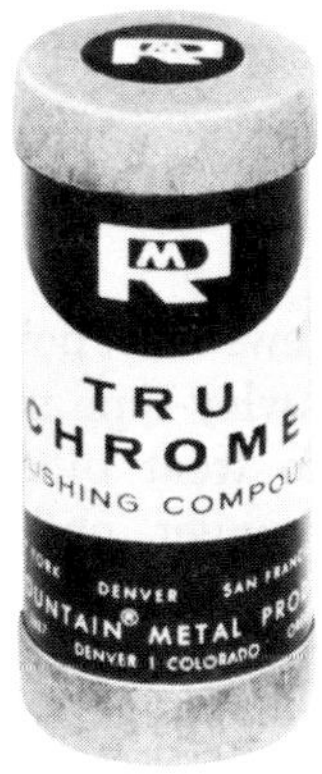

Fig. 14-35. *This hard polishing compound quickly removes discoloration from stainless steel wires and solder points. (Courtesy Rocky Mountain Dental Products Co.)*

C-21 **Bridging wire,** 0.010 × 0.022, 6 ft. roll, Rocky Mountain Dental Products Co., order No. H-30; cost $1.45 per roll.

Soft rectangular-shaped wire that is used to repair broken wires on appliances, for instance, a broken cuspid U-loop on the labial bow of a Hawley appliance. Bridging wire is spot-welded across the break and then soldered, using silver wire solder and the cable tips of the spot welder.

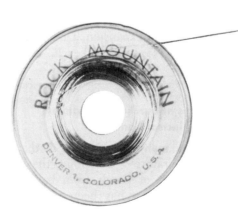

Fig. 14-36. *Bridging wire aids in making repairs on broken appliance wires. This wire is spot-welded across the break and then joined by soldering. (Courtesy Rocky Mountain Dental Products Co.)*

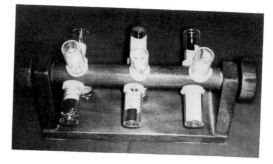

Fig. 14-49. *A revolving display for identifying and dispensing small brackets and attachments may be made by the dentist. It vastly simplifies locating small attachments and helps the dental assistant in reordering procedures.*

Storage of brackets and other attachments

The dentist may find that storage of small but rather expensive brackets and other components poses a problem in his office. It has been found that a small rotating bracket dispenser (Fig. 14-49) can be made of 1-inch dowel material mounted on a stand, using containers obtained from a pharmacist. Small screws attach the caps of each container to the dowel.

Reordering materials

Inside each of the tubes in the bracket dispenser is rolled a slip of paper listing the sources, order number, and cost of the attachments or components. The dental assistant may check the level of supply quickly and easily at the start of each week so that new attachments may be reordered.

Table 18. List of attachments for minor tooth movement

	Attachment	Source	Order No.	Cost
A-1	Horizontal lingual sheaths, 0.036	Unitek	080-210	$3.20/10
	Alternate: Lingual sheaths, 0.036	Rocky Mt.	A-186	3.00/10
A-2	Vertical lingual sheaths, Hotz type	Unitek	080-270	3.50/10
A-3	Vertical plain lingual tube for 0.036 wire (Ellis arch)	Rocky Mt.	A-173	3.20/10
A-4	Round buccal tubes			
	0.040	Rocky Mt.	A-110	3.10/10
	0.036	Rocky Mt.	A-109	3.10/10
A-5	Quik-wing single edgewise brackets, 0.022 × 0.028	Rocky Mt.	A-1	2.20/10
	Alternate: Standard single anterior edgewise brackets, 0.022 × 0.028	Unitek	001-375	2.80/10
A-6	Quik-wing posterior edgewise brackets, 0.022 × 0.028	Rocky Mt.	A-2	2.50/10
	Alternate: Posterior edgewise brackets, 0.022 × 0.028	Unitek	001-376	2.80/10
A-7	Lingual buttons	Rocky Mt.	A-47	2.10/10
A-8	Eyelets, regular	Rocky Mt.	A-38	1.05/100
A-9	Stops, weldable, 1 mm. 0.045	Unitek	519-171	6.00/100
A-10	Weldable double buccal tubes, 0.045 and 0.022 × 0.028	Unitek	048-212	5.60/10
A-11	Connector tubes for sectional lingual arches	Rocky Mt.	A-206	1.80/20

SUMMARY

From the overbundance of instruments, components, and attachments available through orthodontic supply house and other sources, a limited number of materials have been selected and described in this chapter. Alternate choices have been indicated where equivalent materials are available.

Frustration and dissatisfaction will be the lot of the dentist who attempts to accomplish minor tooth movement procedures using poorly selected materials.

It is hoped that by combining the description of how the items are used with illustrations of them, the uses of these materials will be better visualized. The inclusion of the sources, order numbers, and cost should aid the dentist who is not accustomed to ordering these materials. Obviously, the cost of these items may change with the years, but including this factor gives the dentist a method of cost-accounting the fabrication of minor tooth movement appliances in his practice.

Addresses of orthodontic materials suppliers

Rocky Mountain Dental Products Company
P.O. Box 1887
Denver, Colo. 80704

TP Laboratories, Inc.
P.O. Box 73
LaPorte, Ind. 46350

Unitek Corporation
950 Royal Oaks Dr.
Monrovia, Calif. 91016

REFERENCES

1. Graber, T. M.: Orthodontics: principles and practice, Philadelphia, 1962, W. B. Saunders Co., pp. 647-656.
2. Moyers, R. E.: Handbook of orthodontics, ed. 2, Chicago, 1963, Year Book Medical Publishers, Inc., pp. 461-474.

a straw-colored coating. This may be done by flame or by the electric welder action explained later. To *passivate* a wire is to remove all internal stresses from a wire so it is "passive," that is, it exerts no hidden forces against teeth (e.g., an arch wire).

The Elgiloy wires (C-5), whose use is suggested in this book, have some unique properties. A small amount of heat will temper Elgiloy wire so that it produces a stronger spring action. With slightly more heat applied, the wire may be passivated, which removes excess tension from the wire. The same wire, with more heat applied, will become annealed, resulting in a softer spring action, or, in the case of a light wire, no spring action at all. Annealing deadens, or "kills," the spring in the wire.

Operation of the welder

The 660 welder has an upper and lower turret, each containing four differently

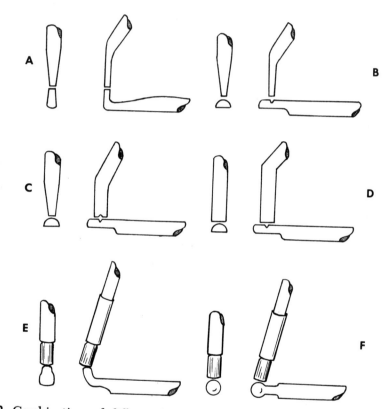

Fig. 15-2. Combinations of different tips of the turrets of No. 660 welder. **A,** *Small round to small round,* used for spot-welding brackets and attachments to molar bands. **B,** *Small round to notched half-round,* used to spot-weld a small wire at right angles to a large wire that is held in the notch. Also brackets may be spot-welded to anterior and posterior bands, using these tips. **C,** *Notched-blade to notched half-round,* used to spot-weld two medium or heavy wires parallel to each other, as when attaching a finger spring to a lingual arch wire preparatory to soldering. **D,** *Large round to notched half-round,* used when spot-welding a heavy wire to a crown or band, as for a crown and loop space maintainer. **E,** *Carbon tip to scoop-blade tips,* used for soldering heavy wire to crown or band, as for a crown and loop space maintainer. Copious amounts of liquid flux must be used when soldering. **F,** *Carbon tip to ball tip,* used for silver soldering heavy wire to crowns or bands. This lower tip is almost interchangeable with scoop-blade tip shown in **E,** when used for heavy soldering, such as soldering crown and loop space maintainers.

shaped electrodes. These electrodes cannot be interchanged with those of other spot-welders made by the same company. This type of welder will render good service for 10 to 20 years *if it is properly cared for and the instruction booklet is followed.*

To weld or solder properly, keep clean all copper, brass, or carbon electrodes. The point of each metal electrode where it touches the metals to be joined should be scrubbed with a brush in hot water and then sanded or filed between each operation to ensure good electrical contact. The carbon electrodes also must be scrubbed with a toothbrush in hot water to clean

away the flux from the previous operation.

Use of turrets holding electrodes. To bring the proper shaped electrodes into position, each upper or lower turret is simply rotated by a spring-loaded device to the desired position. By the matching of the opposing electrodes in varying combinations, a large variety of metal-joining operations may be carried out (Fig. 15-2).

Use of extension cables. There are three holes on the top surface of the 660 welder to insert the plugs for the two extension cables. One insertion point is black, and the other two are white. The *white-black* combination allows about one half the elec-

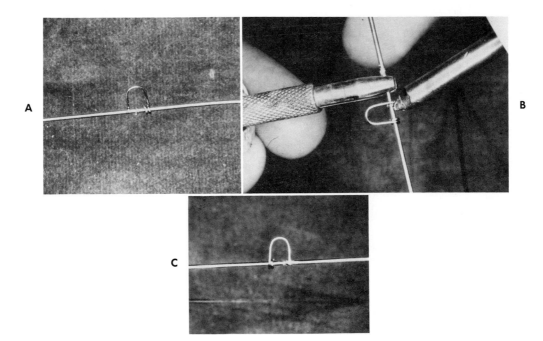

Fig. 15-3. A, Vertical U-loop of 0.020 yellow Elgiloy has been wound around and then spot-welded to the wire, simulating an 0.036 heavy labial arch wire. Before the U-loop is bent (over round jaw of No. 139 bird-beak pliers in position 2), a single ring of solder is slipped over the arch wire, moved along the wire until it is adjacent to the area where the loop end will be spot-welded, and then soldered to the wire. **B,** Area of proposed solder joint is fluxed generously after the alligator tips grasp the larger wire near spot-welded area. The table is locked open on the welder, a setting of about 2 is chosen on the selector-dial, and *white-white* cable inserts are used. The carbon tip is firmly brushed over area to be soldered. The carbon tip must never be left in one place too long or the resulting heat will kill the wire. The whole soldering operation takes about 1 to 2 seconds to complete. **C,** Finished solder joint. The small ring of solder used allows a strong, clean joint and not a cluttery waste of solder solidified on the arch wire.

trical current allowed by the *white-white* combination.

At the working end of the cables are plastic handles holding the variously shaped brass and carbon electrodes, each of which is reversible in the handle. Proper selection of tips can produce the following combinations:

1. Alligator holding jaws—carbon tip
2. Annealing tip—annealing tip
3. Alligator type holding jaws—annealing tip
4. Carbon tip—annealing tip

To use the extension cables for soldering, passivating, and annealing, the turret jaws have to be separated so that no electric current flows through their circuit. To do this, the hinged table to which the lower turret is attached is depressed and locked open by a small spring-loaded pin. A dial on the face of the welder is set for the proper current needed for each operation.

Extension cables plugged into the 660 spot-welder may, by judicious use, enable the dentist to perform the following operations:

1. Soldering. The carbon tip and annealing tip may be used when the wire is stabilized on a model, or the alligator holding tip may be used to hold the main arch wire. (See Fig. 15-3.)

2. Tempering. The annealing tips may be employed to lightly heat the wire.

3. Passivation. The annealing tips may be used while the arch wire is on the model to remove undesirable tensions in the wire.

4. Annealing. With the annealing tips, the wire may be heated red-hot to remove all spring action in the wire.

Use of annealing table. An annealing table (or jack) may also be plugged into the *white-white* holes on the top of the welder. Larger size wires can be held in the grooves for a short period to anneal them. (See Fig. 15-4.) This removes all the original temper from the wire and renders it soft and springless.

FABRICATING FIXED SPACE MAINTAINERS

The following four types of *fixed* space maintainers appear to answer the needs of most dentists in caring for young children:

1. Crown and loop
2. Band and loop
3. Fixed soldered lingual arch (lower arch only)
4. The Nance appliance (upper arch only)

The first two types are used to maintain the space after the loss of *one* deciduous molar. The remaining two types are used when primary molars are lost bilaterally in the same arch.

Crown and loop space maintainers

To fabricate a crown and loop space maintainer, the direct or the indirect method may be used. With the direct

Fig. 15-4. Annealing jack. For use, it is plugged in the top holes of the welder, *white-white* combination. The table is pressed down and locked open. Then the wire to be annealed is simply placed between the jaws of the electrodes of the jack. When the wire reddens, it is annealed.

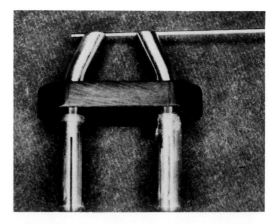

method, the space maintainer is fitted directly in the child's mouth at the chair. With the indirect method, the space maintainer is made on the model in the laboratory.

Materials needed

1. 0.036 blue Elgiloy wire (C-5)
2. Silver bar solder, regular thickness (C-8)
3. Solder flux (C-9)

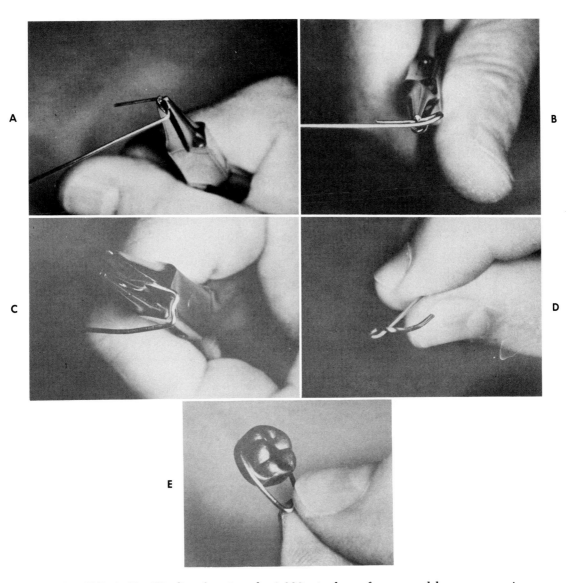

Fig. 15-5. A, No. 53 pliers forming the 0.036 wire loop of crown and loop space maintainer. **B.** No. 53 pliers "squeezing" the wire to produce the gentle curve to allow the loop to approximate the tissue surface of the alveolar ridge. **C,** A deeper grip and a gentle squeeze by the jaws of the No. 53 pliers produce the buccal and lingual bends approximating the wire to the crown or band surfaces. **D,** Finished loop. Wire is now ready to be marked for length and slipped on crown to test fit. **E,** Proper lengths of the wire have been marked with white arch-marking pencil and cut at the marks. Wire has been fitted over crown.

in most cases. Replacing or repairing lost or broken spacer maintainers can occupy a good deal of time in a busy practice. It is much better to make and cement each space maintainer correctly the first time around. (See precautions prior to cementation, in next column and on p. 292.)

Fabricating fixed soldered lingual arches

Occasionally a child will prematurely lose one or more primary molars bilaterally in his mandibular arch. The soldered lingual arch is used as a fixed bilateral space maintainer in the lower arch in the primary dentition. It is a passive appliance, which cannot be adjusted once it is cemented to the second deciduous molars. Although it is possible to make this appliance directly at the chairside, much the best approach is by the indirect method in the laboratory.

Materials needed

1. 0.036 blue or yellow Elgiloy wire (C-5)
2. Two narrow molar bands (C-1)
3. Regular thickness silver bar solder, cut in 2 mm. pieces (C-8)
4. Solder flux (C-9)
5. No. 660 welder (I-1)
6. No. 139 bird-beak pliers (I-3)
7. White arch-marking pencil (I-16)

Procedure (Fig. 15-8)

1. On lower study model, make sawcuts interproximally on each side of the 6-year molars, wet the plaster in molar areas, and carve away plaster so that crowns of molar teeth are well exposed.

2. Fit bands on plaster molars in the same relationship as they have already been fitted in the child's mouth.

3. Contour 0.036 blue or yellow Elgiloy wire in a tapered U-shape with thumb and finger so that the lingual arch wire approximates the lingual surfaces of the lower incisors, cuspids, and bicuspids.

4. Holding the arch wire in place on the model, use white marking pencil to mark the arch wire directly opposite each molar band's lingual groove. Cut wire at these marks.

5. Remove wire from model. Remove bands and spot-weld ends of arch wire so that cut ends of wire are slightly gingival to edge of lingual groove on each band.

6. Slip spot-welded lingual arch onto model and position molar bands in same relation they were fitted in child's mouth. Check relation of arch wire to lingual surfaces of lower anterior teeth.

7. Flux spot-welded areas liberally, then place a 2 mm. piece of silver bar solder on each prospective solder joint. Complete the soldering operation using electric cables of 660 welder (alligator clip and carbon tip).

8. Remove soldered arch from model and scrub with hot water to remove flux, then smooth with Cratex rubber wheel, and polish on lathe.

Precautions to observe prior to cementation

Insides of molar bands must have all discoloration and all remnants of flux removed. This is easily accomplished by using a small green stone point. If allowed to remain, this discolored material may act to dissipate the cement by electrolysis and cause the bands to loosen.

Each molar tooth to be banded must be coated with a film of collodion or cavity varnish *before cementation* of the bands if a zinc phosphate cement is to be used. (See general considerations in fitting and cementing orthodontic bands, Chapter 18.)

Nance appliance

The Nance appliance is used when one or more deciduous molars are lost prematurely in the child's maxillary arch. It is designed exactly as is the lower soldered lingual arch just described except that the anterior portion of the arch wire does not touch the lingual surfaces of the upper front teeth. Instead, the arch wire is contoured against the slope of the anterior portion of the palate approximately 1 cm. lingual to the lingual surfaces of the central incisors.

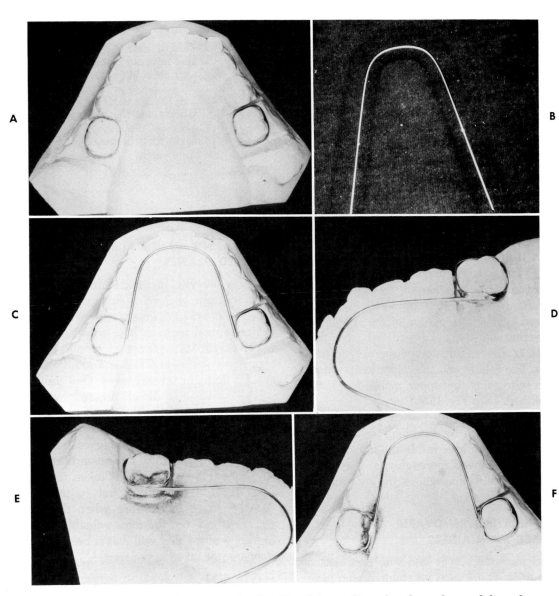

Fig. 15-8. Steps in fabricating a fixed soldered lower lingual arch used as a bilateral space maintainer. **A,** Lower cast with 6-year molars well exposed so that molar bands already fitted in the mouth may be slipped on the plaster teeth. **B,** Lingual arch wire (0.036) is contoured to fit the inside of the lower arch, using thumb and fingers. **C,** Contoured lingual arch wire is fitted into place on the arch, and the wire ends are cut off exactly opposite the lingual grooves on the molar bands. **D,** First one band, then the other is removed, and the corresponding end of the arch wire is spot-welded to each band. The spot-welded appliance is slipped back on the plaster teeth. The spot-welded areas are fluxed; small pieces of bar solder are added to the joint. Shown is the lower right molar, with soldering accomplished using alligator clips and carbon tip. Note cleanliness of plaster. **E,** Spot-welded area on lower left molar was fluxed, small pieces of bar solder were added, and the soldering was accomplished using the blowpipe. Note discoloration of plaster and deteriorative effect on the model. **F,** Note comparison with two methods of soldering (**D** and **E**). Obviously the electric cable extensions can save time and trouble for the dentist or assistant in this operation.

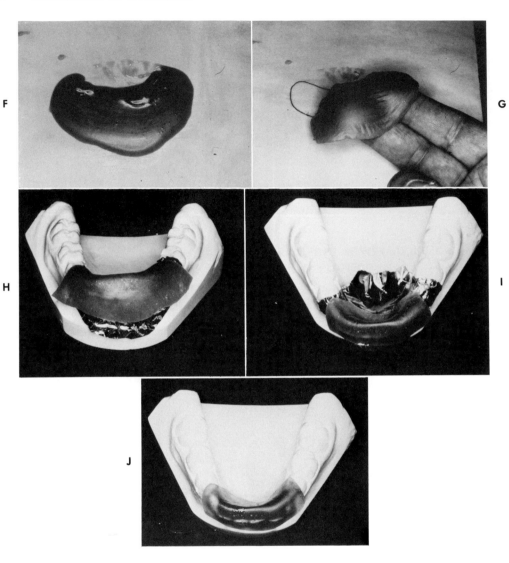

Fig. 15-10, cont'd. For legend see p. 249.

2. Mix in a small paper cup a combination of 2 parts powdered polymer and 1 part liquid monomer of a quick-set, non-slump orthodontic type acrylic. Stir slowly and allow it to thicken to honeylike consistency. This mix thickens rapidly!

3. Lubricate paper mixing pad with film of petrolatum, and onto pad pour honeylike mix of acrylic resin. Allow this to set until it is rubbery and can be picked up with the fingers.

4. Cut the partially set acrylic to the desired "kidney shape" with scissors, then carry immediately to the tinfoiled model. Mold the kidney-shaped acrylic over the foil form, pressing with the fingers to shape the acrylic bite plane into the desired inclined plane configuration.

5. As soon as the inclined plane has been shaped, place in the pressure pot at 20 pounds' air pressure from the laboratory air outlet.

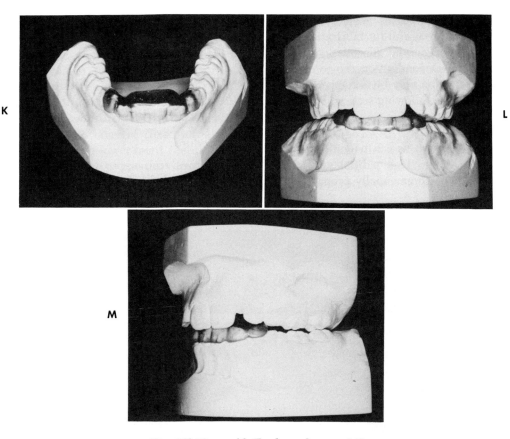

K

L

M

Fig. 15-10, cont'd. For legend see p. 249.

6. When completely set (20 minutes), remove model from pot. Lift off the bite plane with careful pressures to avoid breaking teeth. Peel foil away, and shape with vulcanite or acrylic burs, and polish. Make certain the inclined portion of the bite is at a 45-degree angle to the axes of the roots of the lower central incisors.

NOTE: The appliance is cemented to place with a thick mix of zinc oxide–eugenol (ZnOE) cement to which is added some petrolatum to lessen the cement's adhesion to the teeth and to make the cement more comfortable for the child.

Direct method procedure

To form the acrylic inclined bite plane directly in the child's mouth is usually not the most desirable method. However, it can be accomplished by only slightly modifying the routine followed in the indirect method.

Instead of on the lower model, the dead-soft tinfoil is finger-formed directly over the lower anterior teeth in the child's mouth. This tinfoil form is then removed and trimmed of excess foil. The acrylic is mixed exactly as in the previous instructions; the rubbery kidney-shaped resin is lifted from the pad and finger-pressed over the tinfoil form in the child's mouth. Curing is done in the pressure pot exactly as in the indirect method previously outlined.

CONSTRUCTING ORAL SCREENS

Oral screens are used in malocclusion cases exhibiting protrusion and spacing of upper anterior teeth or in cases where an

16 | Fabricating Hawley and palatal expansion appliances

WIRE-BENDING

Attaining accuracy in the bending of wire is a necessity for the dentist who wishes to fabricate minor tooth movement appliances in his own office. There is great satisfaction to be gained in learning proper methods of wire-bending. However, certain rather fundamental rules must be followed for each appliance to be well fitted and successful. The dentist who is not interested in learning and following these rules should perhaps explore other areas of practice in the spectrum of dentistry.

Value of learning wire-bending

The great value of having learned to bend wires skillfully comes when a dentist finds how easily these skills may be taught to a dental assistant or laboratory technician. In many offices the busy dentist will delegate the responsibility for making appliances to another person on his office staff. By teaching the fabrication of each appliance in a careful step-by-step fashion to his auxiliary personnel, the dentist will find that the resulting appliances will be of a high standard of excellence.

Not only is it necessary to learn to bend wire skillfully, but it is also incumbent on the operator to plan to use *light* pressures against the teeth to move them in the desired directions. The dentist who gets in too much of a hurry to accomplish his goals in minor tooth movement appliance therapy may find he has done more harm than good for his child patient.

Many shortcuts from traditional wire-bending methods are shown in the following pages. Practice, however, is essential. In one sense, there are really no short-cuts to attaining this peculiar skill, which takes care and thoughtful attention to detail.

Learning new methods of bending wire is probably best accomplished by "tell-show-do," in person, with one student learning from one instructor. However, the series of drawings and photographs in this and the following chapters may aid the attentive dentist to gain some new insights into the techniques he is now using. The illustrations that follow should provide a quick review of methods of wire-bending to form the clasps and springs needed for Hawley appliances. Perhaps the most gainful method of reading this chapter is to have a No. 139 pliers in hand and some lengths of 0.020, 0.025, 0.028, and 0.036

wire. In this way an appreciation of some of the shortcuts is gained, and dexterity in handling the several types of orthodontic pliers is increased.

When your assistant has mastered these techniques, she will have increased her value to you, and at the same time you will have helped her to fulfill in greater depth her mission of becoming a more competent dental auxiliary.

General rules for wire-bending

1. The wire must be of the proper *size* and *temper*. It is better to have a wire too large than too small and to have wire too soft than too highly tempered. Entries in Table 17 showing wire sizes and ordering sources should be referred to as the various materials are described in this chapter.

2. Appropriately shaped pliers must be used to accomplish the proper bends.

3. Wire should be bent *around* the pliers by firm pressure with the thumb or index finger, using the pliers as a more or less stationary vise. With larger sizes of wire, this may require considerable pressure by the thumb to control tight bends.

4. Bend the wire in one plane (dimension) at a time. The orthodontist may speak of first-degree bends, second-degree bends, and third-degree bends. This merely describes the dimensions in which he is bending the wire.

5. When a long, complex series of bends is to be made and configurations have to be made at both ends of the wire, as in forming the labial bow of the Hawley appliance, it is usually best to start at the middle and work toward each end.

6. When bending shorter springs and clasps, start by bending the complicated section of the wire first, then bend the easier sections. In bending wire clasps, it is best to first bend the part of the wire that touches the tooth. In bending springs that are to be anchored in the palatal or alveolar acrylic portion of the Hawley appliance, this same rule applies. Only with the helical spring and Hawley labial bow

does this rule not apply. Both of these are started in the middle.

• • •

Although some exceptions can be taken to the above rules, it is perhaps best to try to follow them until experience allows other methods to be applied.

Wire sizes used for springs and clasps

As mentioned previously, the Elgiloy wires have proved to be the easiest wires to work with in the fabrication of springs and clasps for Hawley and palatal expansion appliances. Of the four choices of resiliency, the yellow wires (medium soft) appear to be the best for most purposes. For the sources of these wires, order numbers, and approximate cost please note C-5 in Table 17.

The following Elgiloy wire sizes are listed for making the various springs and clasps used in the upper and lower Hawley appliances described in this chapter:
1. Hawley labial bow
   a. Upper—0.028 yellow Elgiloy
   b. Lower—0.025 yellow Elgiloy
2. Anterior helical or **S** springs—0.020 yellow Elgiloy or 0.018 Australian wire
3. Posterior helical spring—0.028 yellow Elgiloy
4. Adams clasp, molars—0.025 yellow Elgiloy
5. Circumferential (C) clasp
   a. Molars—0.036 yellow Elgiloy
   b. Primary cuspids—0.025 yellow Elgiloy
6. Modified Crozat clasps on molars
   a. Main wire—0.032 yellow Elgiloy
   b. Spring wire—0.25 yellow Elgiloy
7. Modified ball clasps, used between primary molars—0.028 yellow Elgiloy

Important pliers used in bending wires, springs, and clasps for Hawley and palatal expansion appliances

Only four pliers are needed for bending the wires used in the majority of minor tooth movement appliances, although a

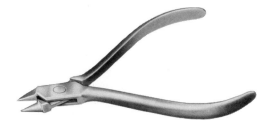

Fig. 16-1. No. 139 pliers, the most versatile instrument available for bending wires.

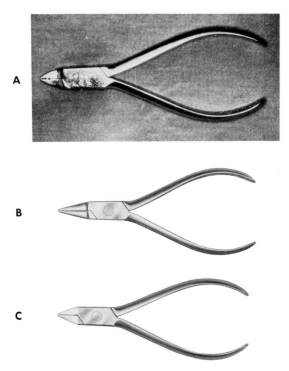

Fig. 16-2. A, Rogers pliers, which may be modified from either the No. 120 Peeso pliers, **B,** or the No. 515 clasp-bending pliers, **C.** Note that the dentist must thin the jaws of the Peeso pliers to a thickness of 2.5 mm. and then cut the grooves in the jaws. (See Fig. 16-4.) The Rogers pliers were designed by Dr. John R. Rogers, an orthodontist in Bellevue, Wash.

fifth is included. The use of No. 53 pliers has already been described in Chapter 15. The use of the No. 139 and the Rogers pliers will be described here. The specific uses of the other two pliers will be described in Chapter 17.

No. 139 Angle, or bird-beak, pliers (I-3) are the most versatile pliers that the dentist can use in minor tooth movement work (Fig. 16-1). They bend both small and large wires with a high degree of accuracy.

The Rogers pliers are used to quickly and accurately form Adams clasps of 0.025 wire and fit them to upper molar teeth. These pliers must be specially modified by the dentist from No. 120 Peeso pliers or other similar pliers such as the No. 515 clasp-bending plier (Fig. 16-2). The grooves in the beaks of the pliers are cut by using a 69 or 169L high-friction grip bur in an air-driven handpiece with *good rest positions* as the plier is held in the dentist's hands during the modification procedure. It is better to make the Rogers pliers from carbon steel, not stainless steel, pliers.

Using No. 139 pliers

Using the No. 139 pliers (I-3), by far the most versatile of any of the four pliers listed here, is made especially easy if the tapered jaws of the pliers are thought of as a three-position vise. This is particularly true when wire bends are made around its *round* jaw. The bends made around its *square* jaw made be made in more than

one position and are not as critical in this regard.

The reason for the three-position vise is made clear in Fig. 16-3 showing the round jaw of the pliers forming some of the wire shapes that are necessary in fabricating Hawley and palatal expansion appliances. In general, the use of each position of the tapered beaks of the No. 139 pliers is as follows:

Position 1 (near tips of jaws)

Forms each bend in the helical spring.

Forms the "indent" for lateral incisors in the labial bow.

Makes the end curls in the portion of each spring that is embedded in the acrylic material.

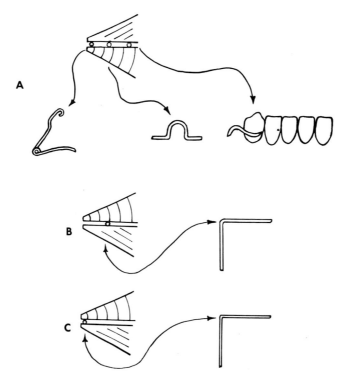

Fig. 16-3. Versatile No. 139 pliers (bird-beak) is used to bend light (0.014 to 0.020) and medium (0.022 to 0.030) wires into most configurations. **A,** It is best to visualize the pliers as having three positions when wire is being bent around the *round* jaw. Position 1 bends helical-loop springs and also the curls used to embed wire ends in the acrylic. Position 2 bends the cuspid adjustment loops on Hawley appliances and the molar adjustment loops in light labial arches. Position 3 bends a C clasp, which nicely fits most primary and permanent cuspids. **B,** When sharp-angled bends are being made in medium or heavy wire, the wire should be held in the position 2 for best leverage, and the heavier the wire, the more rounded the bend that results. **C,** When light wire is being bent, the angle is sharper, and the pliers can grip the wire at the position 1.

Position 2 (middle of jaws)

Forms the U-shaped cuspid loop of the upper or lower labial bow.

Forms the C clasp used on molars.

Position 3 (deepest grip of jaws)

Forms the C clasp for primary and permanent cuspids very accurately.

Using Rogers pliers

The Rogers pliers are the only ones of the five described here that cannot be purchased ready-made from one of the orthodontic supply houses. They must be modified by narrowing the jaws of a No. 120 Peeso or a No. 515 pliers and then cutting grooves in the jaws, using a high-speed tapered bur. Once modified to grasp 0.025 wire tightly, the Rogers pliers will allow the dentist to form Adams clasps easily and quickly (Fig. 16-4).

In Fig. 16-4 it will be noted that the Rogers pliers are used somewhat like the Universal lingual arch pliers, whose use is described in detail in Chapter 17.

FABRICATING HAWLEY APPLIANCES

There are really two kinds of appliances to which the designation of "Hawley" is

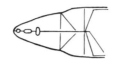

A

commonly attached, the upper and the lower. Of the two types, the upper is the more versatile and more commonly used.

The lower Hawley is used either as a passive retainer after lower lingual arch therapy or as a passive removable space maintainer after premature loss of two or more deciduous molars. It may also be used as an active appliance to distally position a lower 6-year molar. Since this particular type of tooth movement is one of the most difficult of the minor tooth movement pro-

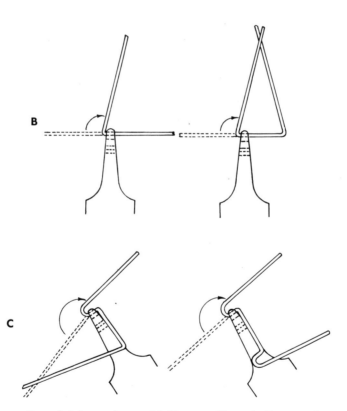

Fig. 16-4. Formation of Adams clasp with Rogers pliers. **A,** Rogers pliers, which must be modified by the dentist from No. 120 Peeso or similar (No. 515 clasp-bending) pliers. Extreme care must be taken to avoid overcutting when the grooves are placed. A high-speed, air contra-angle handpiece with a No. 69 friction grip bur cuts these grooves best. **B,** Adams clasp is started as indicated here. Size 0.025 yellow Elgiloy wire is the best choice. Width of clasp crossbar will be about 5 to 6 mm. **C,** Length of the clasp tip is determined by how far pliers grip below the clasp crossbar. For most children's mouths the high gingival level will necessitate a grip much like the one shown here. **D,** Crossbar of clasp is bent slightly in only two places, once as shown and again on the opposite side of the crossbar. This serves to contour the clasp around the molar. A moderate bend is made to allow the wires to cross the ridge mesial and distal to the molar. **E,** Rogers pliers form all final bends in the Adams clasp, including the palatal curls for embedding the wire in the acrylic.

cedures that may be attempted by the family dentist or pedodontist, the ratio of successful treatment may be expected to be smaller.[2]

Bending clasps for Hawley appliances

Most Hawley type appliances have clasp wires incorporated in them to aid in the retention in the child's upper or lower arch. There is usually a labial bow that aids in the stabilization of the appliance.

The four clasps most used in these appliances are the following:

1. Adams clasp. This clasp is formed of 0.025 wire yellow Elgiloy wire, using the Rogers pliers. It is used best for clasping second primary molars in the primary dentition and 6-year molars during the mixed dentition age.

2. C clasp. This clasp, made from 0.032 or 0.036 yellow Elgiloy wire, is best formed by the No. 139 plier and is used on cuspids, first and second primary molars, and first permanent molars. Since the clasp cannot reach subgingivally for reten-

tion, the use of this clasp should be limited to teeth that have obvious cervical retention areas.

3. Modified Crozat clasp. The main clasp is formed from 0.032 yellow Elgiloy wire, with a length of .025 yellow Elgiloy wire soldered to it to aid retention in the mesial and distal undercut areas. The tips of this clasp may reach slightly subgingivally.

4. Ball clasp. To provide additional stabilization and some increase in retention, a series of ball clasps can be fitted interproximally between the 6-year molar and the second deciduous molar or between the first and second deciduous molars. A modified ball clasp may be formed by tightly doubling the end of a length of 0.028 yellow Elgiloy wire.

The Adams clasp and the C clasp are best adapted over more mature molars, either primary or permanent. The modified Crozat clasp adapts well over partially erupted 6-year molars, the soldered extension wire along the buccal surface of the

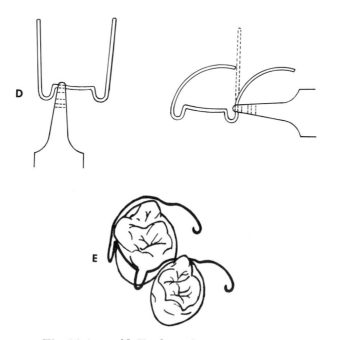

Fig. 16-4, cont'd. For legend see opposite page.

molars permitting the clasp to reach into the mesial and distal undercut areas for better retention. Ball clasps may be fitted wherever posterior teeth are in contact interproximally.

In general, if the child is younger than 8 years of age, the modified Crozat may be the best choice of clasp for 6-year molars. It has the disadvantage of being a soldered clasp, necessitating additional laboratory time to fabricate the appliance on the models. Too, if flame-soldering technique is used, the working model should be poured using a mixture of half orthodontic plaster and half R & R gray investment mix.* This makes a flame-proof cast, and flame-soldering can be more easily accomplished. An additional benefit of this sort of plaster mix is that the heated cast can be immersed in cold water immediately after the flame-soldering procedure to cause the cast to disintegrate and make recovery of the soldered appliance very simple.

The C clasp has been blamed for causing decalcified areas around the gingival area of the clasped tooth. This is rarely the fault of the clasp but stems rather from the lack of good daily oral hygiene on the part of the child. Checking the appliance at 2- or 3-week intervals and the application of topical fluoride treatments every 3 months during minor tooth movement procedures will alleviate much of the problem of decalcification areas along the gingival areas of clasped teeth which has been seen in the past. Stringent rules should be laid down emphatically for the child that no candy or gum be eaten during the whole period of wearing an appliance and that his teeth must be brushed after each meal and before he retires. A "travel toothbrush" given to him from the dental office for use after lunch at school brings good results. *Motivation toward good oral hygiene is absolutely essential for each child in minor tooth movement treatment.*

The Adams clasp[1] has the softest action of any of these clasps on the tooth and causes the clasped molars to undergo the least amount of movement during treatment. Any mesial movement of clasped teeth (loss of anchorage) during treatment is unnecessary and undesirable. This loss of anchorage may take place over a long period of time and is sometimes difficult to detect without measuring. The Adams clasp is clearly the most difficult to bend of the three clasps mentioned here, unless modified pliers are used, such as the Rogers pliers. The Adams clasp can also be converted to a clasp resembling the modified Crozat by spot-welding and then soldering a piece of 0.025 wire to connect each of the U-loops of the Adams clasp along the gingival margin on the buccal surface of the molar. The increased retention that results makes this extra effort worthwhile if retention appears to be minimal in the appliance when conventional Adams clasps are used.[1]

Upper Hawley appliance

The upper Hawley appliance may be used for treating protruding and spaced upper anterior teeth (Class I, Type 2, malocclusion); anterior cross-bites involving the upper central or lateral incisors (Class I, Type 3, malocclusions); moving upper 6-year molars to a more distal position after mesial drift has occurred (Class I, Type 5, malocclusions); and also as a palatal appliance to maintain the positions of the upper teeth after tooth movement procedures (as a full-arch retention device). (See Fig. 16-5.)

Materials needed

1. 0.028 yellow Elgiloy wire (C-5)* (for labial bow or posterior helical springs)
2. 0.025 yellow Elgiloy wire (C-5) (for anterior helical springs and Adams clasps)

---

*Ransom & Randolph Co. products are available through regular dental supply houses.

*Letter-number notations throughout chapter refer to Tables 16 to 18 in Chapter 14.

3. 0.020 yellow Elgiloy wire or 0.018 Australian wire (C-5) (for anterior helical springs)
4. 0.036 yellow Elgiloy wire (C-5) (for C clasps on molars)
5. 0.032 yellow Elgiloy (C-5) (primary clasp wire for modified Crozat clasps)
6. 0.025 yellow Elgiloy wire (C-5) (secondary clasp wire for modified Crozat clasps)
7. Nonslump orthodontic resin, powder and liquid (C-15)
8. Dead-soft 0.001-inch tinfoil
9. Petrolatum

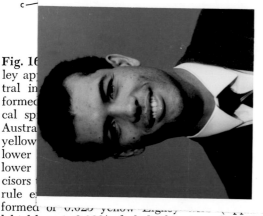

wire sizes will be used
pliance but are included
hecklist for the dentist.

-6)

y appliance used to
spaced upper anterior
oricated with Adams
s. An anterior helical
l lingual to the incisor
intention is to reduce
e.

poratory model needs
m to fabricate a Haw-
o small indentations
to the gingival margin
, one at the distal and
spect of the tooth.
iers are used to form
f 0.025 yellow Elgiloy
tips of which fit into
ed at the gingival mar-

liers are used to form
ow that contacts the
e anterior teeth except
may be in a cross-bite
erwise malposed lin-
be taken that the "in-
bow are placed over
the lateral incisors to prevent a "denture"
smile from developing in the child when
treatment is finished.

The U-loops for adjustment of the labial
bow placed over the cuspids should be designed so that the distal portions of the
springs cross the alveolar ridge onto the

Fig. 16
ley ap
tral in
formed
cal sp
Austra
yellow
lower
lower
cisors
rule e
formed or 0.020 yellow Elgiloy ....
labial bow is 0.028); b, helical spring of 0.018
Australian wire; c, Adams clasp of 0.025 yellow
Elgiloy wire. C, Schematic drawing of lower
Hawley appliance designed to establish full
arch anchorage to distally position the lower
left 6-year molar. a, Labial bow formed of
0.025 yellow Elgiloy wire; b, Adams clasp of
0.025 yellow Elgiloy wire; c, posterior helical
spring of 0.020 Australian wire.

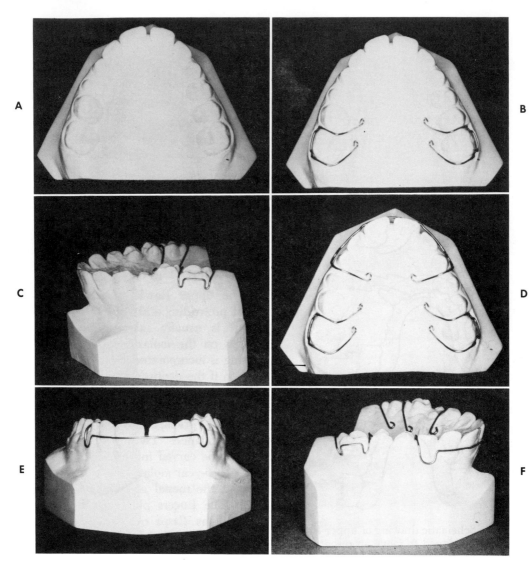

Fig. 16-6. A, Upper model of a Class I, Type 2, malocclusion is shown here, with marked protrusion of the upper incisors. An upper Hawley appliance will be fabricated on this cast. **B,** Adams clasp is bent for each 6-year molar. To help position the clasp tips, cut away a small amount of the interproximal plaster to the mesial and distal of the molar on the buccal aspect. **C,** Adams clasp, side view. **D,** Labial bow wire is carefully contoured, placing indents in the wire over the lateral incisors. **E,** Labial bow from lateral aspect. **F,** All wires in place on cast. **G,** Tinfoil is applied to cast, following instructions in text. Adherence of foil to cast is enhanced by lubricating cast with petrolatum. Wires are shown luted to place, using sticky wax, on buccal and labial areas. **H,** Nonslump orthodontic acrylic is added to cast by drop-and-powder method. Finger is used to smooth final product while surface is still wet. **I,** Cast is placed *dry* in the pressure pot and cured for 20 minutes at 20 pounds' air pressure from laboratory source. **J,** Cured appliance is slipped off cast and tinfoil peeled away, leaving well-finished palatal surface. **K,** Appliance is smoothed and polished with wet pumice and a denture polishing compound. **L,** Upper Hawley appliance polished and placed back on cast ready for fitting. Note lingual relief of acrylic areas lingual to upper incisors. This permits lingual movement of upper incisors when U-loops of labial bow wire are tightened.

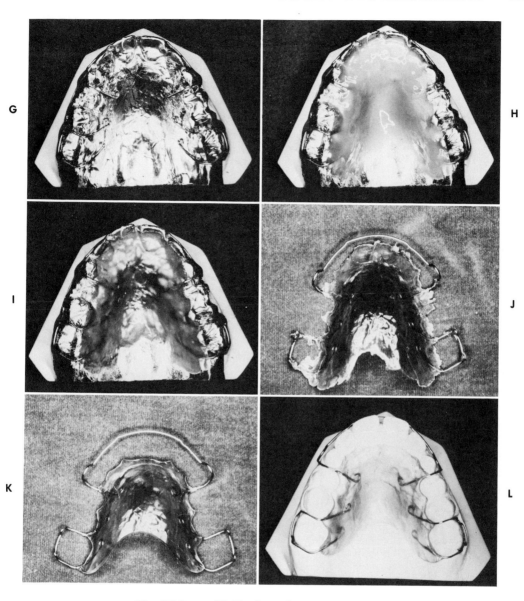

Fig. 16-6, cont'd. For legend see opposite page.

palate between the cuspid and the tooth distal to it. Each wire end is curled so that it may be embedded in the palatal acrylic.

4. The helical loop for the helical spring (for treatment of an anterior cross-bite case) is formed of either 0.020 yellow Elgiloy or 0.018 Australian wire. The helical loop is made with the No. 139 pliers in position 1. The rest of the spring is contoured with the pliers in position 1, but with gentler pressures on the wire. (See Fig. 16-3.)

NOTE: A "step" is incorporated in the spring between the helical loop and the end curl, which represents the transition of the wire from an embedded position in the palatal acrylic to the exposed portion of the spring that acts against the tooth. The helical loop must be left exposed for proper spring action.

5. After the two Adams clasps, the labial bow and the helical spring have been formed and fitted on the cast, they are removed and set aside until tinfoil has been applied to the cast.

6. To properly apply tinfoil to a cast preparatory to applying the acrylic is a necessity in making good appliances. Although tinfoil substitutes have been developed and are widely used, there is really no replacement for 0.001 thickness, dead-soft tinfoil.

To start the application of tinfoil, use a 2½ × 2½ inch square of foil and press it into the palatal area with the thumb (thumb pointing toward the anterior teeth). Hold it there firmly, and smooth the foil over the remainder of the palatal area with the index finger of the other hand. When the foil has been adapted as closely as it can be, remove the foil pattern from the cast and cut with a scissors along the outside of the indentations made by the occlusal surfaces of the posterior teeth and along the incisal edges of the anterior teeth. Leave the foil in the postpalatal area uncut, since it can be pressed down over the heel of the model to help stabilize the foil.

7. Lubricate the cast so that the teeth and palatal surfaces are coated with a fairly thin coating of petrolatum (or silicate lubricant); then fit the tinfoil form back on the cast. It now adheres very well, and the

final burnishing can be done using the fingers and a plastic toothbrush handle smoothed and polished to resemble the spoon-shaped end of the No. 7 wax spatula.

8. The clasps and springs are now refitted to the cast covered with tinfoil and are luted to the cast by the addition of sticky wax melted on the labial and buccal areas. (Sticky wax is also added so that it completely covers the "free" portion of the helical spring, which rests against the palatal side of the central incisor in a case involving an anterior cross-bite.)

9. Using the drop-and-powder method, add the orthodontic resin in increments to the palatal surface of the cast covered with tin-foil to a thickness of 2 mm. or so. When this thickness has been reached, a final coat of liquid monomer is washed over the whole appliance surface and smoothed with the fingers; the cast is placed in the pressure pot at 20 pounds' air pressure. *No water need be added to the pot while the appliance is curing.*

10. After 20 minutes, the dry-cured cast is removed from the pressure pot and immersed in warm water for 10 minutes for final curing. A No. 7 wax spatula is used to slip under the foil at the heel of the appliance to loosen it. The whole appliance should slip easily off the working cast without damage to the cast, which is one of the distinct advantages of the tinfoil method.

11. The tinfoil is peeled off the palatal side of the appliance, starting at the heel. The gingival margins are trimmed, and the palatal surface is smoothed with a flame-

Fig. 16-7. **A,** Upper model showing an upper right 6-year molar that has drifted mesially. Treatment indicated is to distalize this molar using an upper Hawley appliance with a helical spring to generate distal force against the molar. **B,** Modified Crozat clasp is formed and soldered on anchorage molar opposite to mesially drifted molar. **C,** Side view of Crozat clasp showing it is made of a U-shaped wire and a clasping wire soldered together. **D,** All wires contoured and in place. Note helical spring has only one helix located *buccal* to the molar being moved distally. **E,** Tinfoil has been applied to cast, and wires have been luted to place using sticky wax on buccal and labial surfaces. **F,** Drop-and-powder method of applying nonslump orthodontic resin is used. Appliance is cured for 20 minutes at 20 pounds' pressure in pot. **G,** Finished appliance. Note that most of helical spring is free from acrylic.

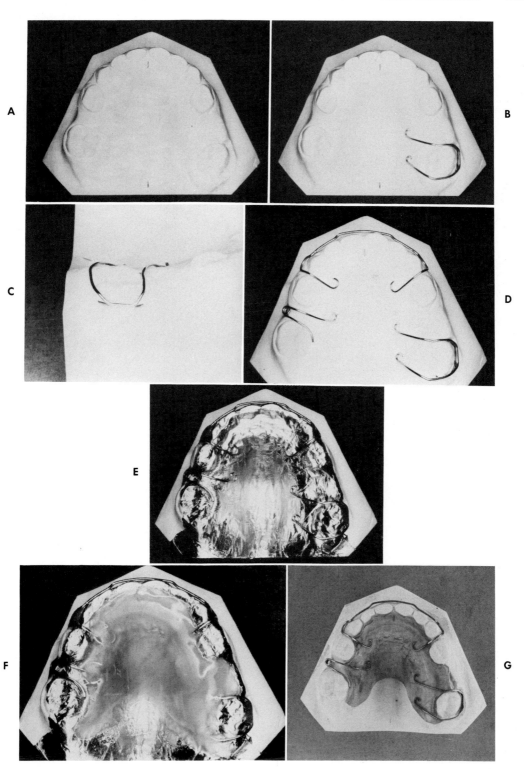

Fig. 16-7. For legend see opposite page.

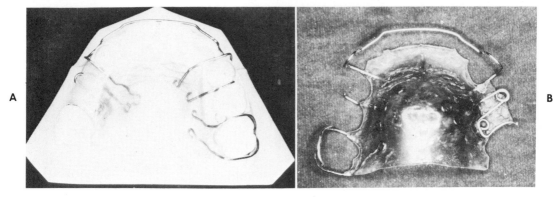

Fig. 16-8. A, Another upper Hawley appliance designed to distalize an upper 6-year molar. In this design a double helical spring was used (0.028 yellow Elgiloy wire). The part of the spring that was to be free was covered with wax to prevent its being embedded in the body of the acrylic. An acrylic shelf was cured over the wax, acting to protect the spring in the child's mouth. **B,** Tissue side view of the finished appliance. Note configuration of double helical spring.

shaped acrylic bur. The wax luting is removed from the clasps and labial bow (and the helical spring areas).

12. The appliance is polished, first with wet pumice and then with a denture polish. It can be placed in a cold sterilizing solution until the patient is available for the final fitting. At this time the final adjustment of spring pressures against the teeth is accomplished.

• • •

The other types of Hawley appliances used in the upper arch are merely variations from the technique just described. Figs. 16-7 and 16-8 demonstrate construction of upper Hawley appliances incorporating single and double helical springs and used to distalize an upper 6-year molar.

Advantages of the tinfoil–dry pressure curing method

Some of the important advantages of the tinfoil–dry pressure curing method for fabricating Hawley appliances are the following:

1. The working cast remains undamaged by the removal of the cured appliance.

2. The tinfoil effectively seals the tissue side of the appliance so that no porosity is present to collect food and cause a discoloration or bad odor during long-term wear by the child. Indeed, made in this way, the acrylic (either pink or clear) is so transparent that fine newsprint can be read through it.

3. The dry curing of the acrylic in the pressure pot prevents bubble formation, and the resulting density (and strength) can surpass that of laboratory–packed and cured denture acrylic.

NOTE: It is sometimes thought that warm water must be added to the pressure pot to immerse the cast during the curing process. To do this only increases the likelihood of incorporating porosity in the acrylic, since the warm water will act to expand the trapped air pockets· Dry curing prevents this. However, as noted in step 10, the cured acrylic is immersed in warm water *after* it is pressurized. This assures final set of the material.

Lower Hawley appliance

The lower Hawley appliance may be utilized to move a lower six-year molar distally to regain lost space (Class I, Type 5,

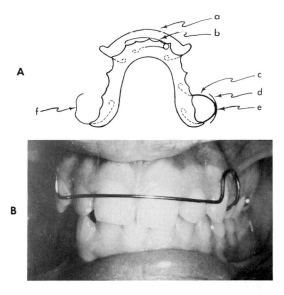

Fig. 16-9. A, Schematic drawing of a lower Hawley appliance designed to reposition all lower incisors more labially. *a,* Labial bow formed of 0.025 yellow Elgiloy wire; *b,* anterior helical spring of 0.018 Australian wire; *c,* clasp wire formed of 0.025 yellow Elgiloy wire, to which is soldered a clasp wire formed of 0.025 yellow Elgiloy to reach into retention areas; *d,* silver solder joint. **B,** Upper Hawley appliance in a child's mouth. Note that the positioning of the labial bow wire should be at the junction of the middle and gingival thirds of the clinical crowns of the central incisors for both upper and lower Hawley appliances.

cases), or it may be used as a full arch retention device after tooth movement procedures. (See Fig. 16-9.)

Materials needed

1. 0.025 yellow Elgiloy wire (C-5) (for labial bow and Adams clasps)
2. 0.032 yellow Elgiloy wire (C-5) (for modified Crozat clasps)
3. 0.025 yellow Elgiloy wire (C-5) (for modified Crozat clasp extension wire)
4. 0.028 yellow Elgiloy (C-5) (for helical spring against lower molar)
5. 0.036 yellow Elgiloy (C-5) (for C clasps on molars)
6. Nonslump orthodontic resin (C-15) (powder and liquid)
7. Dead-soft 0.001-inch thick tinfoil
8. Petrolatum
9. Sticky wax

NOTE: Not all these materials will be used in any one appliance; however, they have been included here as a convenient check for the dentist.

Procedure

The lower Hawley appliance may be used to move a lower 6-year molar distally, incorporating a C clasp or Adams clasp on the molar that is not to be moved. Often these do not supply enough reten-

tion, and a modified Crozat clasp will be used.

1. The lower laboratory cast needs only slight modifications to prepare it for the fabrication of a Hawley appliance. The gingival margin should be carved away a bit on the opposite molar (which is not to be moved distally) so the Crozat clasp (if it is to be used) may be fitted slightly subgingivally.

2. The No. 139 pliers are used to form the two parts of the Crozat clasp. A piece of 0.032 yellow Elgiloy wire is used to form the square U-shaped primary wire clasp against the buccal surface of the molar so that the bottom of the U is slightly above the gingival crest.

A piece of 0.025 yellow Elgiloy wire is used to form the secondary wire of the clasp, which fits gingivally to the U-shaped wire and permits the extension of a retention arm into both the mesial and distal undercuts on the buccal surface. These wires are spot-welded together and then soldered in place on the model, utilizing either the electric cable extensions of the spot-welder or the flame method.

3. The helical spring of 0.028 yellow Elgiloy wire is formed with the No. 139

pliers. The helical hoop is located about 4 mm. to the buccal of the molar, and the distal arm of the spring curves lingually then distally to approximate the mesial surface of the molar. This permits adequate control of the direction of movement of the molar as the spring is activated.

4. The labial bow is formed of 0.025 yellow Elgiloy wire, using the No. 139 pliers. The cuspid loops do not form as great a dimension incisally-gingivally as in the upper Hawley appliance. Also, the position of the labial bow wire must be such that there is no labial interference as the lower incisors close into contact with the upper incisors·

5. After the clasps, helical spring, and labial bow have been fabricated, they are removed from the cast. The dead-soft tinfoil is form-fitted by firm finger pressure, then removed, and trimmed along the occlusal margins. On the lingual aspect an apron of approximately 5 mm. is left below what will be the inferior margin of the appliance. This tinfoil will be turned upward to form a trough to catch acrylic overflow.

6. The fitted tinfoil is removed, the cast is lubricated with petrolatum, and the tinfoil is fitted again and smoothed into place with the spoon-shaped end of the polished toothbrush handle previously mentioned. The clasps and springs are fitted over the tinfoil and attached by sticky wax on the buccal aspect to hold them in place. Then the excess apron of tinfoil is curled up on the lingual aspect, using a No. 7 wax spatula to form a trough.

7. The acrylic is built up using drop-and-power method until a thickness of approximately 2 mm. is reached. Monomer is flowed over the whole surface of the appliance, the surface is finger-smoothed, and the appliance is placed into the dry pressure pot at 20 pounds' air pressure for 20 minutes. When the appliance is removed, it may be placed in a warm water bath for 10 minutes to complete the curing process.

8. Removal of the appliance from the cast is accomplished by levering it loose with the No. 7 wax spatula blade. It is trimmed, smoothed, and polished on the wheel, much like the upper Hawley appliance. Care should be taken not to catch one of the protruding springs in the rag wheel of the lathe during polishing. The appliance can be damaged and the operator's fingers sustain injuries if this should happen.

FABRICATING PALATAL EXPANSION APPLIANCES

Although palatal expansion appliances are "split" acrylic appliances made either with a heavy U-shaped wire curled back on itself or with a jackscrew expansion device incorporated, they are made by essentially the same methods as are Hawley appliances. Most expansion appliances will be made to treat posterior cross-bites, although some will be made to treat genetic lack of space problems.

If the U-shaped wire is used as the expansion adjustment mechanism, the expansion limit of such an appliance is a theoretical 5 to 6 mm. Often during adjustment procedures, however, the U-shaped wire is bent in such a way that the appliance will no longer fit. The appliance must then be remade. The drive on jackscrew expansion devices may extend either 4 mm. or 6 mm. When that limit is reached in treatment, the appliance must be remade to provide further expansion.

Use of modified ball clasps for retention

Because the closing relationships change slightly as the palatal arch expands, the use of modified ball clasps is indicated in many of these appliances. In general, the clasps used are adapted from commercially made ones or constructed from 0.028 wire.

Flattening commercially made ball clasps. Commercially made ball clasps, size 0.028 wire and 0.7 mm. ball tip (C-22 alternate), are most often used. The side next to the tooth, the side away from the tooth, and the tip of the ball are all flattened to create a sort of small rectangle that parallels the side of the arch. This rectangle is inserted into the interproximal area where the papilla between the primary molars has been slightly carved out of the plaster cast. The clasp is then contoured through the interproximal embrasures of the teeth and fitted closely to the palatal slope. A small curl is formed on the palatal end for better retention in the acrylic.

If possible, interproximal clasps shaped the same way are placed between the second deciduous molar and the 6-year molar and also between the cuspid and first primary molar. This is accomplished on both sides of the upper arch, and the result can be startlingly good retention during the full range of treatment.[3]

Bending 0.028 wire end double to simulate ball clasp. One end of the 0.028 yellow Elgiloy wire may be doubled over on itself and squeezed to form a modified ball clasp. The doubled wire end may be fitted interproximally into the embrasure between posterior teeth with its flat side oriented mesiodistally or buccolingually. Usually the latter works best.

The wire end may be bent in a 3 mm. curve with the No. 139 bird-beak pliers, using the beaks in position 1. (See Fig. 16-3.) Then the wire may be squeezed double on its own end by using the tip grooves of the Universal lingual arch pliers (Fig. 17-3). The remaining bends to fit the clasp in the interproximal areas between the teeth and over the ridge onto the palatal tissue area may be accomplished with the No. 139 pliers, again in position 1.

Materials needed

1. 0.028 yellow Elgiloy wire (C-5) (if doubled wire ends are to serve as modified ball clasps)
2. 0.028 wire with commercially made 0.7 mm. ball clasps at the end (C-22 alternate)
3. Expansion screw, spring-loaded, extra

small, expanding 4 mm. (C-23 alternate)
4. 0.040 blue Elgiloy, tempered (C-5) (for the U-shaped wire expansion device if jackscrew is not to be used)
5. 0.001 dead-soft tinfoil
6. Nonslump orthodontic acrylic resin (powder and liquid) (C-15)
7. Petrolatum
8. Sticky wax

Procedure for appliance with jackscrew (Fig. 16-10, *A* to *K*)

1. The upper laboratory model is prepared by carving slight depressions in the interproximal areas where modified ball clasps are to be fitted.
2. Two, four, or six modified ball clasps are fitted and contoured onto the palatal area.
3. 0.001 dead-soft tinfoil, 2½ × 2½ inches, is adapted to the palate and the lingual surfaces of the upper teeth exactly as in the preparation of the Hawley appliance described previously in this chapter.
4. Tinfoil is removed carefully, petrolatum is applied to cast on palatal surface to create adhesion, and tinfoil is readapted and burnished. Excess tinfoil is trimmed away.
5. Ball clasps are luted to place on the buccal interproximal areas, using sticky wax.
6. The expansion screw device comes with a 1 mm. thick vertical metal shield attached to the jackscrew to seal out the acrylic from the drive area in the middle. This shield should be oriented so that it runs anteroposteriorly, with the screw flat against the middle of the palate and midway between the second primary molars. The arrow etched into the top of the screw (away from the plaster) should point *toward* the upper front teeth on the model. This means the lever will be able to be inserted, and when moved toward the incisors, the drive mechanism will be opened about 0.3 mm. by each complete back-to-front lever stroke.
7. The jackscrew is luted to its position

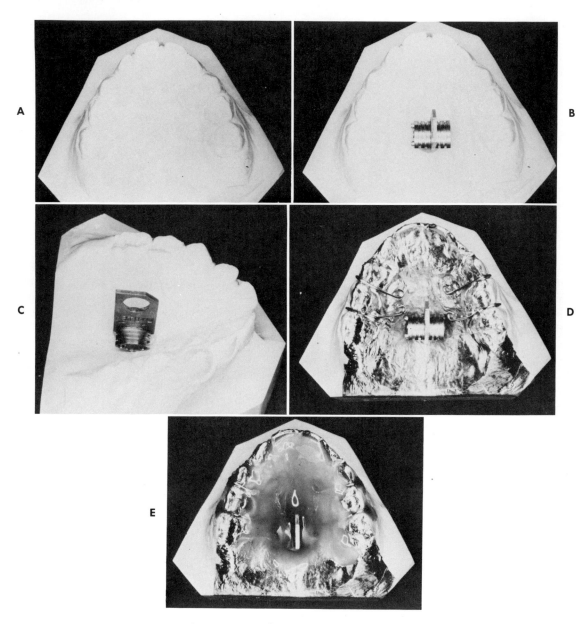

Fig. 16-10. For legend see opposite page.

(see step 6) by using drop-and-powder method of applying nonslump orthodontic resin. The shield must be finger-held for a minute or so while the resin sets enough to act as a glue to hold the jackscrew in place.

8. When the jackscrew has been stabilized, the drop-and-powder method is used to cover the whole palatal surface to a depth of 2 mm. or so. The lingual surfaces of the posterior teeth must be covered adequately with the resin build-up.

9. The wet-surfaced acrylic is finger-rubbed, and the model is placed in the pressure pot *dry*, with the laboratory air pressure run up to 20 pounds. It is left to

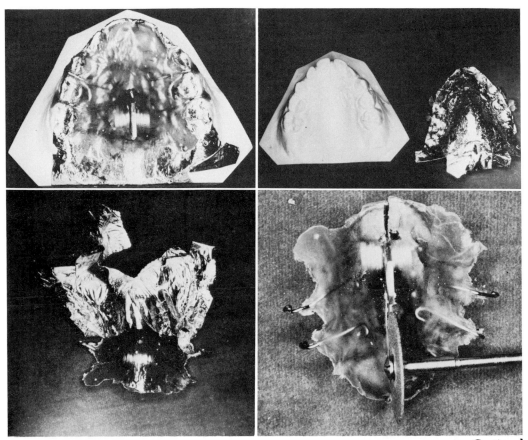

F

G

H

I

Continued.

Fig. 16-10. **A,** Upper cast of 4½-year-old child. He has an expressed unilateral cross-bite, and a bilateral palatal expansion is planned. **B,** Expansion appliance utilizing a jackscrew (C-23) is tentatively placed in the palatal area with the "arrow" on the plate pointing toward the incisors. **C,** Jackscrew and vertical sealing plate shown from the side. The plate seals out the acrylic from the drive mechanism during fabrication of the appliance. **D,** Tinfoil is applied to cast, and jackscrew is luted to place with some of the nonslump orthodontic acrylic. **E,** Remainder of the palate is covered with non-slump orthodontic resin, using drop-and-powder method. The wet surface is finger-smoothed. Cast is then placed in pressure pot *dry* for 20 minutes at 20 pounds' pressure. **F,** Cured appliance is removed from pressure pot. **G,** Appliance is slipped off cast without damage to the cast, which is one of the advantages of this method of fabrication. **H,** Tinfoil is peeled from palatal surface, leaving it highly finished. **I,** Separating disk is used to split appliance, taking care not to cut into metal housing of the jackscrew. **J,** Heavy duty pliers are used to remove the vertical sealing plate. It must be torqued only anteroposteriorly to remove it. **K,** Finished appliance was used to expand the child's upper arch about 4 mm.; to fabricate retention appliance, a new impression was taken *while* appliance was in the child's mouth. Appliance was poured-up in place on plaster model. It was then removed and cleaned, and tinfoil was applied to the cast. After this procedure the wide palatal-split area was filled in with resin and cured in the pressure pot to make retention appliance seen above. **L,** Alternative method for providing palatal expansion is the upper U-loop expansion appliance. This is also a split-acrylic appliance as is the jackscrew one shown in **A** to **K.** **M,** Finished U-loop palatal expansion appliance. Adjustments are made in either the *anterior* or *posterior* loop areas, depending on the direction of forces required. (**L** and **M** courtesy Dr. Theodore R. Oldenburg, Chapel Hill, N. C.)

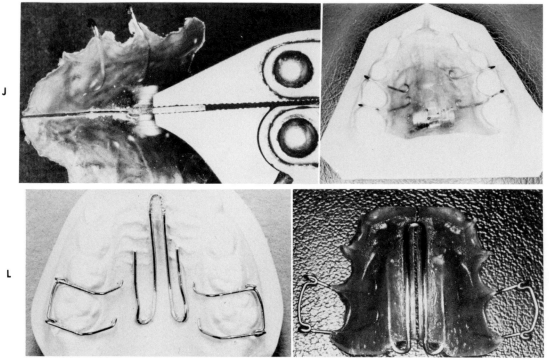

Fig. 16-10, cont'd. For legend see p. 273.

cure for 20 minutes. At the end of this period it is placed in a warm water bath for 5 minutes to complete the curing process.

10. Removal of the appliance from the cast is easily accomplished using a prying action with the spoon end of a No. 7 wax spatula. The laboratory model should remain unbroken after removal. The tinfoil is peeled off the palatal side.

11. A critical step in making the appliance is now at hand. Two things must be accomplished to allow it to act as a "split" appliance.

    a. The metal shield must be removed. This is done best by using a rugged square-nose pliers such as the Bernard pliers or equivalent. Placing one thumb on the front part of the palatal surface and prying or rotating the shield to the rear usually works best. It is not a delicate piece of equipment, so don't spare the horsepower in the use of pressure at this point.

    b. After the removal of the shield, the appliance is "split" by a thin metal or corundum separating disc (⅞ inch), cutting on a line drawn from between the central incisors posteriorly along the midline of the palate. *Extreme care* must be used not to cut or damage the outer edges of the drive-screw device buried in the resin. The resin posterior to the drive-screw must also be cut in the midline so that the two halves of the drive-screw will be freed.

12. For completing the freeing of the acrylic around the jackscrew to allow the appliance to "split," a sharp No. 10 scalpel blade may be used. The lever is inserted and moved *toward* the front teeth to test the freedom of the working of the drive mechanism.

13. Last, the acrylic is smoothed, polished, scrubbed in hot water, and then cold-sterilized until being fitted in the child's mouth.

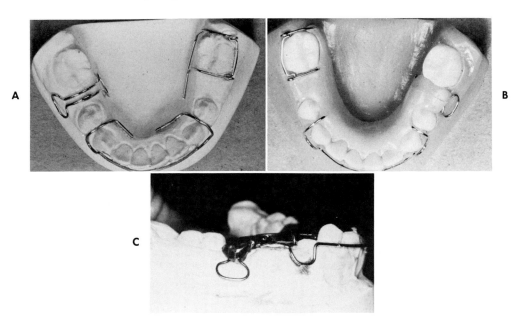

Fig. 16-11. Lower Hawley appliance being fabricated in a 10-year-old child's lower arch. **A,** Lower right 6-year molar is to be distalized by the opening action of the dumbbell spring. An Adams clasp is shown on the opposite 6-year molar. **B,** Finished lower Hawley appliance in place on model of the child's arch. Note split acrylic through middle of dumbbell spring. **C,** Finished appliance, shown from the side on model to demonstrate position of dumbbell spring against alveolus. Cuspid U-loop of the appliance must not touch tissue, which would cause abrasion. (Courtesy Dr. Theodore R. Oldenburg, Chapel Hill, N.C.)

Procedure for appliance with U-shaped wire (0.040) (Fig. 16-10, *L* and *M*)

Since the palatal expansion appliance using the U-shaped wire is made almost exactly as the jackscrew appliance just described, only the bending of the U-shaped 0.040 wire that serves as the expansion mechanism will be described here.

1. The 0.040 wire should be of blue Elgiloy. The U-shape is contoured as if it were bent around a regular-size round pencil. The bottom of the U is bent again so that it fits against the palate about 1 cm. lingual to the lingual surfaces of the upper central incisors. The sides of the U are contoured straight back posteriorly in close approximation to the palatal tissue (plaster cast).

2. Opposite the distal surface of each upper 6-year molar the wire is bent in a small-diameter rounded bend so that it turns 180 degrees and moves anteriorly again for about 1 cm. The ends may be curled laterally to act as a retention device in the acrylic resin.

3. The single anterior U-shape and the smaller posterior U-bends must be waxed out to prevent their being incorporated in the acrylic. This allows adjustments to be accomplished at all three U-bends.

SUMMARY

The fabrication of Hawley and palatal expansion appliances is quite easily accomplished in the dentist's laboratory. Using the tinfoil method of preparing casts saves time, provides highly polished tissue surfaces on the appliance, and avoids the necessity of breaking the cast to remove the cured appliance. The dental assistant who makes these appliances for the dentist will appreciate the added neatness of this procedure.

REFERENCES

1. Adams, C. P.: The design and construction of removable orthodontic appliances, ed. 4, Bristol, England, 1971, John Wright & Sons.
2. Graber, T. M.: Orthodontics: principles and practice, ed. 2, Philadelphia, 1966, W. B. Saunders Co., pp. 760-774.
3. Moyers, R. E.: Handbook of orthodontics, ed. 2, Chicago, 1963, Year Book Medical Publishers, Inc., pp. 540-542.

17 | Fabricating lingual arches

The lower lingual arch has proved to be one of the most versatile of all the appliances used in minor tooth movement. It is described here as an active fixed-removable (F-R) appliance and not merely as a passive holding appliance for the lower arch. The single exception is the fixed soldered arch, which was described in Chapter 15 as a bilateral space maintainer.

MATCHING TYPE OF LINGUAL ARCH TO AGE OF CHILD

Both horizontal and vertical types of lingual arches have been suggested for younger children 6 to 11 years of age. Because of its ease of construction and because it is kinder to the gingival tissues of younger children, the horizontally attached lingual arch will be emphasized here. Beyond age 11 the horizontally attached lingual arch cannot be used as efficiently because of the difficulty of insertion and removal due to the increased curve of Spee and the increased crown height of the lower incisors. However, with younger children it is ideally suited to the shorter clinical crowns they exhibit.

Both the horizontal or the vertical types of F-R lingual arches may be made with U-loops in the bicuspid area (Fig. 17-1).

These loops provide for adjustment of both length and pressures against the molar teeth and may be used for applying reciprocal pressures directed against the lower anterior teeth.

Other springs may be added. These are spot-welded, first, and then soldered to the basic lingual arch appliance. They may be finger springs designed to move the lower incisors labially, S springs to move a bicuspid or cuspid facially, or gathering springs to exert light pressures against the distal surfaces of the lower lateral incisors to move them toward the midline.

For the most part, a lingual arch is considered to be applicable only to the lower dental arch. In some special circumstances, however, a modification of the lingual arch appliance suitable for the upper arch may be constructed. The Porter appliance (or the similar W appliance) is one such modification. It is used primarily to treat posterior cross-bites in the primary and mixed dentition.

BENDING ARCH WIRE FOR A HORIZONTALLY ATTACHED LINGUAL ARCH

Much of the dentist's time can be wasted by inefficient wire-bending methods. Even

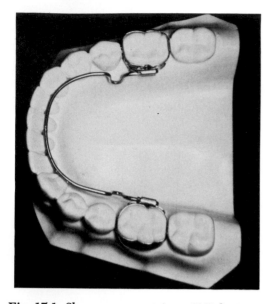

Fig. 17-1. Shown on a cast is an F-R horizontal lingual arch with U-loops for adjustment. The U-loops in the bicuspid area may be used but are not always necessary.

though a pair of pliers may perform only one main task, if they do this task efficiently in a way no other pliers can, then they become indispensable for the dentist. The following two pliers fall into this category when lingual arch fabrication, insertion, and removal are considered:

1. The Universal lingual arch pliers (I-7),* which accomplish only one task—bending double the ends of the 0.036 blue or yellow Elgiloy lingual arch wire so that each end may accurately insert into the horizontal sheaths attached to the lingual surfaces of the molar bands (Fig. 17-2, *A* and *B*). To demonstrate the use of the Universal lingual arch pliers is not as straightforward a task as with most other pliers. Fig. 17-3 shows its use in a stepwise fashion.

*Letter-number designations throughout chapter refer to Tables 16 to 18 in Chapter 14.

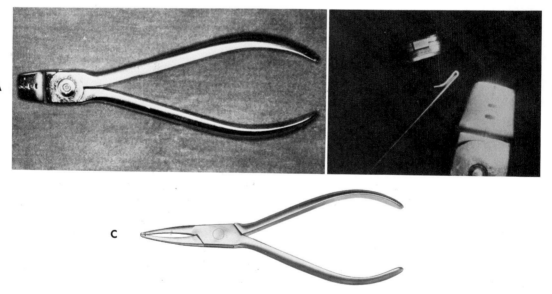

Fig. 17-2. A, Universal lingual arch pliers, which can be used quickly to bend double the ends of an 0.036 arch wire (yellow Elgiloy) to fabricate a horizontal F-R lower lingual arch appliance. **B,** Enlarged picture of the Universal lingual arch pliers. Doubled end of the arch wire is ready to be inserted into the lingual sheath and spot-welded to the lingual aspect of the narrow molar band. **C,** No. 110 How pliers. This instrument is used to insert the horizontal lingual arch into the child's mouth and remove it. The doubled wire-ends fit in the lingual sheaths by friction only.

2. The No. 110 How pliers (I-4), which do not bend wire but instead are used to facilitate the easy removal and insertion of the horizontal lingual arch in the child's mouth after it has been cemented (Fig. 17-2, C). They may also be used to insert or remove other arch wires that fit into tubes, such as light and heavy labial arches fitting into molar buccal tubes.

FABRICATING F-R LINGUAL ARCH WITH HORIZONTAL ATTACHMENTS, SUITABLE FOR MIXED DENTITION

Materials needed

1. 0.036 blue or yellow Elgiloy wire (C-5)
2. 2 horizontal lingual sheaths, size 0.036, (A-1) (to receive doubled arch wire)
3. 2 narrow molar bands (C-1)
4. No. 660 welder (I-1)
5. Universal lingual arch–forming pliers (I-7)
6. No. 139 pliers (I-3)
7. Cratex rubber wheel
8. White arch-marking pencil (I-16)

Procedure (Figs. 17-3 and 17-4)

1. On lower study cast make saw-cuts interproximally on each side of the 6-year molars, wet the plaster in the area, then carve away plaster so that molar crowns are well exposed.

2. Fit molar bands on plaster molars in the same relationship as they have already been fitted in the child's mouth.

3. Contour 0.036 blue or yellow Elgiloy wire in a tapered U-shape with controlled thumb and finger pressure so that the lingual arch wire approximates the lingual surfaces of the lower incisors, cuspids, and bicuspids.

4. Holding arch wire in place on the model, mark the arch wire *exactly* opposite the distolingual cusp of each lower 6-year molar. The accuracy of this mark allows the wire to be bent double at this mark and fit into the horizontal lingual sheath. The sheath will be spot-welded later so that it is exactly centered on the lingual groove of each band on the 6-year molars.

5. Lift the marked arch wire off the model and bend in the slight curve of Spee

that is required, using finger and thumb pressure.

6. Holding the arch wire just above the model, and parallel to it, bend each end of the wire 90 degrees upward exactly at each white mark, using the square beak of the No. 139 pliers.

7. Carefully referring to Fig. 17-3, bend the wire ends double, using the Universal lingual arch pliers. Squeeze the wire-ends successively tighter and tighter together until the wire is tightly doubled against itself. Cut off the turned up portion of the wire, leaving only a long enough piece to act as a stop to prevent the doubled end from sliding completely through the sheath.

8. Smooth the wire ends on the Cratex rubber wheel to remove any sharp projections and smooth the slight bulge at the elbow of each doubled wire. This aids in reducing the tightness of fit as the doubled ends slip into the streamlined horizontal lingual sheaths.

9. Slip both lingual sheaths onto the doubled ends of the arch wire, flange side out. *These sheaths* (horizontal attachments) *will not be removed from the arch wire until the last stages of spot-welding.*

10. Return the arch wire, with both horizontal sheaths fitting snugly over the doubled ends, to the model. The middle of the sheaths should be in exact relationship to the lingual groove of each band. Usually the U-shaped arch must be correctively bent slightly during these manipulative procedures. This is done with pressures exerted by the thumb and finger.

11. Remove one molar band, clean away the loose plaster on the inside with a wetted cotton-bud applicator, and tack-weld (a single spot-weld used to assess alignment) the *distal* flange of the horizontal lingual sheath to the band. The flange should be kept parallel to the occlusal edge of the band, and as explained previously, the lingual groove of the band falls exactly at the middle of the sheath.

12. Return the spot-welded band that has been attached to the arch wire to the

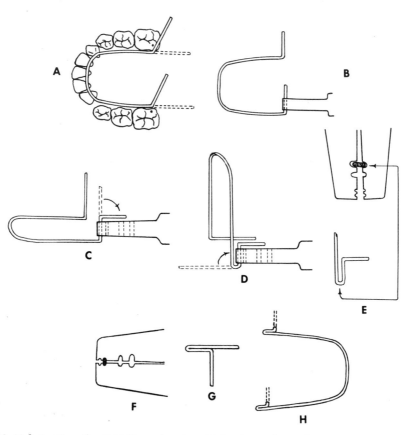

Fig. 17-3. Fabricating the F-R lingual arch with horizontal attachments. **A,** With thumb and finger, the lower lingual arch wire is bent in a U-shape that fits to lingual area of the lower arch. Distolingual cusps of each 6-year molar are marked, and the wire is also marked opposite these cusp marks. Ninety-degree bends are made upward at these wire marks, using the square jaw of the No. 139 pliers. **B,** Wire is grasped snugly in the first grooves of the Universal lingual arch pliers, and the next two bends are accomplished *over the end of the jaws* without shifting the pliers grip. **C,** In the first bend of the wire, made by firm pressure of the *index finger,* the wire is pressed flat against the upper side of the jaws of the pliers. This forms the stop bend. **D,** Then with firm *thumb* pressure, the wire is pressed *over* the jaws of the pliers, *not around the jaws,* to form a 180-degree bend in the wire. **E,** In the deepest grooves of the pliers, the doubled wire is squeezed slowly but firmly. It is then squeezed in the shallower third grooves. This must be done carefully to avoid twisting the doubled wire. **F,** Doubled end is now squeezed in the second grooves. The ends should now be disked *lightly* in the "bulge" areas that are caused by the soft wire's being bent over against itself. **G,** Slightly enlarged view of the doubled wire before the ends are cut just above the stops. **H,** Finished horizontal lingual arch is shown. The cut ends are rounded and polished with the Cratex abrasive rubber wheel. The two advantages of such a lingual arch are that (1) no soldering is necessary unless a finger spring is added and (2) the low gingival-occlusal dimension allows the arch to be fitted in young children's mouths without gingival impingement.

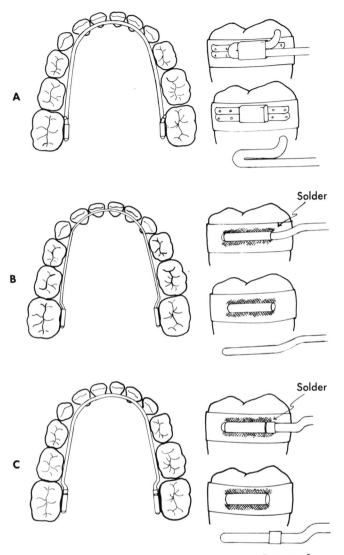

A

B

Solder

Solder

C

Continued.

Fig. 17-4. **A,** Lingual arch in place and the pattern of the spot-welding to the band of the flanges of the horizontal sheath. **B,** In certain instances the choice may be to do a variation of the horizontal lingual arch using 0.036 wire and 0.036 round tubes that are spot-welded and then soldered to the lingual surfaces of the bands. Such a variation is shown here. **C,** Another type of horizontal arch utilizes 0.036 weldable stops to position the 0.036 arch wire inserted into 0.036 round tubes. **D,** Lower plaster cast prepared to fabricate a lower F-R horizontal lingual arch. Note that saw-cuts have been made on each side of the 6-year molars and the plaster carved away to expose the clinical crown of the molars. **E,** Horizontal F-R lower lingual arch has been fitted on the cast. A decision may be made to add a finger spring to move lower anterior teeth slightly labially. **F,** Spring of the same configuration as the main arch wire, but of smaller diameter (0.028 yellow Elgiloy), is bent in a U-shape and cut off at the cuspid area and the bicuspid area on the opposite side. **G,** The spring is spot-welded to place superior to the arch wire. After the spot-welding, 25-gauge solder wire is wrapped around the joint 3 or 4 times. With the use of the alligator clips, generous flux, and a firm electrical contact (brushing motion) of the carbon tip against the solder joint, the wires are soldered.

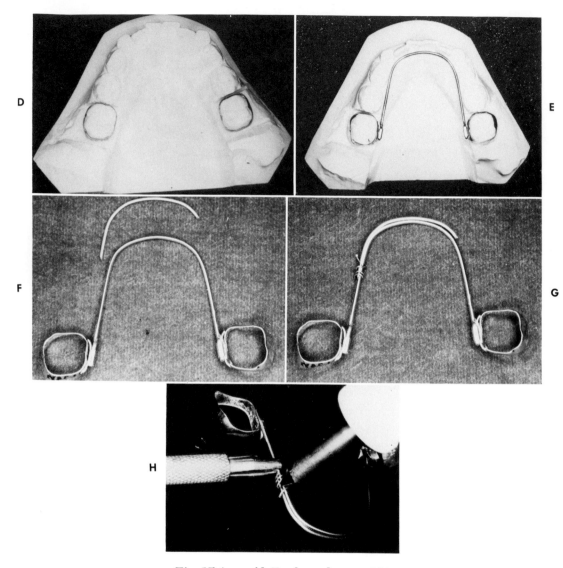

Fig. 17-4, cont'd. For legend see p. 281.

model and press the band into place over the plaster molar. Hold the anterior portion of the U-shaped arch in place against the lingual surfaces of the anterior teeth and note the position of the *opposite* horizontal sheath in relation to the lingual groove of the unattached band. It is to be expected that the middle of the sheath will fall closely in relation to the band's lingual groove.

13. Mark the position of the flange by eye, remove the partially spot-welded arch together with opposite band. Then remove the band that has not been welded. Clean inside of unwelded band with wet cotton bud, and spot-weld flange to band in same relationship as the eye "measured" it on the model. Again it will be seen that the middle of the horizontal sheath falls almost exactly on the lingual groove of the band.

14. Replace the arch on the model,

checking for ease of fit as it slips onto the molars. When quiescent fit has been achieved, remove arch from model and spot-weld all around the distal of the flange on each molar.

15. For the first time, slip the doubled ends of the arch wire out of the sheaths and weld the mesial ends of the flanges, completing the joining of the sheaths to the bands.

16. Smooth the spot-welded areas on each flange with the Cratex rubber wheel and then finish the lingual arch by passivating the wire on the model, using the brass tips of the extension cables. (Refer to welding procedures, Chapter 15.) Polish the wire with Cratex rubber wheel to remove discoloration and then use stainless steel–polishing compound on the laboratory lathe. Clean the *inside* of the bands before cementation, first with a stiff brush in hot water and then with a small green stone. All discoloration must be removed so there are no traces of flux and oxidation residue.

• • •

Although the foregoing explanation may appear somewhat complicated on first reading, the whole procedure—from first sawcuts on the model to the final passivating of the wire and polishing—may be done in as little as 15 minutes. The great advantage of this type of lingual arch is that a dental assistant may learn to accomplish the fabrication of this appliance quite easily.

FABRICATING F-R SECTIONAL LINGUAL ARCH WITH VERTICAL ATTACHMENTS FOR LATE MIXED DENTITION AND YOUNG PERMANENT DENTITION
Materials needed

1. Custom sectional lingual arch set, size 0.036 yellow Elgiloy wire (C-17)
2. 2 vertical plain lingual tubes (same type as for Ellis prefabricated lingual arches) (A-3)
3. Connector tube, size 0.036 (A-11)
4. 2 narrow molar bands (C-1)
5. 25-gauge silver wire solder (C-7)
6. Solder flux (C-9)
7. No. 660 welder with cable extensions (I-1)
8. No. 139 pliers (I-3)
9. Laboratory saw
10. Laboratory knife

Procedure (Fig. 17-5)

1. On lower study model make sawcuts interproximally on each side of 6-year molars, wet the plaster in the area, then carve away the gingival plaster so that molar crowns are well exposed.

2. Fit molar bands on plaster teeth in the same relationship as they have already been fitted in the child's mouth.

3. Remove bands, clean their inside surfaces of plaster, and spot-weld a vertical lingual tube to each band. Be careful that the top of the lingual tube is 1 mm. gingival to the occlusal margin of the band and that each tube is centered on the lingual groove of the molar band.

4. Seat bands with the tubes attached onto the plaster teeth. Bend the anterior portion of one sectional arch wire into a rounded L-shape with thumb and finger and insert the post of the sectional arch into the tube.

5. Note the fit of the sectional arch wire in relation to the lingual surfaces of the lower anterior teeth on the model. Then adjust the curvature of the wire with the No. 139 pliers (rounded jaw).

6. Mark and cut the arch wire exactly opposite the midline between the lower central incisors and disk the wire-end flush.

7. Insert other half of the sectional arch and bend its wire so that it is in relation to the lingual surfaces of the lower anterior teeth. Cut arch wire opposite the midline between the lower central incisors. Blunt the wire-end with a disk.

8. The two wire ends should now appear to be part of a continuous lingual arch extending from molar to molar.

9. Slip double ring of wire solder onto each wire and then slip the connector tube over each wire-end. The arch wires, formerly in two sections, now form a contin-

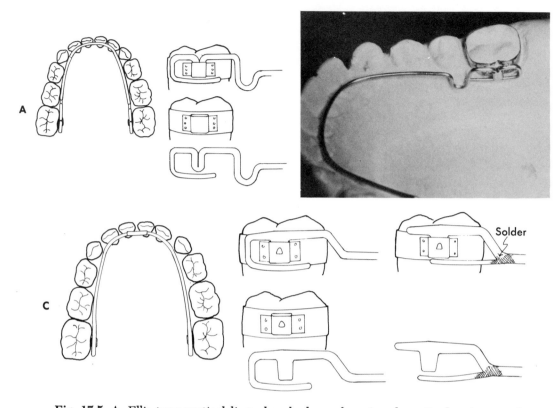

Fig. 17-5. A, Ellis type vertical lingual arch shown here in schematic drawing can be purchased in kits of varying sizes. It is a nightmare to bend from scratch, even with the use of the Universal lingual arch-forming pliers. The bend in the wire immediately distal to the insertion of the post into the lingual tube tends to fatigue and break easily, necessitating soldering a new spring. **B,** Ellis arch shown fitted to a cast. The U-loops are optional but serve to make the arch more versatile in use. **C,** Schematic drawing of a variation of the sectional lingual arch, showing the distal return spring being cut off and a piece of 0.025 wire soldered *mesially* to form the lock spring. Note the connector tube soldered in position uniting the two halves of the appliance.

uous arch, with the connector tube uniting them. Although the connector tube may be spot-welded on one side before soldering, it usually is not necessary.

10. Flux the joint on each end of the connector tube and use the carbon tip–brass alligator clip cable combination for the soldering operation.

11. Bend the distal end of each section of lingual arch down and then forward under the lingual tube to form a spring lock to make the lingual arch fixed-removable. Bend this spring lock with the round jaw of the No. 139 pliers so that the wire

returns as a spring *under* the whole lingual tube to lock the arch wire in place.

12. Remove the arch from the model and scrub it with a brush under hot water to remove the flux. Then thoroughly clean and polish all parts.

Alternative types of vertical lingual arches

There are many alternative types of vertical lingual arches if one chooses not to fabricate a sectional vertical lingual arch. Among the easiest to use are the Hotz preformed lingual arch and the Ellis lingual arch. Because each of these is fitted in

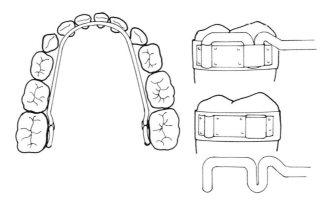

Fig. 17-6. Another popular type of vertically attached lower lingual arch is the Hotz appliance shown here. It is easily fitted on a cast and locks by adjustment of the wire as it inserts into the distal tube. The chief disadvantage in using this attachment is the large size of its lingual tubes, which causes gingival impingement and tongue abrasion in many children.

much the same fashion as the sectional vertical lingual arch described previously, details of fabrication will not be given. Rather, an overview of the advantages and disadvantages of each will be discussed, and illustrations will be used to explore the minor differences.

Hotz preformed lingual arch

The Hotz preformed vertical lingual arch is one of the easiest of all arches to assemble. It comes in assorted sizes in kit form (C-19) and has the distinct advantage that it needs no lingual or gingival locking spring as do most vertically attached lingual arches. The Hotz arch, instead, fits into its vertical sheath by a friction fit, aided a bit by the spring action incorporated into the distal part of the wire as it inserts into its vertical tube.

The disadvantages of the Hotz appliance are that (1) the vertical tube attachment is far too broad in dimension mesiodistally to wrap around a good portion of the lingual surface of the 6-year molar and (2) the appliance has proved to be a real problem as an abrader of tongue margins. This may be due to its bulk but more probably is due to the fairly sharp edges at the tops of the tubes. Smoothing these

edges seems to help appreciably in some cases.

Ellis preformed lingual arch

The Ellis arch is preformed but does not come already bent into an arch shape as does the Hotz arch. Bending the basic arch form and getting the Ellis arch to fit into the vertical lingual tubes can be quite a task. There are two shortcuts that can shorten the fabrication time, however. One is to fit the lingual tubes on the posts of the arch *before bending the arch wire around the arch.* The vertical tubes can act as guides to both horizontal and vertical positioning at the lingual grooves of the molar bands, which is the place where the tubes should be centered for spot-welding. The other shortcut is to *fit the bands on the cast* as in step 2 of fabricating the F-R horizontal lingual arch explained previously in this chapter.

When the arch is reasonably well fitted, one lingual tube should be welded in its proper position. The other tube may be out of position because of stresses still in the wire due to inaccuracy of bending. The tube may be forced into its proper position on the other molar, however, and the arch wire length assessed. If it has been

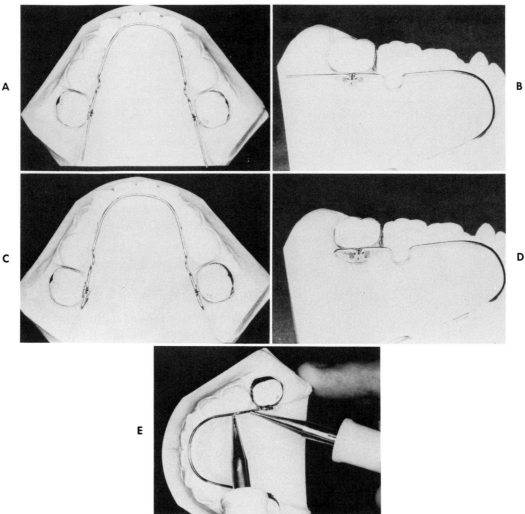

Fig. 17-7. A, An Ellis vertical lingual arch is fabricated on the model which has molar crowns carved away much as in the making of the horizontal arch shown previously. **B,** U-loops for adjustment of the length of the arch may be bent by the dentist or may be purchased that way in kits (C-18). **C,** Spring ends of the arch are bent around gingivally to the vertical attachment to serve as a lock mechanism. **D,** Side view showing lock beneath vertical post. **E,** Lingual arch is being passivated using the cable tips of the 660 welder. With a dial setting of 2 and cables inserted white-black, the tips are "stepped" around the arch passivating about ¼ inch of the arch wire at a time. As soon as the puff of smoke rises from the wire, the arch in that area has been sufficiently heat treated. The resulting color of the wire will be a dark straw color. *The wire must not be reddened during this process.* Heating the wire to a red color will remove all temper from it.

fitted properly, the length will check out all right. The band may be removed, and the last tube spot-welded in its proper position directly over the lingual groove in the molar band. (See Fig. 17-7.)

After the arch has been spot-welded and is an integral unit of bands, tubes, posts, and wire, it can be lifted up and *forced* to place on the model. Then the welder cables can be used to passivate (remove the stresses from the arch wire) causing it to fit in place with no tension exerted against the teeth.

Cementing lingual arches

Cementation of lingual arches should be accomplished much as the discussion of general considerations in fitting and cementing described in orthodontic bands, Chapter 18. Instead of the cementing of each molar crown separately, however, the best method has proved to be cementation of both molar bands at once, so that the appliance is seated to place as a unit.

FABRICATING PORTER APPLIANCE (UPPER)[2]

A fixed-removable Porter appliance for the upper arch is used to treat posterior cross-bites in primary and mixed dentition. NOTE: This appliance requires a fair degree of wire-bending skill to accomplish its construction within a reasonable time. (See Fig. 17-8.)

Materials needed

1. 0.036 blue or yellow Elgiloy wire (C-5)
2. 2 posterior edgewise brackets (A-6)
3. 2 upper narrow molar bands (C-1)
4. No. 660 welder (I-1)
5. No. 139 pliers (I-3)
6. 0.009 dead-soft ligature wire (C-6)
7. Silver wire solder, 25 gauge (C-7)
8. Solder flux (C-9)
9. Laboratory saw
10. Laboratory knife
11. White arch-marking pencil (I-16)

Procedure

1. On upper study model make saw-cuts interproximally on each side of the

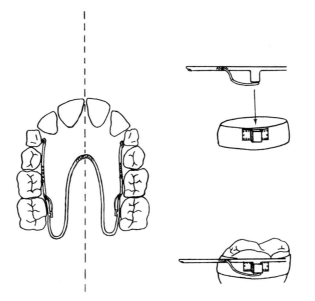

Fig. 17-8. Porter appliance is usually made as a fixed soldered appliance. However, this schematic drawing demonstrates one method of fabrication utilizing parts of a sectional lingual arch, the two halves of which may be soldered at the palatal bend. Result is a highly satisfactory F-R Porter appliance. In some cases the lingual return wires may need to be lengthened by soldering extensions. Another method of fabrication is explained in the text.

6-year molars, wet the plaster in the area, then carve away the gingival plaster so that crowns of the molar teeth are well exposed.

2. Fit molar bands on plaster teeth in the same relationship as they have already been fitted in child's mouth.

3. Using a two-side separating disk, enlarge the slots in both posterior edgewise brackets until 0.036 wire will fit into the grooves.

4. Remove the molar bands, clean their inside surfaces with a cotton bud, and spot-weld the modified posterior edgewise brackets to the lingual surfaces of the bands. Center them on the band, with 1 mm. clearance between the occlusal edge of the band and the occlusal margin of the bracket flange. *Arrange the groove of the edgewise bracket horizontal to the arch* (90 degrees to the axis of the molar tooth).

5. Make a mark on the palate of the plaster model 5 mm. lingual to the slot of the edgewise bracket on each molar. Remove the bands with their spot-welded attachments from the model and bend the 0.036 wire in a U-shape that will approximately accommodate the operator's index finger tip if placed within the U.

6. Place the U-shaped arch wire against the palate of the model so that the anterior edge of the U is approximately at the lingual tip of the incisal papilla. Carefully widen the distal dimension of the arch wire so that each wire passes immediately over the marks on the palate 5 mm. *lingual* to the position of the slot in the posterior edgewise bracket.

7. Using the white arch-marking pencil, mark wire on each side exactly 5 mm. *distal* to the molar (second primary molar in a primary dentition case; 6-year molar in a mixed dentition case).

8. Grasp the wire with the No. 139 pliers at each of these marks and bend a smaller, distal return U-loop around the round jaw. Bend the return wire on each side of the arch so that it will pass accurately *through the slot* of the molar at-tachment. Each of these return U-loop bends is quite difficult to judge because the return wire must be bent to be at a higher level than the main arch wire due to the rising slope of the palate.

9. Contour the return wire so that it continues through the slot mesially and is in close relation to the lingual surfaces of the primary first molar and cuspid (primary dentition cross-bites) or the second and first primary molars (mixed dentition cross-bites).

You will recall from the discussion in Chapter 12 that most posterior cross-bites are in reality *bilateral,* even though they may be expressed in the child's bite as unilateral ones. Therefore the respective lengths of the return wire, which establish anchorage by pressing against the lingual surfaces of the upper teeth, will be the same. These return wires function in the same fashion as the lingual arms soldered to the lingual surfaces of the molar bands in the heavy labial arch appliance. (See Fig. 12-10.)

10. At the ends of each return wire solder a small ball. This is done by wrapping wire solder twice around the tip of the wire, adding flux, and soldering by cable method, using alligator clip–carbon tip.

11. Remove the stress from the arch wire by passivating it with the electric cable tips. Lift the F-R Porter appliance off the model, scrub in hot water, and polish.

12. In the cementing of the appliance, cement each molar band first and then clean each molar tooth of cement. Ligate the F-R Porter appliance to the molar banded brackets with 0.009 ligature wire. Tuck the pigtail (twisted ligature wire) distally under the return wire.

SUMMARY

Three different kinds of fixed-removable lingual arches have been described in this chapter: the F-R horizontally attached lower lingual arch, the F-R vertically attached sectional lower lingual arch, and the F-R upper Porter appliance. In addition, two alternative types of vertically attached lingual arches have been described.

The versatility of the lingual arch is unquestioned in minor tooth movement procedures. And yet, the appliances must be fitted to the age of the child to some degree. The horizontally attached lower lingual arch appears to fit the dentition of younger children (to age 11 or 12) the best, whereas older children are best treated with the vertically attached lower sectional lingual arch.

The Porter appliance described here is best used in the 4 to 9 age group to reduce posterior cross-bites.

REFERENCES

1. Graber, T. M.: Orthodontics: principles and practice, ed. 2, Philadelphia, 1966, W. B. Saunders Co., pp. 657-660.
2. Moyers, R. E.: Handbook of orthodontics, ed. 2, Chicago, 1963, Year Book Medical Publishers, Inc., pp. 495-496.

Fabricating heavy and light fixed labial arches

The mechanics of fabricating a fixed labial arch are fairly uncomplicated. The main arch component is a U-shaped wire that is contoured to approximate the middle of the facial surfaces of the clinical crowns of the incisors and the posterior teeth. The position of the arch wire at the cuspids may or may not be at mid-crown, but this is of slight concern because children younger than 10 years of age rarely need their upper cuspids banded.

In the broader view, neither the heavy labial arch discussed in this chapter nor the light labial arch fall into the classic definition of the "fixed-multibanded appliance" category. Rather, they are better termed *limited fixed labial appliances,* since in some instances the upper 6-year molars alone may be banded whereas in other cases the upper 6-year molars and the upper incisors are banded.[1]

The proper fitting and cementation of bands is a necessary skill to acquire if fixed labial arches are to be fabricated. The following section explores this highly important area and presents some time-saving techniques the busy dentist may appreciate.

GENERAL CONSIDERATIONS IN FITTING AND CEMENTING ORTHODONTIC BANDS

Relatively few dentists have been taught in dental school the proper techniques for cementing anterior and posterior orthodontic bands. In the past there was some justification for this because preformed seamless bands were not available and bands had to be custom-made in the child's mouth. Now this is no longer the case. Many companies make fine kits of stainless steel seamless bands, which may be fitted to the great majority of children's teeth as if they had been painted on the tooth. And this is just the sort of close fit the dentist should have in his mind when he attempts this task.

Bands that are poorly fitted are in the same category as poorly prepared and condensed amalgams—they are unworthy of the efforts of a dentist who desires excellence in his practice. In the following section, some methods of fitting seamless bands are presented that should make the task of fitting an anterior or posterior band no more of a problem than the placing of a well-fitting matrix around a tooth to be restored with amalgam.

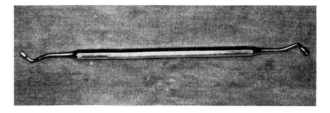

Fig. 18-1. Round, serrated-tip amalgam-plugger used to press bands into place on the teeth.

Fitting anterior bands

The anterior band kits that have been suggested for purchase by the general dentist or pedodontist are narrow central bands (C-2)* and narrow lateral bands (C-3). Each kit is divided into sizes for the right and left central and lateral incisors. To be accurately fitted, the bands must be fitted on the child's teeth at the chair. Those fitted on a laboratory model will usually be found to be too small.

Materials needed

1. 1 kit of narrow upper central incisor bands (C-2)
2. 1 kit of narrow upper lateral incisor bands (C-3)
3. Large round amalgam-plugger with serrated face (Fig. 18-1)
4. Large amalgam-carver such as Hollenback No. 3
5. Crown-contouring pliers No. 114 (I-5) or the No. 800-417 pliers (I-5 alternate)
6. Modified Boley gauge (I-10)

Procedure

Perhaps it is better to start with the assumption that a child is being banded for the fabrication of an upper heavy or light labial arch in the mixed dentition age. In each of these, both central and lateral incisors will be banded. In a later section the banding of the molars will be described.

1. Select from the kit an upper central band and check its measurement with the Boley gauge to be sure it measures mesio-

*Letter-number references throughout this chapter are to Tables 16 to 18, Chapter 14.

distally the same as the tooth to be banded. Make sure a *right central incisor band* is being fitted to a *right central incisor*. Even in a well-run office the bands can get mixed up when they are replaced in the kit from previous fitting procedures.

2. Check the band on the tooth, for size. The size is correct if the band slides easily on the tooth until the incisal edge of the tooth shows beneath the band, then begins to bind.

3. Use the large round amalgam-plugger to press the band gingivally until it is seated so that it occupies the middle third of the clinical crown of the upper incisor (Fig. 18-2). The serrated face of the plugger prevents the instrument from slipping. Apply pressures first in an apical direction against the mesial and distal edges of the band, then firmly along the labial margins, and last, *very* firmly along the lingual margin of the band.

4. When the band is firmly seated, use the sides of the round amalgam plugger to burnish all band margins into place so

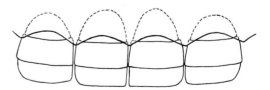

Fig. 18-2. Anterior bands fitted on a child's upper incisors with the gingival margin being shown above them. Note the bands occupy approximately the middle third of the exposed clinical crown.

that the band is adapted tightly with no open margins visible.

5. The last pressure is a very heavy pressure by the amalgam plugger placed against the lingual lug of the band. This accomplishes the final seating pressure for the band. NOTE: All anterior bands do not come furnished with lingual lugs. They must be specified when ordering the kits.

6. Exactly in the center of the labial surface of the fitted band scribe a vertical line, using a sharp amalgam carver. Then slip the band from the tooth so that the anterior edgewise bracket can be oriented and spot-welded in the center of the band. Transfer the band with the spot-welded bracket to a piece of flat beeswax and press it slightly into the wax until time for cementation. In this way the bands can be kept separated into *right* and *left* areas, so that it is less confusing for the dental assistant to fill the proper bands with cement and pass them to the dentist during cementation procedures.

Cementation of anterior bands

Before cementation of bands the teeth must be prepared to receive them.

The child's teeth are cleaned, using a fluoride mix in the pumice material, and a fluoride gel or equivalent is applied for the time suggested by the manufacturer. The child's teeth are then washed and air dried, and cotton rolls are placed under the upper lip to maintain a dry field.

Cavity varnish (or collodion) is painted over the surfaces of all the teeth to be banded, and then they are thoroughly dried. This surface coating prevents any acid-etching from the freshly applied zinc phosphate cement. Teeth treated in this fashion are also extremely resistant to the enamel etching due to plaque accumulation, which sometimes is seen to occur along the margins of bands in the mouth of a child who is not on a good regimen of oral health care at home. *When bands are worn, the tooth-brushing procedures must be constantly reinforced by the dentist!*

Materials needed

1. Bands (with anterior edgewise brackets spot-welded into place) on a flat piece of beeswax, placed in order from right to left
2. Large round amalgam-plugger
3. Large amalgam-carver, Hollenback No. 3
4. Any type of zinc phosphate cement
5. Chilled glass slab
6. Thin-bladed cement spatula

Procedure

1. The dental assistant mixes a *thick,* shiny mix of zinc phosphate cement on a chilled glass slab with a thin-bladed metal spatula, completely fills one band at a time from the gingival side, and passes the band to the dentist. (The bands most difficult to fit are usually seated first.)

2. The dentist presses the band onto the tooth with his index finger as far as he can and then firmly seats the band, using alternating pressures around the margins with the large round amalgam plugger. As the band is pressed into place, cement should be forced out around the gingival margin.

3. While the cement is setting, burnish the margins of each of the bands against the tooth with some pressure, using the side of the amalgam plugger. This prevents "fat-edged" bands and an open cement margin, which invites loosening and the initiation of hypocalcified enamel along the margin.

4. After all bands have been cemented in this fashion, allow the cement to set for 5 minutes, maintaining a dry field. Then scuff away the excess cement with the Hollenback carver blade. All remnants of cement must be cleaned out of the slots of the edgewise brackets. An explorer may be needed to clear the upper and lower ligation areas of the bracket.

NOTE: Bands should remain in place no longer than 6 to 9 months without being removed, checked for leakage, and recemented. During each 2-week check-up the dentist should carefully examine the child for loosened bands. There is no way that

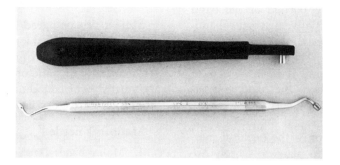

Fig. 18-3. Round serrated-tip amalgam-plugger is compared to Baker (Swinehart) band-driver. Both instruments are used to seat molar bands.

bands can be guaranteed to cause no etching of the enamel surfaces of teeth during treatment, but the precautions listed here will help the dentist avoid this all too common hazard.

Fitting molar bands

Molar bands are fitted with the same careful attention to detail that was used in the fitting of anterior bands. With the stainless molar band kits available today the dentist can accomplish this task in a few minutes.

Materials needed (Figs. 18-3 and 18-4)

1. Kit of seamless stainless steel narrow molar bands (C-1) (divided into upper and lower molars)
2. Baker (Swinehart) band-driver (I-9)
3. Crown-contouring pliers No. 114 (I-5) or No. 800-417 pliers (I-5 alternate)
4. Large round amalgam-plugger with serrated face
5. No. 347 posterior band–removing pliers (I-8)
6. Modified Boley gauge (I-10)

NOTE: Molar bands are never trimmed during the fitting. If they appear in need of trimming, they are usually too small, and a larger size should be tried.

Procedure

1. Select a band size with the same mesiodistal measurement (on the Boley gauge) as the molar to be fitted. Be certain that an *upper molar band* is being

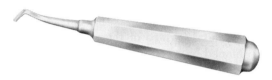

Fig. 18-4. No. 300 band-driver can be a dangerous instrument in untrained hands. It is better to avoid using this, since it can lacerate the gingiva if the driver tip slips off the band while pressure against this band-driver is being used.

fitted on an *upper molar tooth*. NOTE: The groove on the occlusal margin of the band is on the *buccal* of an upper molar band and on the *lingual* of a lower molar band.

2. Finger-press the band on the molar tooth in the child's mouth, then compress the band from the buccal and lingual with the thumb and forefinger. This helps shape the band to the rhomboid outline of an upper molar. Lower molar bands also benefit from being preshaped by the fingers in the same fashion.

3. Using the Baker band-driver, press the band gingivally as far as it will go with careful pressure. Then position the serrated tip of the band-driver on the distal margin of the band and have the child close his teeth on the biting surface of the band-driver. The child cannot injure himself in this way because the band-driver cannot slip onto the gingiva.

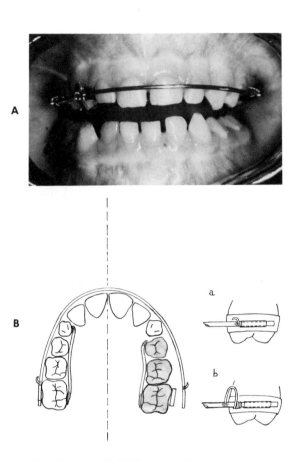

Fig. 18-6. A, Child 5 years old is shown wearing heavy labial arch to reduce a bilateral posterior cross-bite expressed unilaterally as a lingual cross-bite in his primary dentition. Only the E|E's are banded, as a rule. However, in this case the C| was banded to move it labially so that C̅| could be disked to provide a slope and then moved lingually by the pressure of the corrected relationship to C|. **B,** Better visualization of the lingual arms of a heavy labial arch appliance designed to correct a unilateral cross-bite in the mixed dentition stage. The shaded teeth represent the teeth expressed in lingual cross-bite. Note the 0.040 arch wire is activated approximately 3 mm. to the buccal on the cross-bite side. Compare the lengths of the soldered lingual arms and note that greater buccal movement should be achieved on the cross-bite side than on the anchorage side.

Procedure

1. On the upper plaster model contour the 0.040 blue Elgiloy wire with thumb and finger pressure so that the U-shaped wire approximates the shape of the arch formed by the outside surfaces of the teeth.

2. Make saw-cuts interproximally on each side of the second primary molars. Wet the plaster areas with water and carve the teeth down so they are "surgically" exposed. (Wetting allows plaster to be carved without chipping.)

3. Fit onto the plaster teeth the two molar bands that have already been fitted in the child's mouth, preserving the same occlusogingival relationships.

4. Fit arch wire against teeth and mark the positions of the two 0.040 round buccal tubes. (Weldable double buccal tubes may also be used. In this case, the heavy labial arch wire inserts into the larger of the two tubes. Later, if a light arch is used, it inserts into the smaller tube.) Remove molar bands, spot-weld the flanges of the tubes into place (first on the distal end of each flange), and then "sew" each flange to the band with a series of spot-welds. Make sure the buccal tubes are angled to the anterior so that the labial arch wire has proper "draw" to facilitate easy insertion and removal. This can be done by inserting two lengths of straight wire into the tubes and noting that the lengths of wire intersect each other 6 to 12 inches labial to the central incisors.

5. Make final bends in arch wire and cut distal ends of the arch wire so that they may be inserted into the buccal tubes on the molar bands on the model. Adjust the arch wire to clear the anterior labial surfaces of the primary teeth about 1 to 2 mm. Mark the wire on each side exactly 4 mm. ahead of the most mesial buccal tube–opening with white marking pencil.

6. Form the vertical adjustment spring (0.020 wire); spot-weld and solder it at the white mark on the wire. The spring is designed so that the sliding coiled portion goes to the distal, serving as an adjustable

stop against the buccal tube. The shaping of the U-loop to make the spring is done by contouring the 0.020 wire around the *round* jaw of the No. 139 pliers (position 2, see Fig. 16-3) *after* the 0.020 wire has first been coiled at least twice around a length of the arch wire. One precaution to be taken is to attach each vertical adjustment spring so that it angles slightly buccal to the vertical position (using the labial arch wire as a horizontal plane) to avoid having the U-loop impinge on the child's buccal gingiva. (See Fig. 18-7, *B*).

7. Contour two pieces of 0.036 blue Elgiloy against the *lingual* surfaces of the primary molars (and cuspids if the cross-bite extends that far anteriorly). Spot-weld these wires to the *lingual* surfaces of the middle of the molar bands and then solder with the cable extensions of the 660 welder. A small ball of solder may be flowed on

the tip of each lingual arm to avoid trauma to the child's tongue.

8. Scrub the whole appliance in hot water with a stiff-bristled toothbrush to remove the solder flux and then smooth the soldered areas and wire ends with a rubber Cratex wheel. A high polish can be obtained with either stainless steel polish (C-20) or gold rouge on the lathe wheel.

With four anterior bands; for correction of posterior cross-bites in mixed dentition

The discussion in Chapter 12 examines the use of heavy labial arches during the mixed dentition years to reduce posterior cross-bites. Stability of the appliance in mixed dentition is increased by its being ligated to anterior bands as well as inserted into the molar tubes. As in the primary dentition, most of the posterior cross-bites being treated will be expressed as unilateral ones

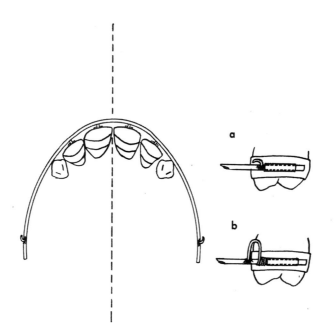

Fig. 18-7. Design of a heavy labial arch appliance to treat a bilateral lingual cross-bite, expressed bilaterally, involving only the 6-year molars. Note the 0.040 arch wire may be activated bilaterally. The four upper incisors are also banded, and the arch wire is ligated to the anterior edgewise brackets for stabilization. *a,* Soldered hooks are used both as tie places and as stops; *b,* adjustable U-loop may be used to act as a movable stop. Note that the sliding coiled portion of the loop is not soldered to the arch wire but serves an adjustable stop against the molar tube.

but are in actuality a bilateral constriction of the palatal arch. (See Fig. 18-7.)

Materials needed

1. 0.040 blue Elgiloy wire (C-5)
2. 0.036 blue Elgiloy wire (C-5)
3. 2 narrow molar bands (C-1); 4 fitted incisor bands (C-2, C-3)
4. Two 0.040 buccal tubes (A-4) or weldable double buccal tubes (A-10)
5. 4 single anterior edgewise brackets (A-5)
6. 0.020 yellow Elgiloy wire (C-5)
7. 25 gauge silver wire solder (C-7)
8. Solder flux (C-9)
9. No. 660 spot-welder (I-1)
10. No. 139 pliers (I-3)

Procedure

1. Contour the 0.040 arch wire around the arch perimeter of the child's plaster model so that it touches the labial surfaces of all teeth. Cut the wire ends distal to the upper 6's.

2. Fit molar bands on the plaster teeth in the same relationship as they were fitted in the mouth and then spot-weld flanges of buccal tubes so that the appliance will "draw" when it is inserted from the anterior. (See step 4 in procedure for arches without anterior bands.) Insert lengths of 0.040 wire into the tubes to check that they intersect 6 to 12 inches in front of the central incisors.

3. The anterior bands need not be fitted on the plaster anterior teeth after being fitted originally in the child's mouth. A scratch line is made vertically on the labial surface of each band while it is fitted in the child's mouth. This will identify the center of the tooth so that the single edgewise anterior brackets can be spot-welded into place on the bands centered on this line.

4. Make the final bends for the fitting of the arch wire with the No. 139 pliers and insert the distal ends of the wire into the molar buccal tubes. Mark the arch wire 4 mm. from the molar tubes to locate the positions of the U-loop adjustment springs exactly as described in making the previous appliance with one exception—the

labial portion of the arch wire must be held 1.5 mm. *labial* to surfaces of the anterior teeth to allow for the added dimension of the anterior edgewise brackets.

5. Form, spot-weld, and solder the vertical adjustment springs (U-loops).

6. Contouring the lingual arms (0.036 blue Elgiloy wire) adjacent to the lingual surfaces of the molars and up to the cuspids is accomplished, exactly as in step 7 of the procedure for heavy labial arch with anterior bands. A small ball of solder may be added to the tip of each of these lingual arms. This protects the child's tongue from abrasion if the tip of the lingual arm should move away from the tissue during treatment.

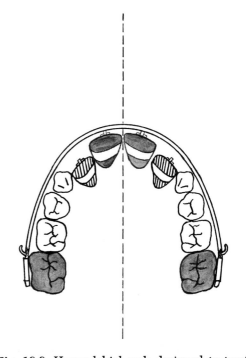

Fig. 18-8. Heavy labial arch designed to treat an anterior cross-bite involving the upper lateral incisors in the mixed dentition. The shaded teeth represent the anchorage units that allow the cross-hatched teeth to move labially into a normal arch configuration. This is a highly effective appliance for treating these fairly common malocclusions. The force generated by ligating the arch wire to the inlocked lateral incisors is distally directed against the banded molars. Ligature wires omitted.

7. Scrub the appliance with hot water to remove flux, smooth it with a Cratex rubber wheel, and polish on the lathe.

Correction of anterior cross-bites in mixed dentition

A heavy labial arch appliance may be used to reduce *anterior* cross-bites involving two maxillary lateral incisors during the mixed dentition years. This appliance may be fabricated in a fashion identical to the one just described for posterior cross-bites in the mixed dentition except for the absence of lingual arm extensions soldered to the palatal surface of the molar bands (Fig. 18-8).

FABRICATING THE LIGHT FIXED LABIAL ARCH

Only a few differences exist between the construction of a light labial arch and that of a heavy labial arch. The light labial arch is made of 0.020 wire instead of 0.040 wire, and the vertical U-loop springs are bent as a part of the arch wire rather than being attached by soldering as in the heavy labial arch. Also, the light labial arch wire fits *into* the grooves of the anterior edgewise attachments rather than *adjacent* to the attachments as the heavy arch does.

The size of the light labial arch wire is usually 0.020 but it may be of a smaller diameter if the dentist chooses a wire with more spring qualities, such as the Australian light wire. Fitting the arch wire into the anterior bracket slots and tying ligature wires around each bracket to fix the arch wire in place makes the appliance a very stable fixed appliance. Its configuration and resiliency allow the positions of anterior teeth to be changed both by tipping and by bodily movements.

There are no hooks or stops to be attached to the light labial arch wire. Gross adjustments are made by bending with the thumb and fingers while the arch wire is held in the hands before ligating it in place. Fine adjustments are made with the No. 139 pliers while the arch is held in

the fingers. The vertical loops adjacent to the buccal tubes on the molars serve as adjustment devices to slightly alter the length of the arch wire and for stops and tying places to hold the inserted wire ends securely in the edgewise tube of the double buccal tubes.

The light-wire arch is considered by many dentists to be more difficult to fabricate because it requires a greater degree of dexterity in wire-bending to obtain a good quiescent fit of the arch wire in all bracket slots. Experience will eventually allow such an arch to be fitted accurately against an upper model in 10 to 15 minutes. With further experience will come the ability to fabricate light labial arch wires so that they may be bent at the chair and fitted directly in the child's mouth. (See Fig. 18-9.)

Arch wires must not be bent carelessly, since this might allow undesirable forces to press against a child's teeth. It is better to start treatment with the more easily fabricated heavy-wire arch and later move to the use of the light-wire arches as confidence in wire-bending techniques is gained. There is less chance of improper arch distortion (and undesired movement of teeth) with the heavy labial arch technique than with the light-wire method.

Use in mixed dentition

The light labial arch is an appliance that, with practice, is easily fabricated and has a high degree of versatility in minor tooth movement in treating certain malocclusions during the mixed dentition.[2,3]

In general, the uses for this appliance are confined to correction of malalignment of one or more of the four upper incisor teeth during mixed dentition. It is an ideal appliance for reducing an anterior cross-bite involving one or two upper incisors. The appliance can be adjusted so that light but constant, labially-directed forces are exerted against any or all of the four incisors. At the same time, of course, a reciprocal force is generated, which is trans-

banded and the arch wire is tied to the edgewise brackets also.

One use of a light labial arch is to treat a case exhibiting an anterior cross-bite involving two upper lateral incisors, with all incisors being banded. In some cases the upper light labial arch should be used in conjunction with a cervical extraoral force appliance to maintain anchorage of the upper 6-year molars.

REFERENCES

1. Graber, T. M.: Orthodontics: principles and practice, ed. 2, Philadelphia, 1966, W. B. Saunders Co., pp. 830-835.
2. Hirschfeld, L., and Geiger, A.: Minor tooth movement in general practice, St. Louis, 1966, The C. V. Mosby Co., pp. 223-230.
3. Moyers, R. E.: Handbook of orthodontics, ed. 2, Chicago, 1963, Year Book Medical Publishers, Inc., pp. 499-504.

19 | Fabricating extraoral force appliances

The methods of making extraoral appliances are many and varied. However, this section will describe only the fabrication of an uncomplicated cervical appliance utilizing a neck pad through which is fitted an adjustable elastic strap. King[2] and others[1,3] have described the construction and use of this type of appliance at some length. The reader is especially urged to read the article by King. It is well written and thoroughly clinical in its approach to the use of extraoral appliances.

Obviously not every dentist will use such an appliance in a general practice situation. It is important, however, to understand the use of such appliances as they are used in the offices of the orthodontist or pedodontist. It is the one appliance described in this book that can have a decided effect on the growth potential of the maxilla if it is used over a period of more than 6 months. Because of this important factor, the extraoral force appliance is better used under the guidance of an orthodontist unless special training in its use has been acquired by attendance at continuing dental education courses taught by recognized authorities in the use of these appliances.

DESCRIPTION OF EXTRAORAL FORCE APPLIANCE

Basically, the extraoral force appliance consists of two sections. The first is a face bow made of two wires soldered together: the extraoral bow and the intraoral arch wire. The other part is composed of a neck pad and an elastic band that slips through the neck pad and attaches to the two hooks of the outer bow of the face bow. When put together, the whole appliance consists of the intraoral arch wire (which fits inside the mouth), an extraoral bow wire (which fits around the face) ending in hooks, an elastic band stretching from one hook to the other, and a neck pad to cushion the pull on the neck. Inside the mouth the ends of the intraoral wire slip into double buccal tubes spot-welded or soldered to the buccal surfaces of bands on both upper 6-year molars. (See Fig. 19-1.)

The adjustments are usually made once a month by tightening the elastic strap to a tension of 4 to 8 ounces. The strap may need to be shortened to maintain its tension as often as once a month. The loosening of the strap results from wear and fatigue of the stretched rubber components in the neck strap, not from the molars' having been moved distally.

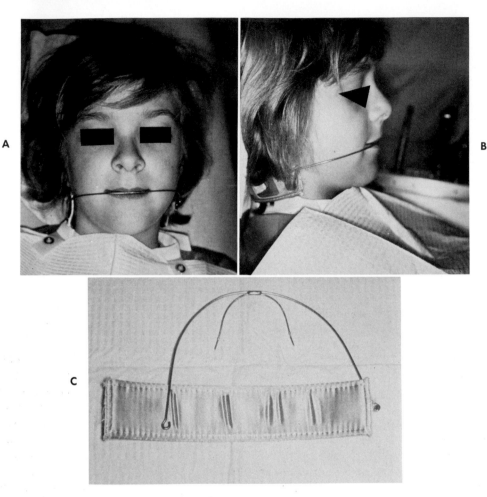

Fig. 19-1. A and **B**, Girl, 10 years of age, wearing a cervical extraoral force appliance. Note that the face bow bisects the commissure of the lips when it is properly fitted. **A,** Front view. **B,** Right view. Note ¾-inch elastic cervical strap is pulled through the loops on the outside surface of the neck pad. **C,** Appliance pictured in **A** and **B** has just been removed from the girl. Note the stops on the intraoral arch wire, which serve to position the wire end in each large round tube of the double buccal tubes, and the hook at each end of face bow.

FABRICATING EXTRAORAL FORCE CERVICAL APPLIANCE

The following sequence of steps in the construction and fitting of an extraoral cervical appliance designed to distally position one or both upper 6-year molars to correct mesial drift (3 mm. or less) may vary somewhat due to the training or technique of an individual dentist. However, these steps should serve as a starting point in considering the least complicated method of fabrication. *It is important to remember that the face bow is fitted with the outer bow at a lower angle than the intraoral arch wire.* For the face bow used in Fig. 19-1 the difference in angulation between the inner bow and outer bow is 15 degrees.

Materials needed

1. Extraoral force plain face bow (C-10)*
2. 2 narrow molar bands (C-1)
3. 2 double buccal tubes (A-10)
4. No. 660 welder (I-1)
5. No. 139 pliers (I-3)
6. 1 mm. stops (as needed) (A-9)
7. Foam rubber neck pad (C-11)
8. Elastic cervical traction brace (C-12)
9. White arch-marking pencil (I-16)

Procedure (Fig. 19-2)

Fitting the upper molar bands. The upper molar bands are fitted in the child's mouth at the chair either at the same time the impressions are taken or at a subsequent appointment. (See section on fitting molar bands, Chapter 18.) The bands are not left on the teeth during the impression taking. Rather, they accompany the impressions separately to the dentist's laboratory to be fitted on the molar teeth of the working casts exactly as in the procedure described for making a lingual arch (Chapter 17).

Laboratory preparation of the model

1. On the child's upper model make a saw-cut interproximally on each side of the upper 6-year molars. Then carve the plaster away, exposing the crown of the tooth so that the already fitted molar bands will slip on and off fairly easily.

2. Using the spot-welder, tack-weld to the band the *distal* flange of the double buccal tube attachment. Fit the attachment so that the large round tube is *toward the occlusal* and the lumen of the large tube bisected by the occlusal edge of the band.

3. Check the alignment of the tubes by inserting wires (lengths of 0.036 wire will do) into the tubes. The wires should form an isosceles triangle by meeting about 10 to 12 inches in front of the anterior teeth. To allow the tubes to diverge or converge too much from this angulation will cause real difficulty later when the child inserts the ends of the intraoral bow into his mouth to wear the appliance. When the

*Letter-number references throughout chapter are to Tables 16 to 18, Chapter 14.

buccal tube alignment is satisfactory on both sides of the arch, complete the spot-welding of the tubes by spot-welding around each flange in at least six places.

Contouring intraoral arch wire

1. Place the arch wire on the child's upper model and note the position of the wire in relation to the outer perimeter of the dental arch. Using the 139 bird-beak pliers to hold the solder joint firmly in one hand, contour the arch wire to approximate the perimeter of one side of the child's dental arch with the thumb and fingers of the other hand. Repeat with arch wire on the other side.

2. Position the contoured arch wire so that the solder joint is a full 3 mm. *anterior* to the labial surfaces of the central incisors. This will allow 3 mm. of distal movement of *both* upper molars before an adjustment has to be made in the dimensions of the arch wire ends that fit into the buccal tubes.

3. Measure the arch wire. Cut the ends of the intraoral arch wire so that about 2 mm. of wire is allowed to protrude from the distal end of each tube. This allows for adjustment in arch wire length later on during treatment. Polish the wire ends.

• • •

The foregoing steps are all that may be accomplished in the laboratory. The remainder of the fitting must be accomplished with the child seated in the dental chair.

Cementation of molar bands. Review carefully the section on the fitting and cementation of molar bands in Chapter 18.

Fitting intraoral arch wire

1. Bring the partially fitted face bow to the child's mouth, and insert *one end* of the intraoral arch wire into a buccal tube. A right-handed dentist may well begin with the upper left tube. Check the relationship of the other wire end on the right side to see if it is parallel and reasonably close to being able to fit into the tube on the right side.

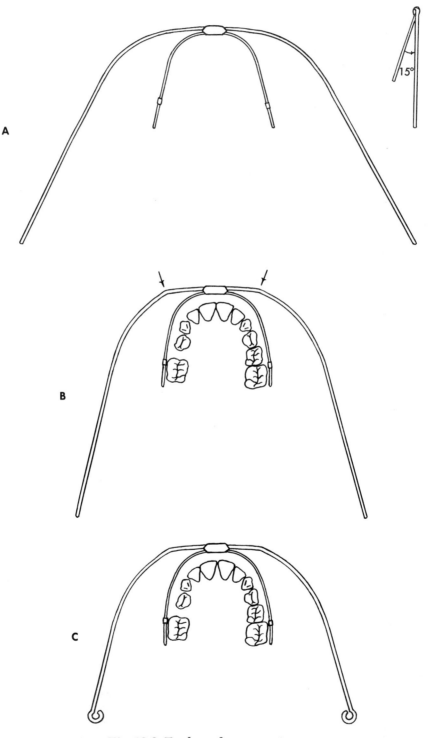

A

B

C

Fig. 19-2. For legend see opposite page.

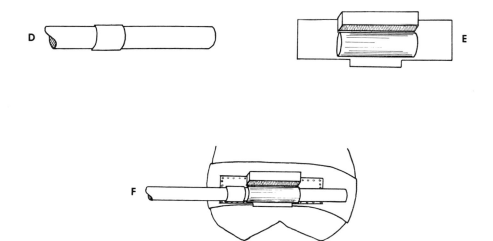

Fig. 19-2. **A,** Basic face bow described in this chapter is the simplest of all the head gear and cervical appliances that are used to establish extraoral force to distally position upper 6-year molars. In some cases U-loops may be bent in the inner arch wire to serve both as stops and adjustments in the length of the inner arch. *Insert,* 15-degree difference in angulation between intraoral wire and extraoral wire. **B,** Intraoral wire has been contoured to fit approximately 3 mm. labial to surfaces of upper central incisors. The ends have been cut so that they protrude about 1 mm. distal to 6|6's. Each weldable stop has been slid up the wire until it is approximately opposite the mesiobuccal cusp of each 6-year molar. Outer bow has been contoured slightly inward, as shown by arrows, with No. 139 pliers. **C,** About 1¼-inch pieces have been cut off the ends of the outer bow. With the annealing table on the spot-welder, each heavy wire end is annealed for one inch, polished, and bent into a hook with No. 139 pliers. **D,** Sliding weldable stop is moved mesially, and the molar bands are fitted on the model. **E,** Weldable double buccal tube is positioned on each band and spot-welded so that the round tube is toward the occlusal aspect of the tooth, parallel to the occlusal margin of the band. **F,** Appliance is now slipped into the buccal tubes. After the 3 mm. clearance labial to the central incisors has been checked, the weldable stops are slid distally until they touch the buccal tube. They are not spot-welded, however, until the appliance is finally fitted in the child's mouth.

2. Slight corrective bends in the arch wire may need to be made with the round jaw of the 139 bird-beak pliers. These should enable the ends of the arch wire to be slipped fairly easily into the tubes and pressed distally until each arch wire end protrudes from the distal end of the tube about 2 mm.

3. Slip back with the fingernails the weldable stops on each side of the arch wire until they both touch against the mesial opening of each buccal tube. Check the arch wire for the 3 mm. clearance from the labial surfaces of the central incisors present on the model when the arch wire was fitted originally in the laboratory.

4. Remove the appliance from the child's mouth, being careful not to disturb stops. Spot-weld each stop at least three times, then slip a ring of solder onto each end of the arch wire. Flux and solder the stop in place. Scrub and polish each stop area.

5. Incorporate a slight curve of Spee in the intraoral arch wire so that the wire positions itself approximately across the incisal one third of the upper central incisors.

Fitting extraoral wire

1. Now cut the ends of the heavy extraoral bow and add the end hooks at a position such that the 5½-inch elastic cervi-

cal strap can be adjusted with the proper tension. For most children, each extraoral bow wire end is marked for cutting about 1 inch anterior to the ear lobe.

2. Smooth the cut end and then bend a hook at each wire end to create an attachment for the elastic cervical strap.

3. To assemble the appliance, slip the cervical elastic strap through the loops of the neck pad and engage the left (child's left) hook in the ring at the end of the elastic strap. Tighten the wire hook so that the ring cannot slip out. Leave hook open on right side (toward the dentist as child sits in the chair) so it will be convenient for adjustments.

4. Adjust elastic strap at 2- to 4-ounce pull after the appliance has been fitted on the child. After 1 week use 6 to 8 ounces.

ADJUSTING THE APPLIANCE

Before the discussion of adjusting the tension of the elastic band, perhaps a review by King[2] will help explain why the exact amount of tension cannot be measured more explicitly when extraoral force appliances are fitted. He explains that the amount of elastic pull to use in the cervical strap may be determined by the response of the patient over a period of time. Several devices are available for measuring the pull of the elastics to achieve a precise amount; however, the patient himself will provide a better guide to this. Tissue response to the pressure applied varies so greatly from individual to individual that what is correct for one child is not at all adequate for another. It is better to ask the patient to aid in determining the proper adjustment of the elastic.

Bimonthly adjustment. Start the child out with a light pull. Each time he comes in, at intervals of about 2 weeks, adjust the elastic slightly tighter until at a subsequent visit the patient indicates that the maxillary molars are slightly tender when he arises in the morning but that the tenderness quickly goes away after appliance has been removed. This amount of tension,

whatever it may be—or slightly less—apparently is correct for that individual child.

Subsequent adjustment by adding stops. Other adjustments are necessary in addition to the regular bimonthly adjustments already mentioned. It will be seen within a period of 3 or 4 months that the original 3 mm. anterior clearance labial to the upper central incisors has lessened substantially. Within 6 months or less, the inner surface of the solder joint of the face bow may begin pressing against the central incisors. When this occurs, additional 1 mm. weldable stops may be added to one or both ends of the intraoral arch wire. At this time the dentist should realize that he has gained 3 mm. *on each side of the upper arch,* or a total of 6 mm.

Unilateral pressure added against one molar. Occasionally, the dentist will wish to exert a distally directed force against one upper molar but not against the opposite molar. By putting an additional weldable stop on *one side only,* the molar on that side receives most of the distal pressure when the cervical appliance is worn. There are other methods of adjusting the cervical appliance so that it applies unilateral pressure on one molar, but these variations are clearly outside the scope of this book.

The finished appliance. The finished extraoral force appliance should be comfortable for the child to wear, whether he is watching TV or sleeping in bed. If it is not comfortable, the chances of its being worn exactly as the dentist suggests become less than good.

Repairs of appliance during treatment. Occasionally the cervical appliance will break while in use. Almost always it will be at the point on the intraoral arch wire where the stops have been spot-welded. Some operators solder these stops to the wire (as described in step 4 of procedure for fitting intraoral arch wire), but this seems to weaken the wire even more than regular spot-welding.

Most often, it will be found to be easiest to remake and refit a new face bow rather than to attempt to repair the broken wire end. With some practice a face bow can be refitted in about 20 minutes at the chair.

SUMMARY

The uses of extraoral force appliances in orthodontic treatment are many and varied. However, the cervical strap appliance discussed here is proposed for only one situation in minor tooth movement—distally positioning of one or both upper 6-year molars that have drifted mesially. A further limitation is imposed in that it is suggested that no more than 3 mm. of space can be expected to be regained in either upper quadrant over the projected 6 months of treatment. The appliance is worn only at night (12 to 14 hours daily). It must be checked by the dentist every 2 weeks, and the tension of the cervical strap adjusted once a month.

REFERENCES

1. Graber, T. M.: Orthodontics: principles and practice, ed. 2, Philadelphia, 1966, W. B. Saunders Co., pp. 850-864.
2. King, E.: Extraoral appliance treatment: the neckband, Dent. Clin. North Am., pp. 479-488, July, 1966.
3. Moyers, R. E.: Handbook of orthodontics, ed. 2, Chicago, 1963, Year Book Medical Publishers, Inc., pp. 506-510.

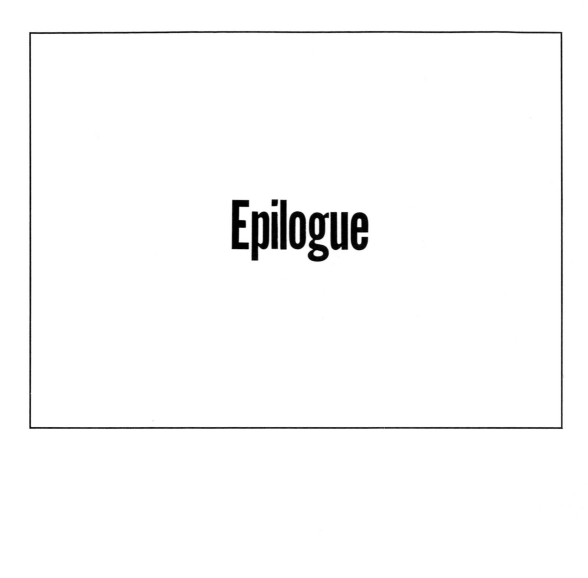

Epilogue

20 | For the parents

Probably you are reading this chapter because your family dentist has recently examined your child and has concluded that he or she will benefit from interceptive orthodontic treatment. This will involve having your child wear certain appliances or braces especially designed to move or straighten younger children's teeth. Many times, the early interception of a problem of this kind may resolve it or lessen considerably the effect on the child.

Using his training and experience in diagnosis, your dentist may have already informed you of the extent of your child's bite problem (malocclusion). Just as you might classify children according to the color of their eyes—blue, gray, or brown—he classifies them by the manner in which their teeth fit together—Class I, Class II, or Class III (Fig. 20-1). The bite problem, or malocclusion, of your child could be partly inherited from you and partly the result of how he uses his tongue, lips, and chewing muscles. Habits seen in your child, such as thumb- or finger-sucking, may also be affecting the positions of teeth, and your dentist may want to help your child correct them. Usually, to have serious consequences, these habits must be continued over a period of several years.

TREATMENT OF MAJOR MALOCCLUSIONS

Of the three large families of malocclusions, Class II and Class III contain more of the *severe, or major, malocclusions*.

Children with Class II malocclusions may have upper front teeth that protrude too much for them to properly close their lips (Fig. 20-1, *B*). Some people might term these "buck teeth" or speak of an "Andy Gump" chin. Although it may seem to you that such a child has crooked teeth only in the front of his mouth, the problem usually starts from the 6-year molar teeth, which grow out of position first and then later force other teeth toward the front to be out of place.

Class III malocclusions are almost the opposite of Class II bites, since in this type of malocclusion it is the *lower* front teeth that seem to stick out too far (Fig. 20-1, *C*). In fact the whole lower jaw appears to have grown too far forward. In these children also, it is the 6-year molars that could be out of their correct positions.

Children exhibiting these *severe* types of malocclusions (Class II and Class III) will probably be referred to a dentist who specializes in orthodontic care. For some of these boys and girls certain permanent

313

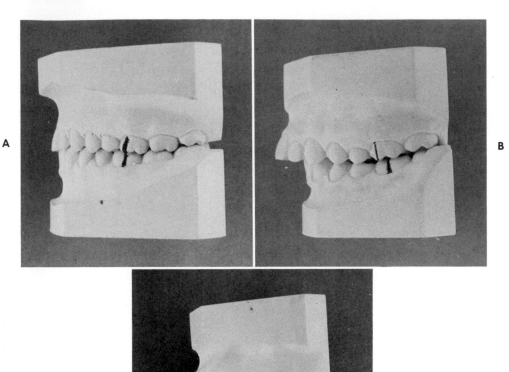

Fig. 20-1. Models of three classes of major types of malocclusion have been marked to indicate bite relationship. **A,** Class I malocclusion. Marks line up to show what is considered to be normal tooth and jaw relationships. **B,** Class II malocclusion. Note that lower jaw seems to bite *too far back* when it closes against upper jaw. **C,** Class III malocclusion. Note that lower jaw seems to bite *too far forward* in its closed position against upper jaw.

teeth may have to be extracted to provide proper space for good alignment of the remaining teeth for a healthy bite and nice smile. If this procedure is necessary, your dentist will want the orthodontist treating the malocclusion to carefully outline on a referral slip the exact teeth to be extracted and will ask you to return this slip to him. The family dentist usually will extract the designated teeth himself, although some-

times he may refer your child to a dentist specializing in exodontia or oral surgery.

Some orthodontic treatment programs to straighten the teeth of children who have the more severe, or *major,* Class II or Class III malocclusions may take 2 years or longer. In extremely difficult cases as much as 4 years of specialized appliance therapy (wearing braces on teeth) may be necessary.

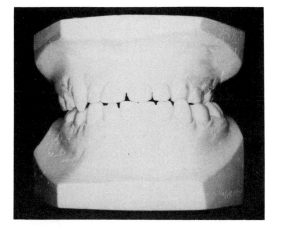

Fig. 20-2. Example of a minor malocclusion—posterior cross-bite in primary dentition (5-year-old child). Note how the child's upper left teeth in the back of his mouth seem to bite *inside* of the lower teeth, rather than in the proper bite as seen on the child's right side.

TREATMENT OF MINOR MALOCCLUSIONS

The treatment of *minor* malocclusions in children may be much simpler and less time consuming than that of major ones, particularly if the diagnosis is accomplished in the young child. Sometimes such a treatment program may be started as early as 4 years of age, although most *minor* malocclusions are treated best when the child is between the ages of 7 and 10.

Most of these *minor* malocclusions come under the type that your family dentist may call Class I malocclusion (normal 6-year molar bite). In general, these malocclusions show a fairly normal molar bite but may have such deviations as open-bite, cross-bite, or a critical loss of space in the back of the dental arch. *Open-bite* is present when there is an opening in the front of the mouth causing the front teeth not to touch when the back teeth are closed together. *Cross-bite* indicates that the front or back teeth are locked sideways out of position when the child closes his mouth (Fig. 20-2). This could be on one side (unilateral) or both sides (bilateral). *Loss of space* may be caused by the too early loss or extraction of deciduous (baby) teeth. Your dentist will explain to you the specific problems that are present in your child's mouth, since it is possible for your child to have a combination of two or more of these problems. As a parent you should understand that if these malocclusions are allowed to persist until the teens, the treatment of *minor* malocclusions becomes, in many cases, as costly in time and effort for the orthodontist as that of the *major* malocclusions. To treat these minor problems early before they become complicated is a splendid example of the proverb concerning "a stitch in time."

Philosophy of treating minor malocclusions

Although it is unethical to provide a guarantee of any sort when rendering dental care, it may be assumed that many of the children whose *minor* malocclusions are treated early will not have a recurrence of the malocclusion for which they were treated. Some children, however, may erupt other teeth in malocclusion, and a second stage of treatment may be necessary at a later time.

In general, however, the bite may be corrected in *minor* malocclusions using relatively uncomplicated appliances (braces) worn for a short period of time on the child's teeth. This is true, provided there are only a *few* teeth out of position and provided there is space enough in the dental arches to permit the teeth to be moved into their normal positions. After the bite has been corrected, the pressures exerted by the lip and tongue muscles and by the force of the opposing bite will help hold the straightened teeth in their new positions. In some cases, the dentist may want your child to wear a retainer (removable) or night appliance for several months to assist in holding the teeth in the corrected positions.

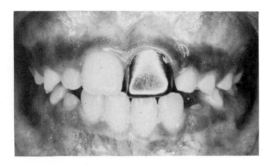

Fig. 20-3. Second example of a minor malocclusion—anterior cross-bite involving one upper front tooth. This is being corrected by a stainless steel crown cemented on backwards to provide an inclined plane in the bite. When the child bites down on his lower teeth, the upper tooth is forced to move out toward the lips into its proper place.

Advantages of early treatment

Several advantages are seen by your dentist in planning to solve problems of minor malocclusions at a younger age, such as the following:

1. The permanent teeth may be moved through younger, immature bone more easily and in less time than with the older child.

2. If a cross-bite (locked bite) exists, early correction allows the biting pressure on the rest of the teeth to be normalized, as well as preventing abnormal wear on the surfaces of the teeth in cross-bite. The pull of the facial and chewing muscles can help the child's facial bones and jaws to grow in a more normal fashion. (See Fig. 20-3.)

3. If a loss of dental arch space has occurred because the 6-year molar has drifted forward, this lost space can be more easily regained in a younger child than in an older child. (See Fig. 20-4.)

4. If a damaging habit is present, such as prolonged thumb- or finger-sucking, tongue-thrusting, or excessive pressure of the lower lip muscle during swallowing, the habit is more easily corrected in the

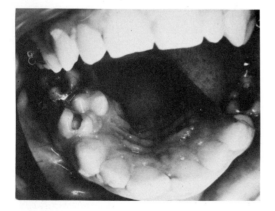

Fig. 20-4. Third example of a minor malocclusion (mirror picture of upper teeth)—loss of space in posterior portion of dental arch. The erupting tooth had no place in the arch in which to erupt, so it was forced to the palatal side. Incidentally, it also has rotated, so that it is now backward to its proper position.

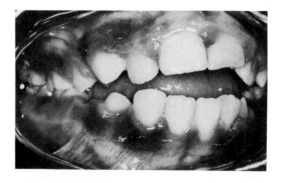

Fig. 20-5. Fourth example of a minor malocclusion—anterior open-bite caused by prolonged finger- or thumb-sucking. The child may also have developed a bad swallowing and speech pattern.

younger child than later during the years of adolescence. (See Fig. 20-5.)

5. Children younger than 12 years of age seem to cooperate better by wearing their appliances more diligently and keeping their teeth cleaner during the course of treatment for minor malocclusion than do some of the older children. Teenagers sometimes balk at the idea of wearing braces on their teeth.

Disadvantages of early treatment

Some disadvantages will also be explained by your dentist regarding the early treatment of minor malocclusions, such as the following:

1. When a younger child is treated for a minor malocclusion, all his permanent teeth may not have erupted. There is always the possibility that one or two of the remaining teeth may erupt in an improper position and will have to be corrected at a later time.

2. Occasionally a relapse, or movement of teeth back to their original positions, occurs after the treatment has been completed and the retainer brace (if one was needed) has been removed. This also may occur after teen-age orthodontic treatment in some children.

3. If the family dentist treats the first stage of a two-stage treatment of a malocclusion, the second stage may later have to be done in the child's teens by an orthodontist.

• • •

After weighing the many factors involved in your child's dental health, your family dentist will advise you as to which course of treatment he feels will be best for your child. If in his judgment, early treatment in his office is indicated for a younger child, you may be assured that in addition to diagnosis, he has considered the time, effort, and cost factors in detail. He will be most happy to answer your questions in this regard.

Making the decision to have minor tooth movement treatment for your child

Your family dentist will usually ask *both* parents to come to his office, even if they must come one at a time, for a conference before he begins treatment for minor malocclusions. By doing this he can be certain that the valuable information he gives concerning the child's malocclusion is understood by both parents. At this conference the dentist will probably have the child's fullmouth x-ray films, plaster casts of his teeth, and examples of the appliances he may be asked to wear. The dentist will discuss with you the approximate length of treatment and will present some sort of cost estimate. This may involve your paying an initial fee and then a monthly treatment fee until the treatment has been concluded, although some dentists prefer to charge a fee for each visit.

The time intervals between visits to check your child's teeth and adjust the orthodontic appliances may vary from 2 to 6 weeks. It may be necessary for the dentist to schedule some of your child's appointments during school hours, especially the two or three more lengthy ones. He will reserve the short after-school appointments for the routine adjustments of appliances. The dentist has provided for this in many cases by arranging with the school authorities for your child to return to school with a signed slip noting the time the child was seen in his office.

The family dentist's responsibility

The family dentist has the responsibility of carefully observing the children in his practice as they grow and develop. When he sees a malocclusion developing in a child, he will make a decision as to whether it is a minor or a major malocclusion. If it is a minor malocclusion, he may choose to treat it himself. If it is a major malocclusion, he may refer the child to a dentist specializing in treating major malocclusions (orthodontist).

Your dentist will avoid starting a treatment program when a specialist trained in orthodontics might be the best choice to render treatment. He will explain the differences in treatment at your request.

Treatment by a pedodontist

A pedodontist is a specialist in pediatric dentistry (dentistry for children). Often he will have had the experience and training to treat more difficult malocclusions than his colleagues in general dental practice. He will see in his practice a larger number of children who need treatment for minor malocclusions, as a rule. For the major malocclusions the pedodontist will also refer his child patients to the orthodontist. In some cases the two specialists may work together at solving a particularly difficult problem in a growing child.

Types of appliances used for treating minor malocclusions

In general, there are four kinds of appliances that fit on, over, or around your child's teeth to provide the necessary light pressures to permit healthy movement of teeth. These are removable appliances, fixed appliances, muscle action appliances, and retainer appliances. (See Fig. 20-6.)

A short explanation of each of these appliances as they are used in treating minor malocclusions is offered for parents who hear these terms used by the dentist or his assistant but have never had a professional explanation of them.

Removable appliances. These appliances are removable by the child and are worn inserted over the teeth. Springs made of tiny stainless steel wires help to move the

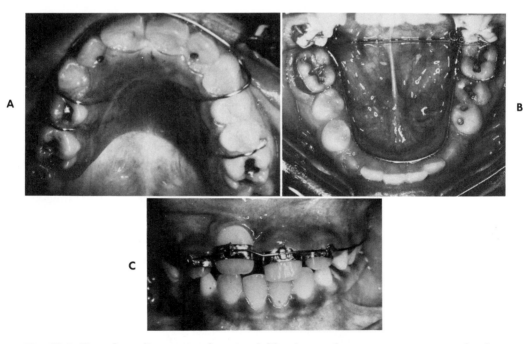

Fig. 20-6. Dental appliances in place in children's mouths to correct minor malocclusions. **A,** Hawley appliance. This is a plastic and wire appliance and is removable by the child. **B,** Lower lingual arch appliance. This is a fixed appliance, cemented to the child's 6-year molars. It is removable in the dental office for adjustments. **C,** Light labial wire appliance. This is a fixed appliance worn to change the positions of upper front teeth. The dentist leaves the bands cemented to the teeth during treatment but unties the arch wire for adjustments when the child comes in for check-ups (every 2 or 3 weeks).

teeth to new and more acceptable positions. The child usually may remove this type of appliance to eat, and while he wears it he must keep it and his teeth clean at all times. This means brushing after each morning and evening meal and rinsing carefully after lunch at school. In many cases it also means *no candy or gum* during the entire treatment period. The accuracy of fit and the spring effect of the wires must be maintained carefully, so the child must avoid damaging the appliance by chewing these hard, sticky foods.

NOTE: *These appliances can be lost unless care is used, and the dentist usually charges to replace a lost appliance!*

Fixed appliances. A few types of malocclusions are treated better with fixed appliances. These are usually constructed of metal bands cemented onto the teeth, with wires running through the bands. Some children call these appliances "railroad tracks." Although occasionally a tie-wire may loosen, the appliance cannot be lost or easily bent by the child. Some dentists will prefer to do certain kinds of malocclusion treatment with this kind of appliance because they may feel it gives more control over movement of the teeth.

Fixed appliances demand more of the dentist's time to construct, but in some cases they may result in a shorter treatment program for the child. Children who are older than 9 may more often be fitted with this sort of appliance.

Muscle action appliances. There are a few appliances whose action depends on a biting force, a swallowing force, or a lip

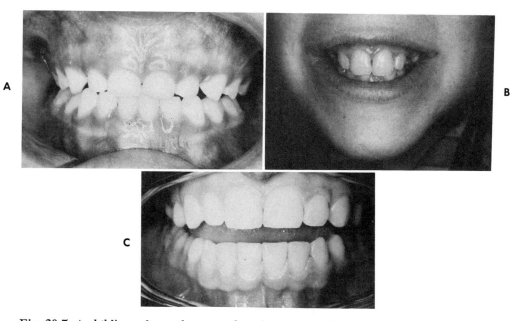

Fig. 20-7. A child's teeth are shown as they change through the years from the deciduous dentition (baby teeth) to the permanent teeth of a young adult. A, Young child's smile—deciduous dentition (baby teeth). B, Nine-year-old boy's smile during mixed dentition (part baby teeth, part adult). Note how large the front teeth appear to be in relation to the size of his face at this stage of growth. C, Young adults's smile. The goal of your dentist is to help each child to have healthy teeth and as nice a smile as possible.

muscle force. These are called muscle action appliances and may be fitted by the dentist to treat certain malocclusions, as well as certain poor lip or swallowing muscle habits. He may also use one of these appliances as a helping, or auxiliary, appliance while the child wears another main appliance.

Retainer appliances. After a child's minor tooth movement treatment has been completed, the dentist may require that he wear a retainer appliance to hold the teeth in their new positions. This may have to be worn for a certain number of hours each day over a period of 3 to 6 months. It is essentially a removable appliance, which is close-fitting but free of any pressures against the teeth. Occasionally, however, your dentist may add one or two springs to the retainer to accomplish additional minor tooth movement.

SUMMARY

As you have read these pages, you as a parent may have been surprised at the advances in treating dental malocclusions in younger children that have come about since you were growing up. Some parents have themselves undergone orthodontic treatment of some sort. Most have not, perhaps because of a combination of lack of opportunity and because of cost.

Your dentist realizes that more than 30% of the children whom he sees in his office have some sort of malocclusion that requires correction for good dental health. He knows that early treatment in many cases will help avoid later, more severe problems caused by the development of a poor bite, bad chewing habits, and possible periodontal disease (pyorrhea). In addition, there is the factor of your child's appearance. Sometimes the happiness of a child is measured by his own acceptance of the way he smiles (Fig. 20-7).

In this day and time, if a child has good teeth, there is really no valid reason why he cannot have a reasonably nice smile and a healthy bite. If there are measures that you feel should be taken to help him have a healthier and nicer-appearing mouth through the treatment of a minor malocclusion, ask your family dentist for guidance. The satisfaction he derives from his dental practice is increased tremendously when he joins you in caring for your child's malocclusion. He is deeply interested in your child's dental health and appearance. A final thought for all parents—an investment made in our children's future is certainly the finest investment of all.

Index*

A

Abnormal arch patterns, 28-47; *see also* Malocclusions

Abnormal habit forces; *see* Oral habits

Alveolar growth, 99

Anchor teeth, 102

Anchorage, 102

Anchorage units, **103**

Angle, Edward, 28-29

Angle's classification, 29-31

  Class I, 29

    Dewey-Anderson modification, 31-47

  Class II, 30-31

    divisions, 30-31

      subdivisions, 31

  Class III, 31

Ankylosis, 105-116

  of primary molars, 99

Annealing, 240

Anterior crowding, 126-141

  from genetic lack of space, 130

    appliances, 134-137

  from mentalis muscle, 35, 74, 131

    appliances, 74, 137-140

Anterior open-bite; *see* Open-bite, anterior

Antimere, 115

Appliance(s); *see also* specific appliances

  active, 71, 72, 169-174

  construction; *see* Fabrication of appliances

  expansion, 73-74, 81, 135

  fixed, 135

    soldered, 136

  fixed-removable, 136

  for anterior cross-bite, 164-174

Appliance(s)—cont'd

  for anterior open-bite, 149-159

  for Class I, Type 1, malocclusions, 72-75, 135-141

    expansion, 73-74, 135

    F-R lower lingual arch, 74-75, 136

    lower Hawley, 75, 135

    oral screen, 149-151

  for Class I, Type 2, malocclusions, 75-77

    extraoral force, **157**

    fixed labial arch, 155-156

    habit retraining, 153, **154**

    lower Hawley, 77

    oral screen, 77, 149-151

    upper Hawley, 75-77, 146-148

  for Class I, Type 3, malocclusions, 77-81, 164-174

    banded metal incline, 169

    inclined plane, 78, 166-167

    reversed stainless steel crown, 78, 167-169

    tongue blade, 78, 165, **166**

    upper Hawley, 75-77, 169-171

      with bite plane, 79

    upper heavy labial arch, 81, 171-172

    upper light labial arch, 81, 172-174

  for Class I, Type 4, malocclusions, 81-82, 183-194

    bands, hooks, and elastics, 81, 183-184

    palatal expansion, 81, 185-188, 190-192

    Porter (or W), 82, 190

    upper heavy labial arch, 82, 188-190

  for Class I, Type 5, malocclusions, 83-85, 197-209

*Entries in boldface refer to pages with illustrations or tables.

Appliance(s)—cont'd
  for Class I, Type 5, malocclusions—cont'd
    extraoral cervical force, 84, 197-198, 201-207
    F-R lingual arch, 85, 197, 200-201
    lower Hawley, 85, 197, 198-200
    space maintainers, 83, 112
    upper Hawley, 84, 198
  for ectopically erupted 6-year molars, 207-209
  for expansion of lower arch buccally, 134-135
    lower Hawley with jackscrew, 135
  for minor tooth movement, 11, 71-85
    fixed
      acrylic inclined plane, 11
      crown (band) and loop space maintainer, 11
      lower lingual arch, 11
    removable
      clasped space maintainer, 11, 71
      Hawley, 11, 71, 75, 77, 79-81, 135, 146-156
      Kloehn extraoral force, 11
      oral screen, 11, 71, 146-151
  general considerations, 71-72
  passive, 72, 165-169
  selection, 69-85
  to correct protrusion, 75-77, 146-149
  to move 6-year molar distally, 197-209
  to reposition lower incisors, 139-140
  to retrain swallowing pattern, 139-140
  to tip incisors labially, 135-136
  types, 11, 71
  younger child and, 93-94
Appliance attachments
  brackets, 234
  buttons, 234
  eyelets, 235
  lingual sheaths, 233
  list of, **236**
  stops, 235
  storage, 236
  tubes, 233, 235
Appliance components
  acrylic, 227
  band material, 224
  bands, 223-224
  clasps, 230, 257
  elastics, 227
  expansion screws, 230
  face bows, 226
  habit control screens, 227
  lingual arches, 228, 229
  list of, **231-232**
  neck bands, 226
  orthodontic impression trays, 50, 228
  polishing compound, 229
  selection, 214, **231, 232**
  solder, 225
  solder flux, 225

Appliance components—cont'd
  traction braces, 226
  wire, 224-225
Arch(es), dental; *see also* Fixed labial arches;
    Lingual arches
  constriction of, **180**
  distortion in cross-bite, 41
  expansion of lower, buccally, 132-133
  expansion of upper, **180**
  form
    abnormal development, 111-116
      ankylosis, 115
      caries, 112
      cross-bites, 115
      ectopic eruption, 21-23, 114
      environmental effects on, 20-22, 111
      eruption patterns, 16-27, 118-121
      extractions, 112
      genetic, 114
    effects of axial inclination, 118-119
      preventive treatment, 34-45, 118
      significance of hyperactive mentalis muscle, 35, 118
    measurement, 109, 117-118
    normal development, 16-21, 110, 118
    preservation, 109-125
  ideal, Class I, Type 0, 45
  increase in width, 18, **180**
  lack of space, 43-44
  length, effects of abnormal eruption, 128
  maintainance of lower, 11, 126-131
  ovoid shaped, 127, **129**, 131
  perimeter, 137, 138
  position of teeth in, 16
  space
    analysis, 61-66
      combination, 63-66
      malocclusion chart, **54**
      Moyers, 61-63
      radiographic, 63
    gain from extraction of permanent teeth, 35
    loss, 43-45, 128-130
Arrow rule, 25, 58
Axial inclination of teeth, 118-122
  F-R lower lingual arch appliance to prevent, 119, **132**

B
Banded metal incline, 169, 174
Bands
  and hooks and elastics for posterior cross-bite, 183, 192-193
  orthodontic, 223-224, 290-295
    anterior
      cementation, 292
      description, 223-224
      fitting, 291
      order list, **231**
    considerations, 290

Bands—cont'd
  orthodontic—cont'd
    molar and incisor
      advantage of seamless, 230
      cementation, 292, 294
      description, 223
      fitting, 290, 291, 293
      order list, **231**
BBC segments, 130, 195
Bite(s)
  closed, 122
  cross-bite; *see* Cross-bites
  open-bite; *see* Open-bite
  overbite, 59
    negative, 59
  overjet, 59-60, 147
  planes, 79, 81, 148
  wax, 51
Blocked-out teeth, 44
Boley gauge, modified, 33, **56, 59**, 62, 187, 219
Bone response to forces, 105
  mandibular and maxillary, differences in, 105
  root erosion and, 106

C

Caries, 44, 112, 195
Case presentation, 86-95
  closing, 89
  equipment list, 87
  explanation of treatment, 88-89
  fees, 94-95, 317
  parents' understanding, 87, 317
  where to hold, 86
Casts, 51
  trimming, 51-55
Clasps, orthodontic
  Adams, 257, 263
  ball, 270
  "C", 257
  circumferential, 257
  modified ball, 257, 270, 271
  modified Crozat, 257, 269
Class I malocclusion, 28-47
Class II malocclusion, 29-31
Class III malocclusion, 31
  referral, 164
Classification of malocclusion
  Angle's, 29-31
  definition, 29
  etiologic, 37, 41-42, 44
  timing, 28
Cross-bites, 115
  anterior, 9, 38-39, 162-174
    appliances, 164-174
    diagnosis, 38-39, 163-164
    summary of treatment, **174**
  arch distortion, 41
  buccal, **180**, 193
  dental, 193

Cross-bites—cont'd
  description, 38-39, 162, 178-182
    former designation, 178-179
    measurement in diagnosis, 182
    measurement table, **180**
    new system, 179-182
  ectopic eruption, 42, 195; *see also* Eruption, ectopic
  genetic, 178-179
  locked bite, 38, 42, 162
  posterior, 9, 39-42, 175-194
    appliances, 81-82, 182-194
    Boley gauge measurements, **180, 187**
    buccal, 40-41, **180, 181**
    complete lingual, 40, 181
    description of molar relationships, 176
    diagnosis, 40, 176
    etiology, 41, 175, 179
    expansion, **180**
    first permanent molars, 41, 42
    functional and genetic, 40, 41, 178-179
    lingual, 40
    prediction, 176-177
    primary cuspids, 42, **178**
    six combinations, 182-194
    summary of treatment, **194**
    treatment timing, 177
    unilateral or bilateral, 40-42, 179-182
    untreated, 177-178
  reduced, 164
  treatment, general, 43, **180**

D

Dental arch; *see* Arches, dental
Dental concepts
  Angle's classification of malocclusions, 29
  community attitudes, 4
  dentists' attitudes, 4
  future needs of profession, 7
  related to minor tooth movement, 4, 315
Dental cross-bite, 193
Dental growth factors, 5, 16-27
Dentition
  Angle's classification, 29-31
  changes in spacing, 24, 109, 195-210
  Dewey-Anderson modification, 31-47
  eruption; *see* Eruption
  mixed, 10, 117
    early, 143
    middle, 143
    space control, 116-117
  normalized, 10
  permanent, 18-20
  primary, 10, 18, 117
    timing of space control, 117
  primate spaces, 18
  spaced, 18, **110**, 143
  unspaced, 18
Deviation; *see* Midlines, dental

Dewey-Anderson modification, 28, 31-47, 57
  Class I, Type 0, an addition to, 45
  Class I, Type 1, 33-36
  Class I, Type 2, 36-38
  Class I, Type 3, 38-39
  Class I, Type 4, 39-43
  Class I, Type 5, 43-45
  diagnostic review, **46**
Diagnosis
  considerations, 46
  Dewey-Anderson modification, 31-47
  diagnostic quadrangle, 48-61
  general problems, 12
  malocclusion analysis chart, **54,** 66-67
  mixed dentition analysis, 61-66, 117-118
  normal and abnormal occlusion, 7, 110
  of malocclusion, 48-55, 69
Diagnostic quadrangle, 48-68
  cuspid relationship, 57
  molar relationship and type of Class I, 57
  position of midline, 57-59
  presence of oral habits, 59-61
Diastemas, 122-125
  closing, 9, 124
  developmental factors, 122-124
  prediction for closure, **123,** 124
  treatment to close, 124
    bands and wire, 124
    Hawley appliance, 124
    light labial arches, 124

E

Ellis prefabricated lingual arches, **232,** 285-287
Eruption
  ectopic, 21-27, 44, 114, 121, 207-208
    causing shift of dental midline, 23-25
    definition, 21, 121
    environmental factors, 25
    lower permanent lateral incisors, 23
    treatment, in 6-year molars, 121-122, 207-208
      Humphrey appliance, 122, 208
      ligature wire, 121
    upper first permanent molar, 22
  pattern, 16
    normal, 16
    permanent teeth, 18-20, 127-128
      ages of, **20**
    primary teeth, 18
Expansion appliances; *see* Palatal expansion appliance
Expansion therapy, 132-133
Extractions
  permanent teeth, 35
  primary cuspids, 129
  serial, 34
Extraoral force appliance, 84-85, 102, 201-207, 303-309
  adjusting, 308
  bow wire, 303

Extraoral force appliance—cont'd
  Class I, Type 5, malocclusion, 84-85
  components, **231**
  description, 303
  distalization of 6-year molars, 201-207
  intermittent force, 102
  precautions, 207

F

Fabrication of appliances
  extraoral force appliances, 304-308
  fixed space maintainers, 242-248
    band and loop, 244-246
    crown and loop, 242-244
    fixed soldered lingual arch, 246
    Nance appliance, 246-248
  Hawley appliances, 259-262
    lower, 268-270
    upper, 262-268
  heavy fixed labial arches, 295-299
  light fixed labial arches, 299-301
  lingual arches, 71, 279-289
    F-R with horizontal attachments, 279-283
    F-R with vertical attachments, 283-287
  palatal expansion appliance, 73, 270-275
  Porter, 287-288
  removable space maintainers, 248-255
    acrylic inclined planes, 248-251
    oral screens, 251-255
Fees, 94-95
Finger-sucking; *see* Thumb-sucking; Oral habits
Fixed labial arches
  heavy, **80,** 81, 295-299
    fabrication, 290-299
    for anterior cross-bites, 81, 171-172
      in mixed dentition, 81, 299
    for cross-bites in mixed dentition, 297-299
    for cross-bites in primary dentition, 295-297
    for posterior cross-bites, 82, 188-190
    upper, 81, 82
    use in Class I, Type 3, malocclusions, 81
    use in Class I, Type 4, malocclusions, 82
  light, 299-310
    for anterior cross-bites, 172-174, 299
      in mixed dentition, 299-301
    for closing diastema, 124
    upper, 81
    use in Class I, Type 3, malocclusion, 81
Fixed space maintainers; *see* Space maintainers, fixed
Forces
  biomechanical, 102-103
    anchorage, 102
    continuous, 102
    intermittent, 102
    interrupted, 102
  bone response to; *see* Bone response to forces
  eruption, 97
  mesial vector of, 98, 99

Forces—cont'd
  muscle, 97
  natural, 96-102
    abnormal, 100-102
      lip habits, 101
      oral play, 101
      thumb- and finger-sucking, 100-101
      tongue thrust, 100
    normal, 96-100
  root response to, 106
  tissue response to, 103-106
  tongue, 97
Forensic dentistry, 35
4-handed dentistry, **4, 49**
F-R lingual arch; *see* Lingual arches, fixed-removable

G

Generalist, 14, 48, 111
  language barrier, 7
Growth and development
  comparison of, in mandible and maxilla, 209-210
  correction of malocclusion, 20-21
  of arch, 110-111
  stimulation of, in mandible or maxilla, 209

H

Hawley appliance
  additions to, 148
  as retainer, 77, **148**
  bending clasps for, 216
  lower, 75, 77, 268-270
    for expansion of lower arch, 134-135
    for repositioning lower incisor, 139
    to move 6-year molar distally, 198-199
  removable, for closing of diastema, 124
  upper, 75, 77, 84, 262-268
    correction of protrusion, 77, 146-148
    for anterior cross-bite, 169-171
    to move 6-year molar distally, 198
    to regain space when 6-year molar erupts ectopically, 207
    use in Class I, Type 1, malocclusion, 75
    use in Class I, Type 2, malocclusion, 75-77
    use in Class I, Type 3, malocclusion, 79, 81
    use in Class I, Type 5, malocclusion, 84-85
    with bite plane, 79, 148
Holding arch, lingual, 136
Hotz preformed lingual arch, **232,** 285
Humphrey appliance, 22, 122
  and ectopically erupted 6-year molar, 208

I

Iatrogenic malocclusion, 13, 44
Impressions, 50-51
  trimming casts, 51-55
Inclined plane, 78-79
  for anterior cross-bites, 166-167
  for Class I, Type 3, malocclusion, 78-79

Inclined plane—cont'd
  lower acrylic, 78
  reversed stainless steel crown as, 78
  tongue blade, 78
Indent in labial bow, 77, **147**
Instruments, orthodontic
  band driver, 219
  Boley gauge, modified, 219
  bow divider, 221
  list of, **222**
  marking pencil, 221
  selection of pliers, 213, 216-218, 220
  serrating file, 220
  spot-welder, No. 660, 215
  tension gauge, 221
Interceptive orthodontics, 9; *see also* Minor tooth movement; Preventive orthodontics
  limits, 9
  recognition of minor malocclusions, 10

J

Jackscrews; *see* Palatal expansion appliance

K

Kloehn cervical extraoral force appliance, 102, 201, **202;** *see also* Extraoral force appliance

L

Labial arches; *see* Fixed labial arches
Labial frenum, 122
  surgery of, 122
Ligature wire, 121, **231, 300**
Lingual arches
  bending arch wire, 277-279
  cementing, 287
  Ellis preformed, **232,** 285-287
  fixed soldered, 135-136, 246
  fixed-removable (F-R), 12
    lower, 75
      for repositioning incisors, 139
      to increase arch length, 74-75, 200
      to maintain lower midline, **138,** 139
      to move 6-year molar distally, 200-201
      to regain space when 6-year molar erupts ectopically, 208
      to tip incisors labially, 135-136
    upper, 82
      Porter appliance, 82, 190, 287-288
      with horizontal attachments, 279-283
      with vertical attachments, 283-287
    for late mixed and early permanent dentitions, 283-287
  for mixed dentition, 279-283
  general types, 135
    fixed, 135, **136**
    fixed-removable, 71, 75, 135, **136**
  holding, 136
  Hotz preformed, **232,** 285
  matching to child, 277
  use in Class I, Type 1, malocclusion, 74-75

Lingual arches—cont'd
   use in Class I, Type 4, malocclusion, 82
   use in Class I, Type 5, malocclusion, 85
Lingual holding arch, 136

M

Malocclusions
   abnormal habit forces, 100, 131, 143
   Angle's classification, 29-31, **31**
   dental, 163
   Dewey-Anderson modification, 28, 31-47
      Class I, Type 1, appliance, 72-75
      Class I, Type 2, appliances, 75-77
      Class I, Type 3, appliances, 77-81
      Class I, Type 4, appliances, 81-83
      Class I, Type 5, appliances, 83-85
      diagnostic consideration, **46**
      summary of, 57
   diagnosis, 48-68, 69
      analysis chart, **54**, 66-67
      arch space analysis, 61-66
      diagnostic quadrangle, 55-61
   establishing limits, 9
   minor treatment, 9-10
   parents' understanding of, 87
   pseudo–Class III, 39
   recognition, 10
   resulting from periodontal disease, 12
   self-correction, 20
   skeletal, 163
   treatment timing chart, **91**
Mandibular plane; *see also* Tweed's 90-degree rule
   tongue blades to establish, 61
Mandibular shift, **40, 179**
Mentalis muscle, 20, 26, 35, 97-98, 101, 114, 116
   appliances for correcting arch distortion by, 74-75
      F-R lower lingual arch, 75
      lower Hawley, 75
   significance in axial inclination, 119
   treatment of crowding due to, 137-141
Midlines, dental, 23-25, 58
   arrow rule in determining changes in, 25, **58**
   checking with dental floss, 24, 57
   deviation, 58
   early recognition, 25
   shifting, 23, 58
Minor tooth movement
   appliances, 70-71
      types of, 71, 318-320
         fixed, 11, 71, 313
         muscle action, 148-151, 319-320
         removable, 71, 318
         retainer, 320
   case presentation, 86-95
      health service emphasized, 89
   consensus of orthodontists, 6
   definition, 4
   diagnosis, 69-70

Minor tooth movement—cont'd
   orthodontic "prime time," 10, 11, 194
   retention, 70
   treatment, 70
      timing of, 10, 194
Mixed dentition analysis, 61-66, 117-118
   space measurements, 117-118
Molar drift, 195-197
   and crowding, 134
   from carious attack, 195
   from early extraction, 195
   from ectopic eruption, 195
Moss' functional matrix theory, 146, 177
Muscular envelope, 146
Muscular imbalance, 131

N

Nance appliance, 246-248
Neck strap, **231;** *see also* Kloehn cervical extraoral force appliance

O

Occlusion
   diagnosis, 7
   lower arch form, 11, 110
   normal, 7, 18-20
      distal step, 20
      late mesial shift, 19
      mesial step, 19, 20
      terminal planes, 19-20
   perfect, 45
Open-bite, **46,** 59, 149-161
   and tongue thrust, 159
   anterior, 10, 37, 59, 149-159
      appliances, 149-159
      dental, **144**
      etiology, 37
      skeletal, **144**
Oral habits, 37, 43, 59-61
   diagnosis, 37
   examination for, 145-146
   facial profile, 145
   lip habits, 101
   movement of teeth, 37, 100
   oral play, 101
   thumb- and finger-sucking, 100
   tongue force, 97, 100
      scalloping of tongue edges by, 101
   tongue-thrusting, 35, 100, 155-157
      retraining, 38, 43
Oral hygiene, 103-104
Oral screens, 77, 148-151, 251-255
   acrylic, 76, 252
   adjusting, 254
   fabrication, 251-254
   for open-bite, 149-151, 251
      spaced, protruding upper incisors, 36, 149
      unspaced upper incisors, 37, 149
   overall functions, 151

Oral screens—cont'd
plastic, 253
Plexiglas, 253
precautions in fitting, 254
Rabinowitch, **231, 252**
rubber, 252
to correct protrusion, 148-149
to retrain swallowing pattern, 140
use in Class I, Type 2, malocclusion, 77
Orthodontic casts, 51-55
Orthodontic treatment
anterior cross-bites, 39
full mouth (corrective), 6
genetic Class I, Type 1, 33-34
loss of space, 45, 126-141, 195-210
oral hygiene during, 103-104
posterior cross-bites, 43
pseudo–Class III, 39
serial extractions of deciduous teeth, 34
timing; *see* Treatment, timing
Orthodontist, 15
extraction rule, 35
referrals to, 13, 90, **180,** 194
letter, 14
Osteoblastic action, 102, **105**
Osteoclastic action, 102, **105**

P

Palatal expansion appliance, 73-74, 81-82, 270-275
split-palate
for posterior cross-bite, 185-188, 190
jackscrew, 191
U wire spring, 191-192
jackscrew, 73, 185
use in Class I, Type 1, malocclusion, 72-75
use in Class I, Type 4, malocclusion, 81-82, 185-188
U wire spring, 73, 187
Palate-splitting, 185
Palmer system of tooth notation, **21,** 40
Parents' information, 5, 86-93, 313-320
Pedodontists, 6, 318
Periodontal membrane response to force, 104
Philosophy, treatment, 315-317
Pliers, orthodontic
description, 216-220
four most important, 257
modification, 258
order list, **222**
use in wire-bending, 257-262
Porter appliance, 82, 287-288
for posterior cross-bite, 190
Preventive dentistry, 3, 47
Preventive orthodontics; *see also* Minor tooth movement; Interceptive orthodontics
limits, 12
maintenance of lower arch, 11
Protrusion and spacing of upper teeth, 36, 143
Pulpotomics, 113-114, **113**

R

Rabinowitch habit appliance, 140, **231;** *see also* Oral screens
Radiographs in space analysis, 63, 66
Referrals in Class III malocclusions, 39; *see also* Orthodontist, referrals to
Retention, 13, 70
during mixed dentition, 13
of expansion of lower arch, 137
of repositioned lower incisors, 140-141
Retruding, 13

S

Scalloping of tongue, 101-102
Soldering, 239
Space
existing, **54,** 62, 67
genetic lack of, 33-34
diagnosis, 130
treatment, 131-137
loss, 116-118
environmental factors, 112
estimate to regain, 197
from caries, 116
from change in axial inclination, 116
from premature loss of anterior teeth, 116
timing control measures, 117
in mixed dentition, 117
treatment to control, **116**
needed, 62
preservation, 9
Space maintainers
fixed, 83-84, 242
band and loop, 83, 244-246
crown and loop, 83, **113,** 242-244
Nance appliance, 246-248
soldered lingual arch, 83, 246
removable, 11, 83, 248
acrylic inclined plane, 248-251
after extraction of primary teeth, 112, **113, 117**
use in Class I, Type 5, malocclusion, 83
Spee, curve of, 18, 54, **145**
reverse, **145, 150**
Speech
articulation, 37
factors, 159-161
Rathbone-Snidecor articulation test, 160
Spot-welder, No. 660, 215, 238
operation, 240-242
use of annealing table, 242
use of cables, 241-242
use of turrets, 241
Spot-welding, 239
and soldering, 239
conditioning of wires, 239-240
molar tubes, 294
Springs
double finger, **136**

Springs—cont'd
  double helical, **268**
  dumbbell, 275
  "gathering," 138
  helical, **79**, **168**, 198, 263-264
  labial bow, 269
  lock, **284**
  s, 170
  single finger, 136-137, **281**
  U-loop, **80**, **278**
  W, **79**, 170
Stainless steel crown, 167, 169; *see also* Space
        maintainer, fixed, crown and loop
  reversed for anterior cross-bite, 167-169
"Step," 265-266
Super—Class I relationship, 176, **202**
Supraeruption, 97
Swallowing
  development, 158
  retraining, 139, 158-159
  therapy, 35, 160-161

T

Teeth; *see also* Dentition
  abnormal habit forces, 100
  ankylosis, 45, 99
  anterior, 36-38
  anterior cross-bite, 38-39
  axes, 16
  axial inclination of, 118-122
  blocked-out, 44
  crowding of, in lower incisors, 9
  drifting, 97
  environmental factors, 16
  eruption of incisors and molars, 127
  flared and spaced, 10
  identification, **21**
  injuries to, **144**
  interdental spaces, 37
  lingually blocked-out lateral incisors, 13, 114
  loss of space, 43-45; *see also* Space loss
  mesial migration of 6-year molars, 9
  mixed dentition
    role of cuspids, 120
    role of incisors, 119
  molar drift, 43, 195-197
  Moyers probability chart of widths, **64**
  natural forces on position of, 96
    eruption, 96
    muscle, 97
    tongue, 97
  occlusal tables, 99
  permanent, 18-20, 127-129
    bicuspid, 20
    cuspids, 20, 128
    first molar, 41-42
    incisors, 20, 119
    molars, 18-20, 121

Teeth—cont'd
  permanent—cont'd
    Moorrees chart of mesiodistal crown diame-
        ters, **66**
  primary, 16
    cuspids, 42, 120
    incisors, 118
    molars, 121
    Moorrees chart of mesiodistal crown diame-
        ters, **65**
  protruded and spaced upper, 36, 143
  spaced, 36
  supernumerary, and arrow rule, 59
  trauma to, 16, **144**
  unspaced, 149
Thumb-sucking, 100, 151-152
Tissue responses to natural and biomechanical
        forces, 96-106
  by bone, 105
  by gingiva, 103
  by hard tissue, 104
  by periodontal membrane, 104
  by root structure, 106
  by soft tissue, 103
Tongue blades, 78, 133, 165, **166**
  use in anterior cross-bite, 165
  use in establishing mandibular plane, **61**
Tongue screens for thumb- and finger-sucking,
        153, 155-157
Tongue thrust, 150; *see also* Oral habits
Treatment
  failures, 153-155
  for abnormal swallowing, 140, 151, 158
  for crowding due to overactive mentalis muscle,
        137-141
  for genetic lack of space, 73, 131-137
  general problems, 12-15
  of anterior cross-bite, 162-174
  of anterior open-bite, 77, 149-159
  of axial inclination, 74, 118-122
  of closure of diastema, 124
  of ectopically erupted 6-year molars, 83, 121-
        122, 207-209
  of major malocclusion, 313-315
  of minor malocclusions, 10-12, 315-320
    decision for, 317
    dentist's responsibility, 317-318
    early
      advantages, 10, 316
      disadvantages, 317
      philosophy of, 10, 315
    generalist, 14, 48, 111
    pedodontist, 6, 318
    types of appliances, 318-319
  of posterior cross-bite, 43, 175-194
    timing, 43, **46**, 90, 177
  of spaced, protruding upper incisors, 143-149
  of thumb- or finger-sucking, 151

Treament—cont'd
  timing
    and referral, 90
    chart, **91**
  to control arch space, **116**
  to move 6-year molars distally, 197-207
  to regain small space loss, 208-209
Tweed's 90-degree rule, 60, **61,** 133

W

W appliance; *see* Porter appliance
Williams diagnostic line, 133-134, **134**
Wire(s)
  bending, 256
    general rules, 157
    important pliers, 257-259
      No. 139, 258
      Rogers, 259

Wire(s)—cont'd
  bending—cont'd
    sizes, 257
  conditioning
    annealing, 239
    "killing," 239
    passivating, 240
    tempering, 240
  Elgiloy, 224
  separating, 198, 208-209
    to regain lost space, 208-209

X

X-rays; *see* Radiographs in space analysis

Z

Zero defects, Class I, Type 0, 45